Accent Variation in Indian English

VARIOLINGUA
NONSTANDARD - STANDARD - SUBSTANDARD

BAND 53

PETER LANG

Giuliana Regnoli

Accent Variation in Indian English

A Folk Linguistic Study

PETER LANG

Bibliographic Information published by the Deutsche Nationalbibliothek
The Deutsche Nationalbibliothek lists this publication in the Deutsche Nationalbibliografie; detailed bibliographic data is available in the internet at http://dnb.d-nb.de.

Library of Congress Cataloging-in-Publication Data
A CIP catalog record for this book has been applied for at the Library of Congress.

Zugl.: Heidelberg, Univ., Diss., 2020

The present monograph was accepted as a co-tutelle doctoral dissertation submitted to the University of Naples "L'Orientale", Italy, and the University of Heidelberg, Germany, in 2019, entitled "Language Attitudes, Ethnic Identities and Metalinguistic Awareness: An Accent-based Study of the Indian Transient Student Community of Heidelberg".

D 16
ISSN 1430-6778
ISBN 978-3-631-85742-7 (Print)
E-ISBN 978-3-631-86414-2 (E-PDF)
E-ISBN 978-3-631-86415-9 (EPUB)
DOI 10.3726/b18804

Peter Lang – Berlin · Bern · Bruxelles ·
New York · Oxford · Warszawa · Wien

This publication has been peer reviewed.

www.peterlang.com

A mio padre e mio fratello

Table of Contents

Map of India

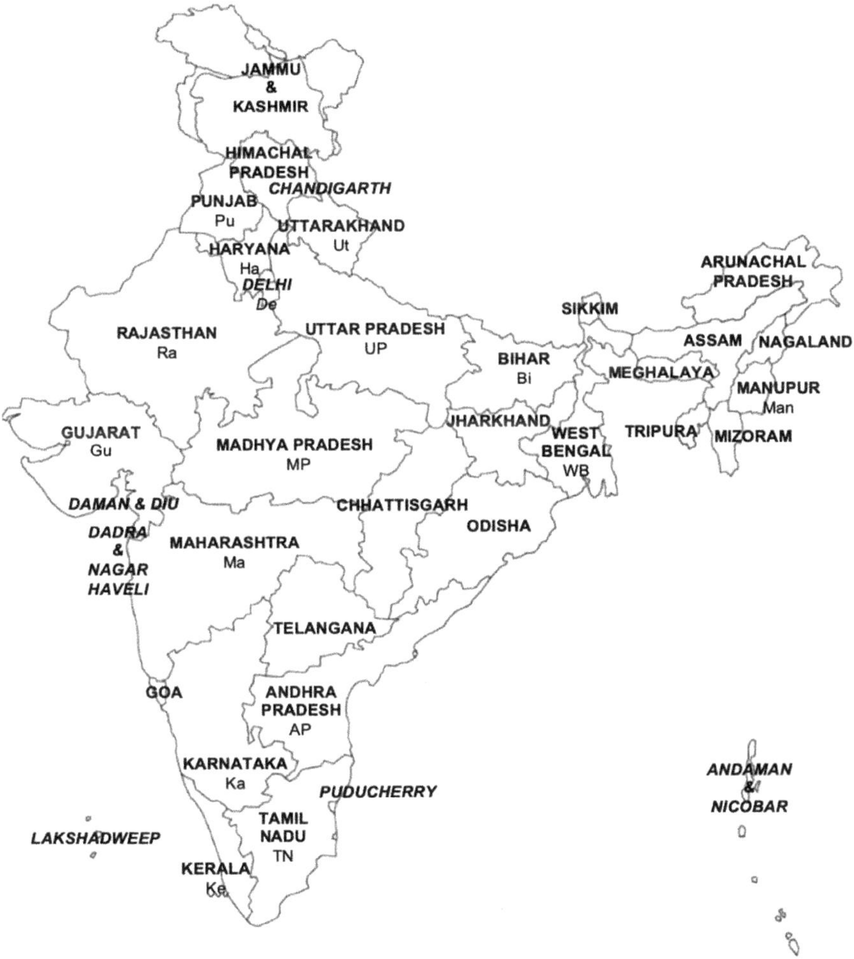
JAMMU
&
KASHMIR
HIMACHAL
PRADESH
CHANDIGARTH
PUNJAB
Pu
UTTARAKHAND
Ut
HARYANA
Ha
DELHI
De
ARUNACHAL
PRADESH
SIKKIM
RAJASTHAN
Ra
UTTAR PRADESH
UP
ASSAM
NAGALAND
BIHAR
Bi
MEGHALAYA
MANUPUR
Man
GUJARAT
Gu
JHARKHAND
WEST
BENGAL
WB
TRIPURA
MIZORAM
MADHYA PRADESH
MP
DAMAN & DIU
CHHATTISGARH
ODISHA
DADRA
&
NAGAR
HAVELI
MAHARASHTRA
Ma
TELANGANA
GOA
ANDHRA
PRADESH
AP
ANDAMAN
&
NICOBAR
KARNATAKA
Ka
PUDUCHERRY
TAMIL
NADU
TN
LAKSHADWEEP
KERALA
Ke

Acknowledgements

First and foremost, I wish to express my gratitude to the students of the Indian community of Heidelberg, without whom this study would not exist. Their warm welcome in 2016 and 2018 made me feel part of their 'home away from home' while I was away from home myself. Their friendliness, their dedication to my project and their cooking skills contributed to making my fieldwork an unforgettable experience. I would also like to thank the members of the Heidelberg Indian Students Association (HISA) for their kind support throughout my fieldwork.

Many people have helped me at various stages of the project. I am very much indebted to Maurizio Gnerre (University of Naples "L'Orientale") and Edgar Radtke (University of Heidelberg), who took an interest in the study from the very first planning stages in 2016 and offered many valuable ideas and comments which flew into the research design and methodology of my doctoral thesis. I would particularly like to thank my supervisors, Katherine E. Russo (University of Naples "L'Orientale") and Beat Glauser (University of Heidelberg) who were encouraging when I needed it and firm when they had to. Thank you for your precious comments and invaluable life lessons. I am grateful to the Cluster of Excellence *Asia and Europe in a Global Context* (University of Heidelberg) which provided an important platform for discussion, and in particular to Jule Nowoitnick. A special thanks to Hans Harder (University of Heidelberg) for challenging my ideas about language and India during the 2018 Bengali summer school held at the University of Heidelberg and over many coffee conversations. I wish to thank Gurdeep Singh (University of Heidelberg) for his help in coming to grips with statistics in general and cluster analysis and bubble matrices in particular. I am grateful to Thorsten Brato (University of Regensburg), who welcomed me to the English linguistics team at Regensburg while I was working on the present book. Thank you for your insightful comments and useful suggestions. It is a privilege to work with you.

Further, I would like to thank Rita Calabrese (University of Salerno), Robert Fuchs (University of Hamburg), Gerhard Leitner (Freie University Berlin), Olga Maxwell (University of Melbourne), Elinor Payne (University of Oxford), Frank Polzenhagen (University of Koblenz-Landau) and Britta Schneider (Europa-Universität Viadrina) for their helpful suggestions. Thanks also go to the members of the research network *New Englishes, New Methods* for lively discussions on the topics raised in my project.

Heidelberg, May 2020 *Giuliana Regnoli*

List of Figures

List of Tables

List of Abbreviations

0.1–1	Informant who has been living in Heidelberg for up to 1 year
1.1–5	Informant who has been living in Heidelberg for up to 5 years
AmE	American English
BAMF	German Federal Office for Migration and Refugees
BrE	British English
BW	Baden-Württemberg
CGI	Consulate General of India, Munich
DESTATIS	German Federal Statistical Office
DIGs	Indo-German societies (Deutsch-Indische Geschellschaften)
EFL	English as a Foreign Language
ELF	English as a Lingua Franca
ENL	English as a Native Language
f	Female informant
HISA	Heidelberg Indian Students' Association
ILOSTAT	International Labour Organization database
IndE	Indian English
L1	First Language
L2	Second Language
LFC	Lingua Franca Core
LP	Linguistic Perception
m	Male informant
MEA	Ministry of External Affairs, Government of India
N	Northern informant
NLM	Native Language Magnet
NRIs	Non-Resident Indians
NUEPA	National University of Education, Planning and Administration
PIOs	People of Indian Origin
RP	Received Pronunciation

S	Southern informant
SIT	Social Identity Theory
UN DESA	United Nations Department of Economic and Social Affairs
VOP	Vowel Onset Point
VtoV	Interval between two consecutive vowel onset points
%V	Percentage of total utterance duration composed of vocalic intervals

Transcription Conventions

_	untimed (brief) pause, within and between utterances
(pauses)	untimed (long) pause, within and between utterances
()	noises, kinds of talk, comments
:	length
↑	global rise
↓	global fall
,	continuing (list) intonation (a slight rise or fall followed by a short pause, not based on grammatical considerations)
?	rising (question) intonation (followed by a noticeable pause, not based on grammatical considerations)
/ /	phonemic transcription
[]	phonetic transcription
[...]	omitted material from the same conversation

1 Introduction

> *It's simply dangerous not to know what real people believe about language and how they respond to it – dangerous to general linguistics, dangerous to applied linguistics, and even debilitating to the desire for a complete account of language and its users.*
>
> (*Niedzielski/Preston 2003:xiv*)

In the world outside linguistics, people who are not engaged in any study of language talk about it all the same. The study of folk beliefs about language is among the many ethnographies of a culture. Just like ethnobotany seeks to uncover a culture's beliefs about "the naming of, relationships among, and uses for plants" (Niedzielski/Preston 2003:xvii), ethnolinguistics points to the intrinsic complexity of language and its attendant beliefs by setting the latter in the large(r) framework of the culture under investigation. From a scholarly perspective, however, folk beliefs about language are, at best, innocuous misunderstandings or, at worst, the basis of prejudice ultimately leading to the reiteration of social injustices. Yet, a close examination of the latter reveals an underlying and subtle complexity arising from the apparent mismatch between belief and use in language and provides evidence that the field, as well as folk beliefs, deserve careful consideration.

The present work is an account of *stankos*, a term Leonard Bloomfield used pejoratively to describe the linguistic beliefs of laypeople. It deals with folk beliefs about accent variation in Indian varieties of English. However, the context under investigation is not India or the Indian subcontinent, but a transient speech community of Indian university students in Heidelberg, Germany. What triggered the interest in this area in the first place was the lack of research into three main linguistic subdisciplines: (i) Indian diasporic communities located in non-anglophone settings; (ii) the peculiar configuration of transient multilingual speech communities and (iii) accent perceptions and attitudes to variation from the perspective of folk linguistics and perceptual dialectology.

With respect to (i), it is striking that very little attention has been given to the Indian diaspora in EFL countries, i.e., countries where English is a foreign language. While the regional spread covered by Indian diasporic studies ranges from the US via Africa and the UK to Singapore, the Caribbean and the

South Pacific, non-anglophone contexts are still underresearched. The present work endeavours to shed some light on Indian communities using English as a *lingua franca* (rather than as an L1 or an L2) in Germany. Recent research has emphasised that Indian migration to Germany is momentous. At present, the Indian diaspora is the major minority ethnic population among the two other South Asian diasporic communities of subcontinental India residing in Germany, i.e., Pakistan and Sri Lanka (DESTATIS 2016). In 2016, India was the most important non-EU country of origin of high-skilled migrants and the second-most significant sending country of international students (Burkhart *et al.* 2017). However, very little is known about Indian speech communities in Germany from a linguistic point of view. In a country where people know neither West Bengal nor Bengalis, but would recognise all Indian ethnic identities as one, being and acting as a Bengali is only possible *within* the Indian community in question. It is only here that the kaleidoscope of ethnic identities acquires social significance (Regnoli 2019b). The present work deals with an Indian community of university students located in Heidelberg, a university town home to around 150.000 people of 160 nationalities, and, among them, almost 47.000 with a migration background (Stadt Heidelberg 2017). Though small, the Indian local community is quite active and mainly comprises IT professionals and university students.

Some communities exist in relation to specific social practices, activities, and relationships (Lave/Wenger 1991). Because of this, their members are typically aware of their role and relationship with other communities as part of normal functioning. However, as Morgan (2004:13) points out: "[e]ven when members are aware of the values, attitudes, and norms [...] of a speech community, their positive standing is not always guaranteed, especially when regular travel and transmigration are the norm". Diasporic settings are interesting contexts with respect to the development of language attitudes, identity and ethnicity in speech communities (Alam/Stuart-Smith 2014; Leung/Deuber 2014). Recent debates about the Indian diaspora have started to address questions of what internally heterogeneous diasporic speech communities look like and how community boundaries and emerging identities affect attitudes (Hundt/Sharma 2014b). This leads to the second research area which has been neglected so far: transient multilingual speech communities. Although work on Indian diasporic stable communities has received wide recognition, only a limited number of studies have examined the peculiar configuration of transient communities, i.e., dynamic language scenarios in which people from diverse sociocultural and linguistic backgrounds come together for a limited period of time around specific shared activities. In such relatively short-lived contexts, norms and attitudes tend to be less stable and more negotiable than in other settings and challenge much sociolinguistic theory, which traditionally is more concerned with the study of stable communities. This fluidity in terms of linguistic norms and attitudes entails a constant renegotiation with respect to language choice and the social meaning which is associated with different ways of speaking (Mortensen/Fabricius 2014). In the present work, the speech community/community of practice under consideration will not be defined beforehand but will rather result from the study. In the context of the Heidelberg Indian social group, factors such as the respondents' knowledge of accents and dialects, their comments about their own identities, their attitudes and their network integration are important. Such concepts will provide insight into the speakers' perception of their community from a folk linguistic and perceptual dialectology perspective (iii).

During my first stay in the community in 2016, I started to experience its complexity as well as the importance that its members attributed to IndE accents and ethnic identities. I soon learned how vitally important it was for them to have a local and situated English accent in particular language domains and sociolinguistic circumstances. At that time, I was collecting data for my master's thesis research, which was mainly focused on the relation between indexicality and contextualisation (Regnoli 2016). Then, as now, both perspectives – much of the research on which has focused primarily on phonological variants and associated aspects of styles (the former) as well as on intonation and discourse markers (the latter) – were intertwined in order to shed light on the folk metalinguistic awareness of the community members. The results from the pilot study emphasise two major aspects: (i) Northern Indian students seem to have stereotypical views about themselves and the South and (ii) Southern Indians are perceived to have a higher competence in and better command of English in syntactic constructions in spite of their perceived heavily accented English. This was when I first began to consider the possible impact of ethnicity on the attitudes and beliefs of the community members.

Shortly after arriving in Heidelberg to begin fieldwork for the second time in 2018, I was invited to a very informal dinner by V.M., my female privileged informant. As we were waiting for the vegetarian *biryani* to be cooked, a new acquaintance – who later became one of my male informants – leaned over to me and, indicating my privileged informant and another female guest said: "they always stress every word, don't they?".[1] Though it was clear that he was commenting on them as typical Southern Indians, I have to admit that I did not

1 *Biryani* is a mixed rice dish popular in the cuisines of South Asia. There are as many variants as regions in the subcontinent and its ingredients usually vary according to the type of vegetables or meat used.

really know what to say. He clearly knew I was working on a related topic and wanted proof that what he was saying was true. He began to laugh and explained that "it is not a big deal", because *they* (Southerners) *know* that they cannot pronounce specific consonant clusters. Taking this at face value, I spent the next few weeks trying to learn everything about perceived Southern Indian accents. Yet, the more I looked into it, the more I talked to people, the more my earlier understanding was contradicted. For instance, I rarely heard Southern Indians talking about a Southern Indian accent, but rather, about multiple, regional Southern Indian accents. In addition, the more Northerners focused on Southern-accent 'markedness', the more Southerners focused on Southern grammatical correctness. Spending more time in the field and getting to know my informants better, I came to realise that the linguistic situation is extremely more complex than the way it had been described to me previously. Accents are perceived not only as an individual identity affirmation, but also as an ethnic one.

The above description was only possible because time spent with each single participant during our sessions, over dinners and while watching football matches enabled me to develop an understanding of the meaning that these accents and dialects carry within the community. This is the kind of insight only a participant-observer approach to language can provide since it favours the most frequent patterns and notes common variations based on contextual factors.

The study addresses a gap in the research on Indian diasporic communities located in non-anglophone contexts and investigates accent perceptions and attitudes to variation in a range of Northern and Southern Indian English (hereafter IndE) varieties. In order to present a detailed description of IndE perceived variation, the data set is based on the speech of educated speakers from two typologically distinct language groups, the Indo-Aryan one, which comprises languages spoken primarily in Northern India, and the Dravidian one, i.e., languages spoken in Southern India. In the present work, the terms Northern and Southern Indian will be used as reference points. While there is a possibility that some of the linguistic aspects of the former group may be applicable to the latter one, the study does not assume that IndE is a monolithic variety. On the contrary, it endeavours to provide an account of IndE as a complex multifaceted variety of South Asian English and to stress the need for further research on the phonetic and phonological features of IndE in order to expand the current state of knowledge of the range and depth of variation (Kachru [1986] 1990). In this light, the accent perceptions and attitudes to variation of the community members towards the following IndE varieties are investigated: Bengali English, Marathi English, Punjabi English, Uttar Pradesh English (belonging to Northern

IndE) and Tamil English, Kannada English (L1 Kannada), Kannada English (L1 Konkani) and Telugu English (belonging to Southern IndE).

The testing aims of the present study are multiple: exploring the connection between dependent and independent variables, gaining insight into intercorrelations within the community and detecting possible crucial factors resulting from the transient character of the community. The first aim of the study is to test whether the folk beliefs regarding accent variation of the community members share a common ground with ascertained linguistic beliefs. Specifically, the study aims at undertaking an ethnolinguistic reflection upon the elaboration of mental maps and border perceptions regarding regional varieties of IndE. The second aim is to record attitudes towards the IndE varieties mentioned above in relation to the participants' self-stated ethnic identities and linguistic consciousness, i.e., to outline the similarities of and differences between these varieties with respect to perceived accent variation. The third aim is to investigate whether network integration plays a role in the attitudes and the identities of the community members, i.e., to provide an account of the intra-group social factors influencing dialectal variation. These testing aims may be summarised in the following research questions:

1. How are different IndE accents perceived by the members of the speech community?
2. Do differences in L2 phonological characteristics index local and situated ethnic identities?
3. How do different IndE accents affect language consciousness, attitudes and behaviour?

The study adopts an experimental design combining both quantitative and qualitative methods in what is generally referred to as a 'convergent parallel design' (Creswell/Plano Clark 2011), where quantitative and qualitative data are collected independently and concurrently. Yet, sequential timing was preferred during individual tasks, beginning with a quantitative strand. Following this 'explanatory sequential design' (Abbuhl *et al.* 2013), the quantitative strand received the greatest emphasis, and the results were followed up by a qualitative phase. The combination of methodologies has been deemed important since this field has not been explored in the past.

The structure of the study is the following. The literature review in Chapter 2 provides an overview of the linguistic fields and subfields that are relevant for the present study as well as a definition of the main key terms. In particular, it gives a brief account of the role of language in society and the main principles of sociolinguistic theory (Section 2.1). Considering the relevance of the transient character of the speech community at issue, the chapter addresses the debate on the concept of 'speech community' and its centrality to the interpretation and representation of societies marked by diversity, globalisation and transmigration (Section 2.2). The subsequent overview of folk linguistics and perceptual dialectology provides insight into folk metalanguage (Section 2.3) and lays the foundation for the discussion of language attitudes and identity (Section 2.4), which are investigated in the framework of the Indian diaspora (Section 2.5). Sections 2.6 and 2.7 deal with the relation between L2 accent and identity, with a major focus on IndE accents.

Chapter 3 outlines the current state of knowledge about the history of the Indian population in Germany and in Heidelberg (Section 3.1), its demographic characteristics and socioeconomic profiles as well as its sociocultural and political integration (Section 3.2).

Chapter 4 outlines the methodology used in the present research. It describes the experimental design that is applied in Chapter 5. It has been deemed important for the interpretation of the results and for further theoretical implications to describe the advantages and disadvantages of quantitative and qualitative methods. The operational definition (Section 4.1), the research methods (Section 4.2), the data collection, i.e., the fieldwork (Section 4.3) as well as the statistical methods applied (Section 4.4) are also provided.

Chapter 5 constitutes the analysis of the data. It consists of two main subchapters dedicated to the quantitative analysis (Section 5.1) and the qualitative one (Section 5.2). Section 5.1 provides an account of the extraction and the coding of the extralinguistic variables and further characteristics of the sample (Section 5.1.1), such as their language background and language use in Heidelberg as well as their network bonds and network affiliations. Moreover, it deals with the ethnic identities of the respondents and their identity development (Section 5.1.2). As one of the main parts, Section 5.1.3 deals with the participants' attitudes towards different IndE varieties. These results are followed up with the qualitative phase. The topics for the qualitative part are prepared and analysed by using a bottom-up approach in order to let the data 'speak for themselves' and by applying a revised version of the qualitative content analysis developed by Mayring (2014). The section is concerned with the analysis of two main topics: indexicality (Section 5.2.1) and metalinguistic awareness (Section 5.2.2) and aims to supplement and expand the interpretation of the results from Section 5.1.

Chapter 6 presents a summary of the findings addressing the research questions presented at the end of Chapter 4. It also highlights the implications of the present study and names aspects for future research. References and appendices follow the concluding chapter.

2 Theoretical Foundations: A State of the Art

2.1 Language in Society: Principles of Sociolinguistic Theory

Language is a form of social behaviour. Social and linguistic aspects of language are coextensive in the sense that societal structures influence language, language variation and the status of languages in groups of people. This means that social pressures are constantly operating upon language as "an immanent social force acting in the living present" (Labov 1972a:3). Like every social construct, language is bound to change and varies from person to person and group to group. Addressing language variation and change entails investigating three separate areas: the origin of language variation, the spread and propagation of linguistic change and the regularity of linguistic change. Such variations may be induced by processes of assimilation or differentiation, borrowing, fusion and contamination.

Ever since Schuchardt's ([1885] 1972:48) pioneering insights into variability ("the pronunciation of the individual is never free from variation"), passing through Sapir's ([1921] 1949:38, 147) epigrammatic awareness of the loose ends of his linguistic analysis ("[u]nfortunately or luckily, no language is tyrannically consistent. All grammars leak [...] [e]veryone knows that language is variable"), Fischer (1958:47–8) is the first to provide the most fundamental impetus for sociolinguistics, and the basis for sociolinguistic analysis:

> '[f]ree variation' is of course a label, not an explanation. It does not tell us where the variants came from nor why the speakers use them in different proportions, but is rather a way of excluding such questions from the scope of immediate inquiry. Historically, I presume that one could investigate the spread of one of these variants into the territory of another through contact and migration, and this would constitute one useful sort of explanation. However, another sort of explanation is possible in terms of current factors which lead a given child in given circumstances to produce one of the variants rather than another.

More than a decade later, William Labov (1972a:2) writes: "[n]ot all changes are highly structured, and no change takes place in a social vacuum. Even the most systematic chain shift occurs with a specificity of time and place that demands an explanation". In claiming that variability is systematic, patterned and orderly, he argues that the understanding of the development of a language change goes hand in hand with that of the social life of the community in which it occurs.[2]

---

2 The variable as a structural unit represents a momentous innovation in linguistics. If hitherto all linguistic units were considered invariant, discrete and qualitative, with

Before sociolinguistics became recognised as a discipline, Sturtevant (1947:74–84) had already outlined a theory of the spread and consolidation of language change which was consistently imbued in its social dimension: "[b]efore a phoneme can spread from word to word [...] it is necessary that one of the two rivals shall acquire some sort of prestige". This points to the role of language as an identity marker since it allows individuals to express their identity in various facets and their membership to a particular group as well. Individuals reveal a lot about themselves – their backgrounds, their characters, their predilections – in the simplest verbal exchange, and the multitude of inferences they make when they are engaged in a conversation (cf. Section 2.4).

As can be seen, language has social functions; it is used as an emblem of overt or covert prestige and, consciously or unconsciously, to express group membership. The fundamental role of social interaction in linguistic change is expressed in those cognitive processes related to social categorisation, identity, acceptability and attitude formation that are, in turn, connected to specific contexts and settings. Hence, while the focus of early sociolinguistics was primarily on the "correlation of dependent linguistic variables with independent social variables" (Chambers 1995:xviii), theoretical frameworks from the social sciences and social psychology were later applied in order to explore the relationship between language and identity in a social context and to grasp a social reality in which identity, language attitudes and language behaviour interact (cf. Section 2.4). The application of such theories is important to obtain a comprehensive image of those ideas and values within a given society, particularly in a complex situation, such as that of a transient community of Indian university students located in a non-anglophone setting.

General orientations to the structural analysis of language depart from the not unproblematic 'Saussurean Paradox' as expressed by Labov (1972a:186) and stated thus: "the social aspect of language is studied by observing any one individual, but the individual aspect only by observing language in its social context".[3] They agree with the conclusion that the object of linguistics must ultimately be language used by the speech community. The study of language in its social context entails investigating variation rather than uniformity, contact rather than isolation, heterogeneity rather than homogeneity. In addition, several problems are to occur when dealing with speech, including the 'ungrammaticality' of

---

the inception of modern sociolinguistics, the variable has become variant, continuous and quantitative. For further details cf. Labov (1994, 1966b).

3 For a detailed discussion of the 'Saussurean Paradox' cf. Sanders (2004).

speech and the variation in speech and the speech community (cf. Sections 2.2 and 2.3).

Ever since Weinreich *et al.*'s (1968) call to take the study of empirical reality in language variation and change seriously, sociolinguistic theory has endeavoured to model the relationship between social structure and language variation, expanding the scope of the principles of linguistic analysis as to incorporate the social context (Sharma 2017). However, none of these principles is ever assumed to be entirely correct and thus requires continual reduplication and testing. As Labov (1972b:98) puts it: "to be right on a matter of general principle is certainly difficult in the extreme, a slim change at best, but the reward is that the work may form part of the continued construction of linguistic theory for a long time to come".

Although the social significance of language variation is only one aspect of sociolinguistics, for the purpose of the present study attention will be mainly given to the social correlates of language variation and change, i.e., to accents and dialects as emblems of an individual's gender, class, ethnicity, style and peer influence. Such social attributes are general and widely observed principles that continue to form the focus of debates within variationist sociolinguistic research (Chambers 2009; Bell 2001; Labov 2001, 1972b). Virtually, all sociolinguistic studies that include a sample of males and females have assessed a rather predominant linguistic conformity in the speech productions of women. In fact, in the same circumstances, for stable sociolinguistic variables, women tend to show a lower rate of stigmatised vernacular variants and a higher rate of prestige variants than men. Wolfram and Fasold (1974:93), for instance, notice that "[f]emales show more awareness of prestige norms in both their actual speech and their attitudes toward speech", while Trudgill (1983:161) argues that "women, allowing for other variables such as age, education and social class, produce on average linguistic forms which more closely approach those of the standard language or have higher prestige that those produced by men". Holmes (1997:132) discusses "the well-established pattern that, in formal contexts, women use more standard or prestige forms than men [...] [and] the widely accepted belief [...] that women are stylistically more flexible and tend to develop a wider linguistic repertoire than men". Again, Milroy and Gordon (2003:103) claim that "[w]omen seem very generally to prefer supra-local variants, which may or may not be identifiable as prestigious; [...] men appear to favor localized variants, which are often stigmatized".

The notion of social class is "inherently fuzzy" (Chambers 2009:40), especially compared to the relatively well-defined two major social partitions – age and gender. Yet, two main principles need to be observed: (i) 'the Principle of

Uniform Evaluation' and (ii) the 'Curvilinear Principle'. While (i) suggests that a regularly stratified linguistic variable is evaluated uniformly by the speech community, (ii) argues that linguistic change from below originates in a central social group which is located in the interior of the socioeconomic hierarchy. However, (i) and (ii) may merge in the most extreme case of mobility, i.e., the formation of villages, towns or cities where formerly there was nothing (Clarke 1987). In this case, homogenisation is the direct result of geographical convergence.

Paying attention to different styles requires ordering them along a single dimension measured by the amount of attention paid to speech (Labov 1972a). A crucial factor influencing style shifting is the audience since speakers tend to design their style primarily for and in response to their interlocutors.[4] In regard to peer influence, major studies (Eckert 2000, 1989; Lippi-Green 1989; Labov 1972c) have highlighted that classmates and close friends are linguistically more influential than teachers and parents, especially in adolescence. In addition, when parents belong to a different speech community from the one in which their children are raised, the 'Ethan Experience' phenomenon occurs (Chambers 2009). Children are, then, exposed to two different models of dialect transmission, but under normal circumstances they seldom choose that of the parents.

However, many of these principles have been considered rather limited and possibly deriving from narrower empirical bases. As Sharma (2017:235) suggests, "[l]imitations in the empirical base in quantitative sociolinguistics are partly due to the extremely labour-intensive nature of variationist (and related) data collection and analysis". In consequence, some aspects of the principles listed above – mainly focused on monolingual speech communities, Western urban cultures and non-mobile groups – have been modelled in current sociolinguistic research, which is more and more concerned with multilingual, non-Western and mobile frameworks (cf. below).

2.2 Speech Community

The concept of speech community does not simply deal with how groups speak the same language or variety. Rather, it implies that language "represents, embodies, constructs and constitutes meaningful participation in a society and culture" (Morgan 2004:3). It also assumes that a mutually intelligible symbolic and ideological communicative system must be shared among its members. It is within the speech community that identity, ethnicity, attitudes, and ideology are

4 For a detailed discussion of style cf. Labov (1972a).

actualised in societies (Bucholtz/Hall 2004; Kroskrity 2004; Labov 1972a). This is to say that a group of people is not necessarily a community unless they share similar views, activities, practices and beliefs. According to Anthony Cohen ([1985] 2001:12), communities can be understood by their boundaries and are identified by both their uniqueness and difference. As he puts it:

> a reasonable interpretation of the word's use would seem to imply two related suggestions: that the members of a group of people (a) have something in common with each other, which (b) distinguishes them in a significant way from members of other putative groups.

Thus, community membership includes not only mutual awareness of sharing the same system of interaction and symbols, but local knowledge of the way language choice and variation represent locally-situated identities, social relationships, etc. What further emerges from Cohen's observation is that speech communities are recognised as distinctive in relation to other speech communities. In other words, in sharing ideologies, beliefs about language, identity, membership and attitudes towards language use, community members tend to distinguish themselves from other groups due to their differences – be they sociocultural, linguistic or behavioural (cf. Sections 3.2 and 3.3).

2.2.1 Early Definitions of the Speech Community

Linguists have conceptualised speech communities differently according to common beliefs of the time and theoretical congenialities (Wardhaugh 1986:113–26; Hudson 1980:38–43). In addition, they have used many strategies to investigate how people build, seek and thrive in their communities throughout cultures and societies.

Four main criteria have been used to define speech communities: (i) same language, (ii) socio-political boundaries, (iii) interaction, and (iv) attitudes. Early definitions of the speech community, for instance, meet with (i), as in the case of American structuralists. In the words of Leonard Bloomfield (1933:29), speech communities are "group[s] of people who use the same set of speech signals". Reflecting the belief of the time, according to which monolingualism was the canonical example of speech communities (one language = one nation-state), Bloomfield's definition goes hand in hand with that of Hockett (1958:8), who conceptualises the speech community as "[t]he whole set of people who communicate with each other, either directly or indirectly, via the common language". Similar, but much more detailed, is the definition by Kloss (1977:225), who includes sociolectal and dialectal varieties in his conceptualisation of the 'mother tongue': "Gesamtheit der Personen, denen als Muttersprache ein bestimmtes sprachliches Diasystem in seinen verschiedenen Dialekten, Soziolekten usw. Varietäten gemeinsam ist".[5] Fishman (1971:28) adds the criterion of norms of usage to that of sharing the same language. As he points out, a speech community is a group "[...] whose members share at least a single speech variety and the norms for its appropriate use". Fishman's definition is more accurate in sociolinguistic terms since it puts forward the concept of speech variety rather than language and does not necessarily associate the speech community with sharing the same L1. However, sharing a common language is too vague a concept for the definition of a speech community. According to Stanlaw *et al.* (2018), a speech community should be narrowly defined based on characteristics such as pronunciation, grammar, vocabulary, and style.

The second criterion implies the socio-political and socio-geographical background: a speech community is a group of people belonging to a given geopolitical entity who shares the same language. Definitions of this kind include Fasold's (1984:43) comments on Ferguson's (1959) conception of speech community, according to whom the latter is constituted by all those who speak the same 'language' within the borders of a country. This criterion is problematic in that it does not take into account discourses regarding diasporas and ethnicity.

More complex and detailed definitions of the speech community concern the models of interaction. In his works, John Gumperz (1972a, 1972b, 1968) revives the concept by considering the speech community a social construct. Instead of focusing on the single language model – as expressed in (i) and (ii) – he defines it as "any human aggregate characterized by regular and frequent interaction by means of a shared body of verbal signs and set off from similar aggregates by significant differences in language usage" (1972b:219). Gumperz's definition is based on three criteria: the presence of effective interactions, the sharing of language varieties, and a distinctive diversity with respect to other aggregates. As can be seen, Gumperz focuses on interface communication and determines that the notion of repetitive, consistent and predictable interactions is crucial for the existence of a speech community. He argues that, regardless of the linguistic similarities and differences, "the speech varieties employed within a speech community form a system because they are related to a shared set of social norms" (220). This formulation could well incorporate the sociolinguistic research that was taking place at the time since it reframes the notion of speech community

5 A group of people who share a certain linguistic diasystem including all its dialects, sociolects, varieties etc. as their mother tongue (translation G.R.).

to include not only language, but also values, attitudes and ideologies about language (cf. below).

Linguistic anthropologists and sociolinguists who follows Gumperz's line of reasoning have committed themselves to describing the verbal repertoires and linguistic heterogeneity of speech communities, and criticised generativists like Noam Chomsky (1965:2), who suggests that "[l]inguistic theory is concerned primarily with an ideal speaker-listener, in a completely homogeneous speech community". Dell Hymes (1972, 1964), for instance, describes the speech community as a "fundamental concept for the relation between language, speech, and social structure" (1964:385), according to which the question of boundaries is essential in order to recognise that speech communities are not fixed units. While the notion of speech community initially focused on language systems and boundaries – as in (i) and (ii) – it later expands to include social representation and norms in the forms of attitudes, values and beliefs. In other words, the notion that the use of the same language constitutes a speech community has been replaced by the recognition that speech communities also require a code of beliefs and behaviour about language and knowledge of how to use them (Hymes 1972). Yet, while highlighting the potential heterogeneity of speech communities and language use, such scholars look for uniformity on another level, i.e., shared norms for the use of language (cf. below).[6]

The fourth criterion, i.e., the one related to language attitudes, has mainly been mainly applied by sociolinguists and creolists. This is not surprising since sociolinguistics is the study of language variation and deals with the identification of features that differ systematically from other varieties whereas creolists focus on language contact systems in order to determine whether one variety is distinctive enough to be called a language in and of itself (Berruto 2000). Labov's (1972a, 1966a) definition of the speech community, for instance, addresses the question of methodological strategies and focuses on the relation of sociological categories such as gender, age, class and ethnicity to variation in language use. Furthermore, he emphasises the reflection of shared norms of social evaluation and abstract patterns of style shifting. As he puts it (1972a:120–1):

6 Suzanne Romaine (1994:22) defines the speech community as "a group of people who do not necessarily share the same language, but share a set of norms and rules for the use of language. The boundaries between speech communities are essentially social rather than linguistic". For a detailed discussion of the interaction model cf. Silverstein (1996) and Dorian (1982).

> [t]he speech community is not defined by any marked agreement in the use of language elements, so much as by participation in a set of shared norms: these norms may be observed in overt types of evaluative behavior, and by the uniformity of abstract patterns of variation which are invariant in respect to particular levels of usage.

In recalling Gumperz's conceptualisation in relation to the sharing of linguistic and social norms, Labov contrasts the attitudes of a speech community towards linguistic variables and corroborates Hymes' above-mentioned description. In fact, his first basic principle of social judgement is the following: "social attitudes toward language are extremely uniform throughout a speech community", to which he adds: "[i]n fact it seems plausible to define a speech community as a group of speakers who share a set of social attitudes towards language" (1972a:248). Thus, his theory of speech community rests on two premises: that speakers' attitudes toward linguistic variables are the same throughout the community despite differences in the actual use of the variables, and that different social groups use linguistic variables in the same way although not necessarily to the same level (1966a). Thus, members of a speech community do not need to speak only one language but constitute an integral social and geographical unit with shared norms of language use.

In contrast to Labov's unifying view concerning attitudes in speech communities, Rickford (1986) argues that speech acts and attitudes may illustrate both concord and contrast in speech norms of creole vs. standard languages: "[s]ome of a community's evaluative and speaking norms might be contrastive, even conflicting [since] [t]he normative homogeneity and sociographic integrity which our current conceptions of speech community enshrine is mythical". Following this line of argument, Morgan (2014, 1994) maintains that different attitudes may be a norm in some speech communities even though some methodologies may not be able to capture it.

More 'pioneering' definitions of speech communities either recommend abandoning the concept as "an already constituted object of inquiry and instead taking it as "a point of view of analysis" (Duranti 1997:82) or emphasise the perception and the role of members within the community itself, arguing that "[t]he individual creates his system for his verbal behaviour so that they shall resemble those of the group or groups with which from time to time he wishes to be identified [...]" (LePage/Tabouret-Keller 1985:115). Hence, membership in and across speech communities requires the renegotiation of languages, dialects and symbolic systems as part of everyday practice. In other words, "[m]embership in a speech community depends on social or behavioral properties that one possesses[...]. [It has] nothing to say about maintenance or (de)construction of boundaries between categories" (Holmes/Meyerhoff 1999:178–9).

However, whatever the criteria used to conceptualise a speech community, it is fundamental to define it in correspondence with reality (cf. Section 2.2.3). According to Hudson (1996:29):

> [o]ur sociolinguistic world is not organised in terms of objective 'speech communities', even though we may think subjectively in terms of communities or social types such as 'Londoner' and 'American'. This means that the search for a 'true' definition of the speech community, or for the 'true' boundaries around some assumed speech community, is just a wild goose chase.

2.2.2 Practicing Speech Communities

As seen in 2.2.1, the concept of speech community has become less simplistic and more specific over the years, overlapping eventually with that of social group and shifting from more objective criteria, i.e., geo-political space and language, to less objective ones, i.e., attitudes, norms, and values (Berruto 2000; LePage/Tabouret-Keller 1985). While members of speech communities can shape their practices to represent beliefs and values, the ongoing process of globalisation and transmigration continues to test its definition and its viability as a useful concept (cf. Section 2.2.3). As Morgan points out (2004:5): "the concept of speech community often incorporates shifts in attitudes and usage and [...] the notion of language that binds it is constructed around several major theories regarding language as a social construct". Such theories include language and identity, attitudes toward language use, language and power and are key factors in understanding how social actors move within and between their speech communities. In fact, speech communities may be marginal and contested (Bucholtz 1999), some may be part of a dominant culture (Labov 1966a) and others of practices that may encompass all of the above (Mortensen/Fabricius 2014). Yet, members always actively engage these complexities of language and representation. For example, the work of Michael Halliday (1976) on the use of antilanguages in prison reports on identity and the construction of underground and embedded speech communities, providing insight into the effective agency of prisoners in discourse, which is associated with acceptance of their incarceration. Thus, a speech community can be "a symbolic entity that both creates and indexes its existence as a hidden product of society and the institutional structure" (Morgan 2004:15).

The integration and knowledge of different norms of communication and its subsequent negotiation and mediation of power and identity are crucial aspects of speech communities. In the words of Bourdieu (1991:46):

> integration into a single 'linguistic community' which is a product of the political domination that is endlessly reproduced by institutions capable of imposing universal recognition of the dominant language, is the condition for the establishment of relations of linguistic domination.

If language practices regulate the ways in which language is used and establish language hierarchies in which some languages are more valued than others (Foucault 1991; Briggs 1986) and hegemonic practices ensure that people acquiesce to invisible cultural power (Woolard 1985), a speech community represents the location of a group in society and its relationship to power. For instance, Morgan's (2002) work on the development of a hip-hop speech community in New York provides interesting insight into the community's counter language practices, arguing that values and norms are communicated through specific practices and symbols of the wider African American speech community. Thus, the identity of members is tied to the power derived from a shared system of representation. Interestingly, Leung and Deuber's (2014) investigation into a popular stereotype surrounding pitch in a community of Indo-Trinidadians, and Alam and Stuart-Smith's (2014) sociophonetic study of syllable-initial /t/ in a Glaswegian Pakistani community shed new light on how such linguistic realisations index local ethnic identities for these communities (cf. Section 2.5.1).

The concept of speech community delves into the importance of local knowledge and communicative competence so that "members can identify insiders from outsiders, those passing as members, and those living in contact zones and borderlands" (Morgan 2004:18).

2.2.3 Transient Multilingual Speech Communities

Some communities exist in relation to specific social practices, activities, and relationships (Lave/Wenger 1991). Because of this, members are typically aware of their role and relationship to other communities as part of normal functioning. However, as Morgan (2004:13) points out: "[e]ven when members are aware of the values, attitudes, and norms [...] of a speech community, their positive standing is not always guaranteed, especially when regular travel and transmigration are the norm". As briefly mentioned in Section 2.2.2, diasporic settings are interesting contexts with regard to the development of language attitudes, identity and ethnicity in speech communities (Alam/Stuart-Smith 2014; Leung/Deuber 2014). Recent debates about the Indian diaspora have started to address questions of what internally heterogeneous diasporic speech communities are like and how community boundaries and emerging identities affect attitude (Hundt/Sharma 2014b). Although work on Indian diasporic stable communities has received wide recognition (cf. Section 2.5), only a limited number of studies have examined the peculiar configuration of transient multilingual speech communities.

Transient communities represent dynamic language scenarios in which people from diverse sociocultural and linguistic backgrounds come together for a limited period of time around specific shared activities. In such relatively short-lived contexts, norms and attitudes tend to be less stable and more negotiable than in other settings and challenge much sociolinguistic theory which is traditionally more concerned with the study of stable communities (Mortensen/Fabricius 2014). This fluidity in terms of linguistic norms and attitudes entails a constant renegotiation with respect to language choice and the social meaning which is associated with different ways of speaking. In this sense, norm fluidity goes hand in hand with language-ideological-construct-resources since members of transient multilingual communities seem to have diverse ideological ideas about language variation compared to members of more stable communities.

Mortensen and Fabricius (2014:195) investigate language attitudes towards different varieties of English among the transient multilingual community of international university students in Denmark. Considering language ideologies as being constituted by different forms of 'knowledge of' and language attitudes as evaluative orientations to a social object, they argue that they "can be studied empirically, for example when they [speakers] crystallize into metapragmatic talk about language variation and its social significance, but also more subtly, through interactional moves". While stable communities are generally characterised by similar standard language ideologies, such shared assumptions cannot be assumed *a priori* in transient multilingual ones since members may develop their own language ideological beliefs which act as interpretative resources toward different ways of speaking. In this sense, a transient community is similar to a community of practice, which is a social construct different from the traditional notion of speech community, primarily because it is "defined simultaneously by its membership and by the practice in which that membership engages" (Eckert/McConnel-Ginet 1992:96). A community of practice is

> an aggregate of people who come together around mutual engagement in some common endeavour [and within which] [w]ays of doing things, ways of talking, beliefs, values and power relations [...] emerge in the course of their joint activity around that endeavour (Eckert/McConnel-Ginet 1992:96).

As in the case of transient communities, it is the practices of the community and the members' differentiated participation in them that structures the community socially.

In the present work, the speech community/community of practice will not be defined beforehand but will rather result from the study. In the context of the Heidelberg Indian social group, factors such as the respondents' knowledge of accents and dialects, their comments about their own identities, their attitudes and their network integration are deemed important. Such concepts will provide insight into the speakers' perception and structure of their community.

2.3 Folk Linguistics and Perceptual Dialectology

The specifics of bilingual identity tend to affect the kind of variation and change that takes place in language (cf. Section 2.5). For instance, Devyani Sharma's (2005) work proposes that bilinguals can evaluate different levels of their language system very differently, thus actively influencing the direction of change. Her study highlights how metalinguistic comments of Indians living in the US tie grammatical variation to proficiency, whereas phonetic variation is more permissive because it is correlated with identity and does not vary with proficiency but rather with individual attitudes (cf. Section 2.5). In fact, grammatical variation is too risky for identity marking because of its role in signalling competence and ratified status as English users (Sharma 2017). This syntax/phonology split is significant in that it seems to drive the selective retention of phonetic variables only. As mentioned above, metalinguistic comments about the split are defined *stankos*, a term Leonard Bloomfield used to describe pejoratively the language beliefs of nonlinguists. It is no accident that the term recalls a noun form of the past tense of *stink* since Bloomfield held the opinion of lay people in low regard.[7] As Niedzielski and Preston (2003:1) notice:

> [f]rom a scientific perspective, folk beliefs about language are, at best, innocent misunderstandings of language (perhaps only minor impediments to introductory linguistic instruction) or, at worst, the bases of prejudice, leading to the continuation, reformulation, rationalization, justification, and even development of a variety of social injustices.

Bloomfield's account of the social and psychological impulses which influence the beliefs of nonlinguists – his "secondary responses" ([1944] 1970:413) – is rather speculative since he never discovered any sets of folk-linguistic beliefs, but only "imagined" (Niedzielski/Preston 2003:2) them. Yet, recurring to *stankos* not only influences the overt and covert reflections on and reactions to language,

---

7 Robert A. Hall Jr. (1950:122) reports that Bloomfield used to collect these "ignorant or stupid remarks about language" during his fieldworks.

but it also contributes to the exploration of the breadth and depth of language theory. The study of folk beliefs about language is one of the most empowering and illuminating ethnographies of a culture, and it needs to be set in the larger framework of the culture under investigation. It may help determine the shape of language itself, since it would be "unusual to discover that what nonlinguists believe about language has nothing to do with linguistic change" (Niedzielski/Preston 2003:xviii). In this sense, folk theory goes hand in hand with variationist sociolinguistic principles (cf. Section 2.1). Dialectology and variationist sociolinguistics have largely been concerned with the distribution of dialect forms across geographical and social spaces (Chambers/Trudgill 1980; Labov 1972a). The perceptual reality of dialect forms and the distribution of beliefs about dialect variation, on the other hand, have typically been researched in the independent tradition of language attitude studies (Giles/Coupland 1991). In both traditions, there has been a tendency to assume that people generally and fairly recognise localised dialect varieties accurately as part of their sociolinguistic competence. Moreover, instances of language change and language attitudes are said to be profoundly influenced by folk beliefs, and, particularly, by those beliefs about the status of language varieties and their speakers (cf. Section 2.4). Yet, even when there is considerable contrast between scientific and folk information, folk facts still have to be investigated carefully in cases where different languages or varieties are held in different regard by members of speech communities.

Perceptual dialectology is the study of how nonlinguists perceive variation in language and how they believe it functions. It differs from standard dialectology in that it is not concerned with formal linguistic differences among dialects, but rather with how laypeople perceive them (which may or may not correlate with scientific linguistic findings). Because of its focus, it is considered a subset of the study of folk linguistics, as well as part of the general field of sociolinguistics (Berruto 2000). In the words of Preston (1999:xxv), perceptual dialectology represents the "dialectologist's-sociolinguist's-variationist's interest in folk linguistics" and seeks to answer the following questions (adapted from Preston 2010; Niedzielski/Preston 2003; Preston 1999):

1. What do lay people have to say about language variation?
2. Where do they believe language variation comes from?
3. Where do they believe it exists?
4. What do they believe is its function?
5. What are the folk theories of language held by lay people?
6. How can they be extracted from discourses and actions?

Once linguists know these facts, they can proceed by comparing scientific and folk characterisations of social varieties. In doing so, Niedzielski and Preston's (2003) revised version of the role of folk linguistics in the general study of language is a valuable resource for the analysis of folk data, or, in the words of Preston (1993:xxiii), for "[the] many, many ways to skin a linguistic cat". Folk theory assumes that there are basically two ways: *a* and *b* (cf. Fig. 2.3.1).

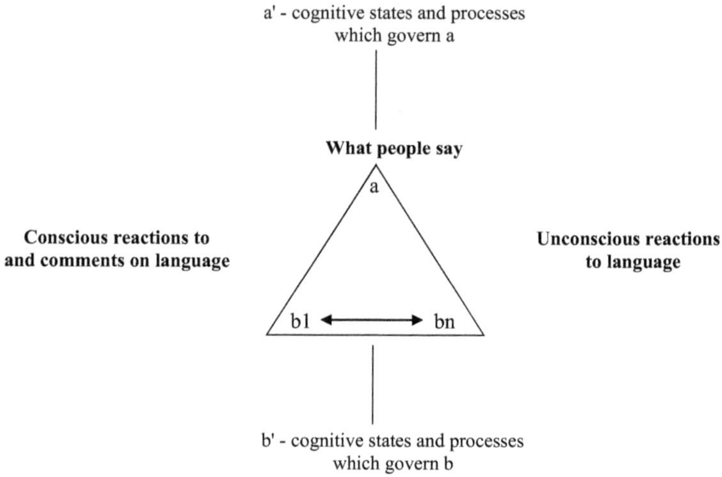

Fig. 2.3.1 Three approaches to language data, revised (Niedzielski/Preston 2003:xi)

The top of the triangle is concerned with the majority of research on language: the investigation of what people say. Not only does language production provide useful insight into the ethnography and social stratification of speech communities, but it also helps classify languages. However, "lurking behind *a*" is crucial in order to unravel the "empowering cognitive underpinnings of language (*a'*)" (Niedzielski/Preston 2003:x) since they shed light on its acquisition, change and use. Some of the underlying explanations in *a'* are related to the social regard that communities and individuals have for one another. This seems to be strongly related to language use. Language beliefs, attitudes and strategies are part of the process and are situated at the two corners on the bottom of the triangle, which are extremes of a continuum (*b1* through *bn*), "one which reaches the most conscious statements about language all the way to the most automatic, least-controlled reactions to it" (Niedzielski/Preston 2003:x-xi). The leftmost (*b1*) corner is the most characteristic territory of folk linguistics although it does take into account other positions along the continuum. Behind such attitudes is an explanatory *b′*, concerned with “facts such as historical relations among groups, psychosociological associations (and the mechanisms that account for them), and a host of other values, beliefs, and cultural stereotypes” (Preston 1999:xxiv). As can be seen, although the study of folk perceptions goes hand in hand with the scholarly characterisations of language variation (Preston 2010), it is important to bear in mind the diversity of the objects of research (i.e., the linguistic facts expressed in *a* and *a′*), the levels of awareness (i.e., the *b*-continuum) and the means of data collection and analysis.

The present study seeks to investigate the most overtly conscious comments about language (i.e., near *b1*) all the way to the most deeply subconscious reactions to it (i.e., near *bn*), recurring to the analysis of cognitive maps, open-end questions and semi-structured interviews to that of the accent identification task (cf. Chapter 4). This diversity of data types, levels of awareness and methodologies suggests that even the data that come from the end of the continuum are worth investigating since they may reveal the folk theory of language held by laypeople.

2.3.1 Historical Background and Earlier Studies

Interest in folk linguistics started to grow from the 1964 UCLA Sociolinguistics Conference and, precisely, from Hoenigswald’s (1966) presentation entitled ‘A proposal for the study of folk-linguistics’. He argues for a broadly conceived plan for the study of language which includes collections of folk expressions and terminologies. Moreover, he suggests that particular attention be paid to folk accounts of correctness and acceptability of linguistic behaviour. As he puts it (1966:20):

> we should be interested not only in (a) what goes on (language), but also in (b) how people react to what goes on (they are persuaded, they are put off, etc.) and in (c) what people say goes on (talk concerning language). It will not do to dismiss these secondary and tertiary modes of conduct merely as sources of error.

However, Hoenigswald’s directions have been objected mainly in relation to the impoverishment of data and their inaccessibility. Labov (discussion of Hoenigswald 1966) raises the impoverishment issue soon after Hoenigswald’s presentation with respect to the Anglo-American context. He argues that the phonological folk linguistic terminology of the latter is inadequate to convey overt remarks about their own language and that this “poverty-stricken” (1966:23) is much more present in the US and in England than in other contexts. Yet, Labov’s judgement of Anglo-American vocabulary impoverishment reflects the focus of his New York City studies (1966a) and is thus connected to the Anglo-American linguistic tradition only. Thus, even though the phonological vocabulary in the Anglo-American context is small, there is no reason to abandon the rest of the field (Niedzielski/Preston 2003). The second critique to folk linguistic research has been the "touted inaccessibility to the folk consciousness of linguistically interesting matters" (Niedzielski/Preston 2003:7). Although there is some evidence of the difficulty in accessing the speakers' ability to bring linguistic phenomena into awareness, other prominent language research traditions investigate the matter. Both general linguistics and quantitative sociolinguistics attempt to discover the hidden organisational principles of language design. While general linguistics has recently turned its interest from the close sets of phonemes and word classes to syntax and semantics, and, hence, circumvented the 'problem' of involving laypeople in language matters, ever since its beginning, quantitative sociolinguistics has made use of attitude studies to measure specific features with scales of social status (Niedzielski/Preston 2003). The only suspicion of folk awareness in quantitative sociolinguistic studies lies in the fact that when people are aware that their speech is being investigated, they tend to monitor it more carefully. This way, the researcher is confronted with the 'Observer's Paradox' (Labov 1972b:113). While most language-attitude studies try to sidestep the problem by recurring to some effective strategies involving the awakening of the vernacular (cf. Section 4.2), folk linguistics seeks to discover the conscious categories and definitions speakers have of linguistic matters.

Generally speaking, the folk believe that language is an idealised construct and that, to some degree, language varieties are different. Such differences are frequently connected to ethnicity, gender and other social subdivisions and most often entail evaluation (Preston 2010). Dialectologists have always been interested in differences in speaker productions and have greatly contributed to shed new light on the principles of language change (cf. Allen/Linn 1986; Davis 1983; Francis 1983; Glauser 1994, 1974; Trudgill 1986, 1983).[8] Similarly, folk linguistic language attitude scholars have included regional variants in their collections of responses to varieties (Coupland *et al.* 1999; Lance 1999; Preston 2010). The regional spread covered by recent folk linguistic studies ranges from Japan to the US, via the Netherlands, Germany, the UK, Ireland and Turkey. However, for the aim of the present study, attention will be solely paid to folk linguistic research in the anglophone settings.

---

8 For a detailed discussion of traditional dialectology and modern dialectology cf. Anderwald (2017).

Although studies of folk perception of regional varieties started in Japan and the Netherlands in connection with dialect production studies, their more recent use has been to supplement work on language attitudes.[9] Moreover, earliest work in perceptual dialectology did not make use of sample voices, and it was rather difficult to match specific attitudes to a particular region when respondents were not asked where they thought the voice was from (Preston 1989). Nevertheless, later work has made voice sample research a crucial part of the discipline and led to the suggestion that "any study of responses to regional speech is an integral part of the perceptual dialectology enterprise" (Preston 1999:xxxviii). This new step has contributed to blurring the lines between perceptual dialectology and language attitude research.

In the first attempt to use hand-drawn maps in dialect studies, Preston (1982) investigates language perceptions and attitudes of Hawaiian students in regard to different American accents. His results provide much helpful information in the understanding of American perceptions of US regional speech and catch the attention of other scholars who work in the field.

Lance's work (1999), for instance, provides a multi-area picture of perceptual maps from numerous regions of the US. Like Inoue (cf. below), he takes pre-set regional areas as the background from which to figure the intensity of perceptual regions. He and his colleagues administer blank maps to students enrolled in the universities of Massachusetts, New York, Ohio, Georgia, Alabama and Missouri and proceed with comparing the results. The most striking feature of Lance's study is the variation in regional identification offered by his regionally differentiated respondents and their representations of the American linguistic situation.

Hartley (1999) also looks at dialect perception, but from the point of view of Oregon residents. Although much work had been done to describe the actual linguistic situation within the US, no research had previously investigated the perceptions of West coast residents towards American English (hereafter AmE) varieties. Her analysis aims to fill the gap in the literature by addressing respondents from one of the major geographical and dialectal areas of the US. The data, collected from a fairly equal number of men and women residing in the Eugene-Springfield area and Portland, indicate that participants view the US as divided into five major dialect regions: Northeast, South, West, Midwest, and Hawaii. While the states of Oregon and Washington are rated highest in terms of correctness and pleasantness, New York City is rated lowest in both categories.

9 For a detailed discussion of earlier work on folk linguistics and perceptual dialectology cf. Mase (1999a, 1999b) and Kremer (1999).

The South, which is the most salient dialect region for the respondents, is rated poorly for correctness, but fairly well for pleasantness. As Niedzielski and Preston (2003:96) notice: "correctness and related affective dimensions, at least in United States English, are notions which, for nonlinguists, have geographical significance".

A similar dimension has been registered in the UK, thus supporting folk theory principles according to which investigating folk perceptions is important since "it represents a set of beliefs both strongly held and highly influential in the linguistic life of large and small speech communities" (Niedzielski/Preston 2003:96). Subjective dialect division, for instance, has been largely investigated by Inoue both in Japan (1977/8, 1995) and Great Britain (1996, 1995). Borrowing techniques from the study of language attitudes, he identifies variety descriptors, uses them to characterise the speech of different areas without voice samples and converts the results to cognitive maps (cf. Section 4.2.3 for further details). His work in Japan and Great Britain (1995) investigates social characteristics associated with dialect image. While 'intellectual'; and 'emotional' are the descriptors used in Japan, the components selected in statistical treatments of labels used in Great Britain are 'rural' and 'standard'. Further information about the treatment of variety perception in Great Britain (Inoue 1996) shows how the multidimensional scaling approach has been applied both to the evaluative labels and to the regions evaluated.

Similarly, the sociolinguistic trend of perceptual dialectology is apparent in the work of Coupland *et al.* (1999). In studying language perceptions and attitudes in Wales, they gather data from secondary school teachers in relation to a wide range of geographical varieties of Welsh English. Their findings show that the labels given to regions correspond with a dialect assessment task and that local varieties of Welsh English that are viewed as more or less Welsh (in a continuum from Welshness to Unwelshness) cannot be linked to any other specific affective or prestige dialect dimension. Drawing on these and other findings (Coupland 1990), Williams *et al.* (1999) further analyse data collected from Welsh secondary school students in relation to the sociolinguistic stereotyping of English in Wales by assessing their perceptions of and attitudes towards these dialects. Specifically, they select fourteen audio-recordings on phonetic and phonological criteria covering six dialects of Welsh English (Cardiff English, North-East English, South West English, Valleys English, Mid Wales English and North-West English) and RP, and compare attitudes of both young adults and teachers. They show that young adults produce lower levels of recognition than teachers as a result of their predictably lower levels of dialect experience. Furthermore, young adults show lower levels of receptive availability, which may be the result of less accurate and detailed cognitive templates of Welsh English sociolinguistic variation. In other words, Williams *et al.* (1999) suggest that even if levels of exposure had been similar between students and teachers, younger people would have still had less experience than older ones in assessing the social significance of Welsh English sociolinguistic differences, also because of their predictably lower geographical mobility.

2.3.2 Metalanguage

A clear conclusion drawn from the above-mentioned survey of folk linguistic works is that if the folk talk about language, they must indeed know (or think they know) about it. Such overt knowledge of and comment about language is termed metalanguage, i.e., language about language. Just like the linguist's metalanguage, folk metalanguage is conscious, hence, "it is not directed to a phenomenon which a speaker is unaware of, but to one which he or she has focused on in some way" (Niedzielski/Preston 2003:302). It is this consciousness requirement that appears to cause severe difficulty in the characterisation of nonlinguists' representations of language facts since language use is itself a largely automatic, hence, covert behaviour:

> [a]n automatic process is characterized by the following properties. It occurs (a) without intention (and is therefore unavoidable), (b) without giving rise to any conscious awareness, and (c) without producing interference with other ongoing mental activities. (Flores d'Arcais 1988:117)

Yet, while there are many occurrences of deliberate language use which are the result of conscious speech monitoring, there is also the possibility of introspection which allows for the retrieval of linguistic material. As seen in Section 2.4.1, under such conditions, laypeople are able to provide linguistic commentary. According to Garrett (1988), folk scrutiny (or awareness) is determined by three main factors: (i) the content one wishes to convey; (ii) the effect one wishes to produce in one's interlocutors, and (iii) the forms permitted by that specific language. While fully conscious reports about what content speakers intend to convey and what effect they intend to produce are most certainly easy for laypeople to give, reflecting on the forms permitted by the language is a rather problematic issue because the levels of language below what is said and communicated are not available to consciousness.[10] These parts of the linguistic system belong to what Jackendoff (1997) defines as the 'computational mind'.

10 Récanati (1991) argues that in the case of sentence meaning, i.e., the result of semantic but not pragmatic processes, only unconscious knowledge on the part of the speaker who is talking can be assumed.

Silverstein (1981) attempts to describe the sorts of linguistic detail which are more likely to be available to folk awareness. He suggests five conditions which enhance such awareness: (i) 'unavoidable referentiality'; (ii) 'continuous segmentability'; (iii) 'relative presuppositionality'; (iv) 'decontextualised deducibility'; (v) 'metapragmatic transparency'. Silverstein illustrates the first condition with the deference versus solidarity pragmatic system of many European languages, e.g., Italian *lei* (deferetial) versus *tu* (solidarity), German *Sie* (deferential) versus *du* (solidarity). These items are unavoidably referential since they both carry the pragmatic meaning of deference and solidarity and the reference to individuals, e.g., *tu* does not just mean solidarity, it also means *you* (2nd sing.). Silverstein argues that the pragmatic meanings of unavoidably referential forms are more likely to be a part of folk awareness since speakers are aware of the pragmatic system symbolised by the two forms of the second-person singular pronoun. Yet, it is possible to think of some exceptions to Silverstein's predictions. With respect to accents and phonology in general, Labov's (1966a) investigation of the presence/absence of non-prevocalic /r/ in New York City speech demonstrates how, at least in the Anglo-American tradition, folk terms for phonological matters lack. Niedzielski and Preston's (2003) study of laypeople's perceptions of American accents seems to confirm this trend when they asked one of their respondents to offer details about her perceptions of the strong Polish accent of her relatives and she could not talk about specifics.

The second condition Silverstein enlists is 'continuous segmentability'. Linguistic units which laypeople are most likely to be aware of are not interrupted by other material. In other words, people are conscious of the fact that in every sentence, each word, phrase or morpheme is segmentable.

'Relative presuppositionality' refers to the extent to which a pragmatic function of language depends on other contextual factors in order to complete its meaning. According to Silverstein, the higher the relative presuppositionality, the higher the chance of folk scrutiny. At the top of the scale are items such as deictics (e.g., *today*) and demonstratives (e.g., *this* and *that*) which only function successfully if they can be connected to a physical reality. At the level of phonology, for instance, the level of relative presuppositionality is rather low since there is nothing like a locus which provides meaning to Labov's (1966a) non-prevocalic /r/. Although the folk are aware of phonological variation, such awareness seems to develop from associated attitudes towards speakers or speech communities which make stereotypes out of linguistic elements.

The fourth of Silverstein's requirements, i.e., 'decontextualised deducibility', refers to those linguistic objects about which the folk can discuss without extensive reference to context. The more elaborate the context in which speakers need to differentiate a pragmatic contrast, the less likely it will be available to folk scrutiny. In other words, laypeople generally provide the contexts in which the use of one particular linguistic form rather than another fits. This approach is most often encountered when the folk need to discuss the meanings of words. Niedzielski and Preston's (2003) work, for instance, highlights the accurate awareness of one respondent regarding the fit between an increasingly specified context (Christmas customs) and the conditions under which two words (*gift* and *present*) are said to occur.

Finally, the last condition emphasised by Silverstein concerns speakers' immediate reproduction of an utterance in metapragmatically transparent performances, i.e., folk awareness seems to focus mainly on direct rather than indirect speech acts.[11]

More recent work on the topic has added a more general account of analysis of folk scrutiny commentary to Silverstein's (1981) considerations, emphasising the unavoidable influence of attitudinal factors, i.e., the social prejudices which create linguistic stereotypes, over the accuracy of folk report. This is mainly because "the straight path from linguistic facts (of any sort, at any level) to folk report is a very rocky one, impeded by the nature of communication itself" (Niedzielski/Preston 2003:16). In order to address the mediating role of language attitudes, Niedzielski and Preston formulate four main principles that contribute to the creation of a valuable folk theory of language (readapted from Niedzielski and Preston 2003; Preston 1996):

1. 'Availability'. As further discussed, not all facets of language are equally available to the folk. They may be, in fact, either *unavailable* – the folk cannot comment on such topics, or *available* – the folk will discuss some matters carefully. Moreover, they may be *suggestible* – the folk will comment on some linguistic facts only if they arise in the conversation – or *common* – the folk will usually describe such topics.
2. 'Accuracy'. Folk reports of every aspect of language may be accurate or inaccurate.
3. 'Detail'. Linguistic facts may be discussed with great or no specificity. Such descriptors may be *global* – as in the case of the lack of terminology for the description of a particular accent that still does not stop the speaker from commenting on it – or *specific* – as in the case of the speakers' detailed accounts of some particular feature of their pronunciation.

11 For a fuller account of examples regarding the present case study cf. Section 4.2.2.

4. 'Control'. In both account and performance, people may or may not control some aspects of the variety under consideration. This principle cuts across the first three characterisations since a speaker who reports on global aspects of an accent only, might, however, give a detailed imitation of it.

Such categories are to be considered as clines of availability ranging along a continuum of detail and lying behind different sorts of unasserted beliefs which members of speech communities share. In other words, presuppositions play a major role in folk theory since they are "what is taken by the speaker to be the *common ground* of the participants in the conversation, which is treated as their *common knowledge or mutual knowledge*" (Stalnaker 1978:320; emphasis in the original). Hence, the deeper the sense of community structure and cultural affiliation, the more presupposed beliefs will play a crucial role. To conclude with Niedzielski and Preston (2003:24):

> the folk awareness of language is not only a matter of degree but also one of mode or type. When one characterizes (however generally, however badly) a linguistic fact, we cannot say that he or she is 'unaware'. Conversely, when one mimics a variety perfectly but cannot provide any overt detail of what it is that one controls in that imitation, we would also not want to say that he or she is 'unaware'. For every act of language production and language perception (including attitudinal as well as 'processing' perception), then, the mode and degree of awareness is an open question.

2.4 Language Attitudes: Attitudes and Identity

Attitudes are rather complex constructs. The term originated in social psychology with the intention of defining "a psychological tendency that is expressed by evaluating a particular entity with some degree of favor or disfavor" (Eagly/Chaiken 1993:1). However, for different reasons, the term has been widely used in linguistic studies for almost a century now. Firstly, it is a "term in common usage" (Baker 1992:9), therefore it functions as a bridge between scientific research and everyday practice. Moreover, attitudes provide insight into overt or covert beliefs and perceptions. According to Ajzen (1988:4), attitudes are of an evaluative nature since they are "disposition[s] to respond favorably or unfavorably to an object, person, institution, or event". They are believed to be relatively stable although new information may alter their evaluation (Ajzen 1988). This relative stability makes attitudes an important object of research in sociolinguistic studies. They are considered to influence behaviour, standing in relation to other attitudes and other influences, such as the situational setting and the personal context. Furthermore, attitudes are not innate but acquired, which means that they must be established by a group and influenced by societal as well as group norms (Eagly/Chaiken 1993). Indeed, they are highly influenced by social norms and social roles – an influence which "often lead[s] people to say things they do not genuinely believe" (Eagly/Chaiken 1993:499). In consequence, in social settings people often seem to represent the attitudes of their group rather than their individual ones, thus marking group membership. The fact that attitudes can be related to certain groups makes them a valuable instrument to distinguish groups and to establish groupness for individuals. This relationship implies that "by measuring attitudes it is possible to get to know about a person's group membership and social identity" (Beinhoff 2013:24).

Attitudes toward languages exist because language fulfils social functions: (i) it helps speakers understand and internalise their surroundings; (ii) it is a group marker as well as (iii) one of the main tools of communication and associated with social groups, thus functioning as a group identifier (cf. Section 2.1). Every type of communication can either be hindered by negative attitudes or facilitated by positive ones which, in turn, can improve communication through an increased willingness to contribute to mutual comprehension and understanding.

The present study, as well as most studies of language attitudes, adopts the so-called mentalist view, exemplified by Allport (1935:810) as follows: "[an attitude is] a mental and neural state of readiness, organised through experience, exerting a directive or dynamic influence upon the individual's response to all objects and situations with which it is related". In other words, attitudes are seen as particular dispositions to respond to some events in a consistent manner (Deprez/Persoons 1987). This means that either directly elicited attitudes or indirectly observed ones can be used, once identified and analysed, to predict speakers' behaviour (Agheyisi/Fishman 1970; Baker 1992; Niedzielski/Preston 2003). Concurrently existing is the behaviourist view of attitudes, which implies that attitudes need to be "located in actual overt behaviour or responses" (Agheyisi/Fishman 1970:138) in order to be investigated, thus discarding the possibility of eliciting them indirectly.

Generally, attitudes consist of three separate but interrelated components: (i) cognition (cognitive); (ii) evaluation (affective); (iii) readiness for action (conative) (Baker 1992; Fasold 1984; Kellermann 2001; Schlieben-Lange 1991). The cognitive component includes beliefs and ideas concerning language, speakers of language and language behaviour. It is the knowledge speakers have about the attitude object- knowledge which is not to be considered as reality as such, but as folk awareness. Hence, these beliefs are always subjective probability judgements and not necessarily factual (cf. Section 2.4). Such a component comprises, for instance, "the assessment of the subject's own broadness of dialect, the knowledge about the vitality of the language or vernacular, the differentiation of the subject's dialect variety from varieties spoken by other groups (geographical, social, or ethnic), and the quality of the variety" (Zwickl 2002:10). It is important to bear in mind that if such beliefs are based on rather incomplete and deficient data, they may be called stereotypes, i.e., hardly differentiated beliefs (Esses *et al.* 1993; Thakerar/Giles 1981).[12]

The second component, the affective/evaluative one, denotes emotional judgements. In this case, emotional values are projected onto the attitude object, revealing, for instance, the consideration of a language, a variety or a particular accent as pleasant or unpleasant, right or wrong, etc. This component is also defined as the "central component" (Deprez/Persoons 1987:126) of attitude because of the pivotal role of the relation between emotions and beliefs. If emotional values are associated with stereotypes, they may be referred to as prejudices. However, Kellermann (2001) points out that the term evaluative is preferable to affective for this component because not all evaluative judgements on language are emotionally conditioned. In consequence, affective attitudes are social and interpersonal in orientation since they may be identified with a particular language group.

Beliefs and evaluation together lead to a predisposition to behaviour or readiness for action (Baker 1992; Fasold 1984). In other words, they are "transformed into more or less specific behavioural intentions" (Deprez/Persoons 1987:126), which are influenced by two main factors: (i) the behavioural beliefs, i.e., those beliefs about the implications of such behaviour, and (ii) the normative beliefs, i.e., speakers' actual or presupposed beliefs about the societal normative expectations regarding such behaviour.

This threefold attitude concept is a valuable tool to describe ideas and beliefs; it allows attitudes to be expressed independently in each of their three components; with the cognitive and the affective elements relating to each other, and the conative component providing the direct connection with the actual behaviour. However, it is important to notice that behaviour and language attitudes correlate very seldom since behaviour seems to be influenced by many other variables besides attitudes (Zwickl 2002). On the other hand, attitudes are closely linked to the assessed functions of language (Baker 1992; Gardner/Lambert 1972). Instrumental attitudes generally relate to "vocational reasons,

12 For a detailed discussion of the impact of stereotypes on inter-group attitudes cf. Spencer-Rodgers/McGovern (2002), Dovidio *et. al.* (1996), Hamilton/Sherman (1994) and Stangor/Lange (1994).

status, achievement, personal success, self enhancement, self actualisation or basic security or survival" (Baker 1992:32).

In the present study, the functions of attitudes are studied from the point of view of the 'Social Identity Theory' (Tajfel 1981) in relation to IndE regional accents as expressed in Heidelberg in order to mark distinctiveness and in-group membership (cf. below). Furthermore, attitudes towards language will not be differentiated from attitudes towards speakers because attitudes toward language always reflect the functions of language, hence the close link with its speakers.

Language in general and accents in particular are often assumed to confer a sense of social identity because they allow their speakers to express their identity in various facets. Accents, for instance, can express regional, national or cultural identity. At the same time, they allow people to perceive and recognise the identities of other individuals, thus playing a fundamental role in the construction of the overall image of other speakers. According to the 'Social Identity Theory' (hereafter SIT), group membership constitutes an individual's social identity (Tajfel 1982, 1981). According to SIT, every individual is a member of different social groups, and "this membership contributes, positively or negatively, to the image he has of himself" (Tajfel 1981:254). Moreover, in order to establish and maintain their social identity, individuals strive for distinctiveness, distinguishing their own behaviour from that of other groups, i.e., the 'out-groups'. This mechanism is defined as 'positive distinctiveness', and it must be acquired through "various forms of relevant social action" (Tajfel 1981:259), which include the so-called 'intergroup comparison'. In consequence, social identity is considered to be "that part of the self-concept that derives from group membership" (Hogg/Vaughan 2002:401) and must be dissociated from personal identity, which, in turn, is based on personality traits and on personal relationships between individuals (Turner 1982). As Hogg and Vaughan (2002:401) argue, although personality characteristics can influence an individual's choice of group membership, the distinction between social and personal identity in SIT is deliberate in that it tries to "avoid explaining group and intergroup processes in terms of personality attributes or interpersonal relations".

Language is supposed to be a major determinant of social identity, and this proposition has often been applied to pronunciation (Setter/Jenkins 2005). The use of language or accent is said to influence the way individuals are evaluated because their languages or accents might be associated with specific social groups (cf. Section 2.2). Accents, in particular, are perceived as one of the main features of a group (Hogg/Vaughan 2002). For instance, an individual speaking with a distinct Geordie accent is likely to be considered as working class and from North East England. In this framework, SIT allows to account for the reason why (i) individuals use specific accents, i.e., to express national, ethnic or cultural identities, and (ii) accents are fundamental in determining a person's identity, i.e., because they are "one of the main features of an individual which is compared to a prototype and then assigned to specific groups according to which the speaker is perceived" (Beinhoff 2013:4–5). However, this conscious or unconscious choice of accent can only be influenced to a certain extent, especially in L2 contexts. Nevertheless, most L2 English speakers are able to speak with a stronger L1–influenced accent whenever they wish to emphasise group membership (Jenkins 2007).

The earliest studies of social identity and attitudinal orientation were conducted by Lambert (1967). They show that members of very differentiated speech communities – in his case, English and French Canadians – evaluate the same speaker very differently depending on the language he or she is speaking (cf. Section 4.2.4). The speaker in question is perceived very positively by English-speaking Canadians when speaking English and very negatively when speaking French. Interestingly, the French Canadians perceive the speaker the same way. Particularly, while English-speaking Canadians are rated 'competent', delineating a quite positive attitude toward the language (and the speakers), French Canadians are judged 'unreliable', thus unravelling quite negative attitudes (Lambert 1967). These responses reveal a fairly good idea of the attitudes of English-speaking and French-speaking Canadians towards their communities of practice.

As briefly mentioned in Section 2.3, research on attitudes towards both L1 and L2 accents of English has mainly focused on the phonetic and phonological aspects of language (cf. Section 2.5 for a more comprehensive account). In Britain, for instance, such studies have almost always delved into the non-regional accent of 'Received Pronunciation' (RP), often referred to as 'Queen's English' or 'Standard British English' (hereafter BrE). The results on attitudes towards this accent are all fairly similar and likely to point to a very positive rating of the prestige and status scales and a fairly negative one in terms of solidarity (Giles 1970; Hiraga 2005). On the contrary, research on British regional accents has demonstrated that they tend to be rated negatively with respect to traits representing the status dimension, but fairly positively in terms of solidarity. With regard to British urban accents, according to Coupland and Bishop (2007:80): "[t]here is some support for the idea that urban vernaculars are systematically downgraded. This is certainly the case with Birmingham, Liverpool and Glasgow, also to a lesser extend with Swansea, Cardiff, Leeds, Manchester and Bristol". Similar results for the Birmingham accent are also reported by Giles (1970) and Hiraga (2005). In this specific case, in-group respondents, i.e., people from Birmingham with a presumable Birmingham accent, downgrade their own accent in some sort of self-stereotyping.

In order to account for the worldwide spread of English, attitudes towards L2 English accents which did not originate in Britain need to be considered as well. For instance, Giles' (1970) investigation of IndE and West IndE accents in the UK registers a slightly more positive rating of these two accents compared to the Birmingham one. In comparison, more than 30 years later, Coupland and Bishop (2007) find that both Asian accented English and the Afro-Caribbean variety are rated similar to the Birmingham accent for prestige, but that the Afro-Caribbean one is perceived more attractive than prestigious. The results from both studies clearly indicate that attitudes toward accents are relatively stable, even across 30 years.

L2 speakers of English tend to be well aware of their accents (Chand 2009; Regnoli 2016; Sharma 2005) and somehow share some characteristics with EFL speakers with respect to attitudinal orientations. In this sense, their attitudes sometimes seem to align with those of English learners who, in turn, are often inclined to changing their accents as well (Beinhoff 2013). Almost half of the participants in a study conducted by Derwing (2003) connect their communication deficiencies to pronunciation problems and regard pronunciation as a key aspect of communication. Yet, unlike learners of English, who do not generally feel that their identity will be threatened if they eliminate their accents or some of their features, L2 speakers seem to build and develop their identities in relation to their English accents as well, due to the colonial heritage and nationalistic issues (cf. Section 2.6). Further issues that come up in Derwing's (2003) study and that are connected with L2 speakers of English as well, concern the intelligibility of their accents and attitudes towards less intelligible accents. Accents which are highly intelligible tend to favour communication whereas less intelligible ones usually require considerable effort from the interlocutor to decode or understand the message. According to Tomokiyo *et al.* (2005:1469) "even highly accented speech can be very intelligible [...] [since] listeners are expending more effort in understanding it". Such additional effort might influence attitudes towards the speaker. However, intelligibility depends on many other factors including the familiarity with a particular accent and may as well pertain to L1 accents of English. In order to shed light on this rather controversial issue, Munro *et al.* (2006) suggest a distinction of speech into intelligibility, comprehensibility and accentedness. As they put it (2006:112):

> [intelligibility is] the extent to which a speaker's utterance is actually understood [...] [comprehensibility is] the listener's estimation of difficulty in understanding an

> utterance [...] [and accentedness is] the degree to which the pronunciation of an utterance sounds different from the expected production pattern.

Although these components are interrelated, this division shows that accentedness does not necessarily hinder intelligibility.

Attitudes seem to be affected by acceptability factors as well. As described by Sharma (2017) and Niedzielski and Preston (2003), acceptability of syntax or grammar is not a problem for L2 speakers of English since "syntactic variation is too risky for identity work because of its role in signalling competence and ratified status as English users" (Sharma 2017:244). On the other hand, acceptability judgements are more concerned with accents as regards social standards. In the words of Beinhoff (2013:37) "[a]cceptability is generally considered to relate to a norm or a mutually agreed standard specified by a particular social group in a certain social context". Thus, it is a subjective evaluation because perceptions toward a specific accent may vary. Just like attitudes, acceptability is created by groupness, and it establishes groupness and identity. Unlike attitudes, acceptability judgements cannot influence beliefs or ideas, but are rather influenced by them. In this sense, people evaluate their attitudes towards an accent before deciding whether it is acceptable or not. In other words, while attitudes influence acceptability, context and social conventions are the only determinants of acceptability judgements.

In short, accents evoke certain attitudes and stereotypes that can either threaten or emphasise an individual's identity depending on whether the person identifies with a particular group or not. Attitudes and stereotypes directly influence behaviour and, in turn, the success of speech acts. This is particularly the case with L2 accents of English, which are identity- and ethnicity-bound (cf. Section 2.6). Moreover, issues of intelligibility and acceptability are likely to play a pivotal role in accent judgement and recognition (cf. Chapter 5).

2.5 English in the Indian Diaspora

The Indian Diaspora today constitutes an important and, in some respects, unique force in world culture. According to India's Ministry of External Affairs, more than 20 million Indians live outside the subcontinent, either as people of Indian origin, i.e., people who have acquired the citizenship of the hosting country (PIOs) or as non-resident Indians, i.e., people living abroad on a temporary resident permit (NRIs). However, this is a rather narrow estimate since it is solely based on the definition of the Indian diaspora as being constituted only by those people who migrated from the Republic of India. In this respect, Skutsch (2005) uses a broader definition so as to include people who migrated from the whole of the Indian subcontinent, i.e., Bangladesh, Bhutan, Nepal, Pakistan and Sri Lanka. As far as scholarly treatments are concerned, aspects of the Indian diaspora have been largely investigated by historians (Lal *et al.* 2006), sociologists and psychologists (Bhatia 2007; Jayaram 2004), anthropologists (Oonk 2007) and economists (Gottschlich 2013; Parek *et al.* 2003), not to mention the wide recognition that literary works have been receiving (cf. the works of authors such as Salman Rushdie, Jhumpa Lahiri and Amit Chaudhuri, to name but a few). Diasporic populations offer unique opportunities for the study of language variation and change. However, it is not until very recently that linguistic studies of Indian primary and secondary diaspora situations have been given much attention. Earlier research on language in the Indian diaspora has focused on the status and maintenance of Indian native languages (Barz/Siegel 1988; Sharma/Annamalai 2003). A great exception has been Mesthrie's work on the Indian diaspora in South Africa which principally examines Bhojpuri Hindi (1991), sociolinguistic aspects of language contact and localised varieties of IndE in the contact situation (1992). With the exception of South African IndE, varieties of English are a fairly recent area of study since research has often been restricted to individual case studies rather than to comparisons of language contact across different diasporic settings (Hundt/Sharma 2014). One such exception is Hallett's (2010) work on the role of code-switching in English-medium newspaper discourse in both the Indian and the Jewish diaspora.

In order to capture language variation in the Indian diaspora, Mesthrie (2008) proposes a tentative schema which identifies three different periods and types of diaspora. The first one comprises movements out of the subcontinent prior to the 17th century, during which migration followed upon trade and settlement by sailing ships in Southeast Asia and East Africa. The second diaspora is more cohesively defined and covers the forced migration of slaves and indentured workers during the period of British imperialism. While places like Kabul and Cape Town were the recipients of large numbers of slaves in the 17th and the 18th century, the Caribbean, Mauritius, South Africa and Fiji received many indentured workers in the 19th and early 20th centuries. During this period, similar Indian communities migrated to Singapore, Malaysia, Suriname, Guyana and Trinidad. The era of indenture is probably the most frequently and best-studied part of Indian diasporic studies. The third diaspora is a direct consequence of decolonisation and globalisation, and the sociolinguistics of Indian languages taken to the UK and the US, Australia, New Zealand and Canada has been widely investigated (Sridhar 2008). In contrast to the indentured workers of the second diaspora, these migrants are well-educated urban Indians who left their mother country in order to further their education or find better positions (cf. Chapter 3).

Regardless of the period or type of diaspora, the role of identity is always crucial to language change. Schneider (2007), for instance, argues that major events may drive change in World Englishes due to the shift to endonormative orientation based on new identities, while Schreirer (2014) uses the framework of World Englishes to refine the understanding of different social roles in koineisation and new-dialect formation. Hence, specifics of bilingual identities may affect language variation (Sharma 2017). This is the reason why recent works on the linguistics of the Indian diaspora tend to provide a more comparative perspective on the topic aiming to deepen the theoretical framework of the studies of language change and language contact, such as the degree of universality in the process of focusing in migration situations (Kerswill/Trudgill 2005), selections of traits from contact feature pools (Mufwene 2001) and interactions between identity, social access and language change (Le Page/Tabouret-Keller 1985). Specifically, they address theoretical and methodological questions concerning issues of (i) endonormativity; (ii) transnationalism; and (iii) community structure, attitudinal orientation and identity development and tend to focus on (socio-)phonetic and phonological variation and on (socio-)lexical aspects of language contact. The regional spread covered by recent studies ranges from Singapore to the South Pacific, via Africa, the UK, the US and the Caribbean.

2.5.1 Phonetics and Phonology

Segmental and suprasegmental research on the English language in the Indian diaspora points to the importance of emergent local identities and the renegotiation of ethnicity. Specifically, it provides insight into the correlation between heritage sources and local contact realisations of linguistic variation by focusing on different variables – from pitch to rhoticity, syllable-initial /t/ and fundamental frequency. For instance, Zipp's (2014) work on the development of endocentric norms in Indo-Fijan English explores language attitudes and use among Fiji's students of Indian descent. In recurring to Schneider's (2007) influential dynamic model of the evolution of new Englishes, she aims to weigh diasporic exonormative effects against endonormative stabilisation. In doing so, she compares data from corpus-based research with evidence from respondents' self-evaluations of attitudinal stances. Her findings support the claim of progressing endonormative stabilisation although "indications for diasporic links to India in the use of English remain weak" (2014:187).

If Zipp's (2014) study in Suva has not proved to be significant, studies of other diasporic settings have given insight into the linguistic effects of transnational network maintenance. One such example is Sharma's (2014) investigation of the extent to which an orientation to Asian norms is maintained over time. The study takes into account network allegiances and attitudinal orientations in the maintenance of IndE phonetic realisations among second-generation Punjabi West Londoners. The impact of transnational relations is examined from the perspective of language use and language ideologies and suggests a pattern of decreasing transnational ties from older to younger second-generation participants. Interestingly, an independent pattern shows that the correlation between transnational activity and the use of retracted /t/ disappears in younger groups. As far as ideological orientations are concerned, her findings are likely to support evidence of overt prestige for Standard IndE, possibly due to positive affiliations of both groups to the mother country since "the variety is not simply reserved for voicing cultural distance or mocking 'parent' or outsider positions" (Sharma 2014:239).

Sharma's (2014) work mirrors other research findings on sociophonetic and language attitude studies in the Indian diaspora in highlighting the development of local meanings for heritage features. Alam and Stuart-Smith's (2014) work in a Glaswegian Pakistani community of practice, for example, explores the emergence of a local ethnic accent with subtle adaptation of heritage features reflecting newly emerging identities. Their detailed spectral moment analysis of syllable-initial /t/ shows a significant correlation between fine phonetic variation and ethnicity for three measures (mean, skew, kurtosis), thus revealing a clear patterning correlated to the social practices and gradience of the participants. The realisation of retroflex stops for the voiceless and voiced coronal plosives /t/ and /d/ is a stereotypical feature of IndE accents, and it is also investigated in many first-generation British-Asian speakers (cf. Bhardwaj 1995; Bhatia 1993; Sharma/Sankaran 2011). Recent research on second-generation British-Asian subjects has revealed that although they show auditorily retracted realisations of /t/ (Heselwood/McChrystal 2000), they usually sound more post-alveolar than retroflex (Kirkham 2011).

Alam and Stuart-Smith's (2014) research is similar to that of Mesthrie and Chevalier (2014) in that the two point to the importance of ongoing social change and emergent local identities in diasporic settings as a crucial factor in "restructuring material originally contributed by Indian languages" (Hundt/Sharma 2014b:3). Comparing evidence from older South African IndE respondents to new data from younger generations, they investigate the variation in the use of the NURSE vowel in South Africa. The results demonstrate that younger South

African IndE speakers move away from the L2 norms of previous generations. Moreover, they align with the findings of Alam and Stuart-Smith (2014) since the phonetic variation in the use of the NURSE vowel points to emergent identities in the post-apartheid era, ultimately highlighting the correlation between gender and class.

Similarly, Leung and Deuber's (2014) case study of fundamental frequency (F0) in Indo-Trinidanian speech proves to be significant as a marker of Indian ethnicity. Despite the commonly held stereotype according to which Indo-Trinidadians have a distinctive speech pattern, very few studies have focused on ethnolects in Trinidad from a phonological perspective (Gooden *et al.* 2009; Leung 2013; Winford 1978). In this light, Leung and Deuber collected data in a survey format among Indo- and Afro-Trinidadians in order to investigate the above-mentioned belief. Recurring to perceptual cues of laypeople who describe Indo-Trinidadian speech as "light, soft, fine, and high in pitch" (Leung/Deuber 2014:13), their findings reveal that F0 is indeed one of the salient cues which Trinidadians rely on to distinguish ethnicity since a high-pitched voice tends to be associated with Indo-Trinidadians.

Rathore (2014) also looks at phonological variation in an East African Indian community located in Leicester. Recurring to major phonological studies of both East African IndE (Schmied 2008; Simo Bobda 2001) – which is still an underresearched variety – and East Midlands English (Hughes *et al.* 2005), her work aims to provide insight into patterns of dialect variation and change in secondary diaspora situations. In order to determine how the complex migration pattern of such speakers, i.e., Asians who settled in Britain via East Africa, has influenced their variety of English and whether linguistic patterns change across generations, she examines variation in the use of non-prevocalic /r/. The results indicate that first-generation speakers have retained IndE forms whereas second-generation subjects show accommodation to the local variety of BrE. As she puts it (2014:80), "the first generation's retention of IndE forms suggests that, even if previous migration to another county results in a strong sense of a separate identity among twice migrant, this does not necessarily lead to linguistic divergence".

2.5.2 Lexicon and Syntax

Lexical and syntactic variation are common areas of investigation in both primary and secondary diaspora contexts and are principally studied in relation to change, adaptation and ethnicity (Hundt/Sharma 2014). A multitude of variables, spanning from article use to imperfectives, semantic shifts and borrowings have been investigated and are often intertwined with studies of phonetic variation. Sharma's (2005) work on Indian communities in a contact situation in the US, for example, explores developing dialectal features along with the concomitant emergence of dialect consciousness. In order to assess the participants' explanatory scope of proficiency, she examines the use of selected phonological variants (rhoticity, /l/ velarisation and aspiration) along with copula use, past marking, subject-verb agreement and articles. Emphasising the respondents' attitudinal stances over proficiency levels, her study points to "the importance of understanding emerging speaker awareness and perceptions of stigma, risk, and value in new varieties of English" (2005:194) and sheds new light on the bilingual continuum of diasporic subjects.

Grammatical variation is the focus of the work by Leimgruber and Sankaran (2014). Investigating the use of imperfectives (including statives and non-delimited habituals) in an Indian Singapore community, they aim to shed new light on the very limited body of research concerning grammatical ethnic variation. Specifically, they analyse and compare the over-extension of the progressive marker *-ing* in the three main Singapore English varieties (i.e., Chinese, Malay, and Tamil) in order to verify whether a substratist explanation could account for any differences. The data, collected from the three main ethnic groups via administration of an online survey, indicate a significant difference in the grammaticality judgements of statives and non-delimited habituals marked with *-ing* between Tamil respondents and Chinese and Malay ones. In other words, they find that the Tamilians rate *-ing* as acceptable significantly more frequently than the two other groups. This is probably due to the grammatical means used in the substrate languages involved, thus supporting earlier work on the topic, which shows a robust over-extension of *-ing* forms in IndE varieties (Sharma 2009).

Marianne Hundt (2014) looks at ethnic variation in article use by comparing the primary diaspora context of Indians in Fiji and the secondary diaspora situation of Fiji Indians in New Zealand. Specifically, she investigates zero or 'null' articles in order to check whether generational patterns differ in the maintenance of transnational ties. While earlier work principally investigate article use in the primary diaspora contexts of Fiji English (Mugler/Tent 2008), American IndE (Sharma 2005) and South African Indian English (Mesthrie 1992), Hundt (2014:132) is the first comparative study to "show whether first-generation migrants are likely to have adapted to the majority ENL [first-language varieties of English] speakers in the secondary diaspora". Her results suggest that article omission decreases with the growing distance from the original diasporic setting and is thus more frequent in first-generation migrants. Moreover, as far as the first-generation is concerned, article omission does not seem to correspond to identity construction, but rather with different degrees of proficiency in English.

Lexical variation in South African IndE has always been central in Mesthrie's work (1992). Having provided a comprehensive lexicographic treatment of the variety, he investigates cultural aspects of lexical retention and variation in the domains of food, music, kinship and clothing (2014). His analysis of borrowings, adaptations, semantic shifts and neologisms indicates that there is a balance between local contact processes and heritage sources and gives "a sense of social history from below" (2014:184).

2.6 The Structure of L2 English Accents: Definitions, Norms and the 'Neutral' Accent

In terms of its formal properties, the notion of 'English' no longer relates exclusively to the seemingly monolithic standard forms and norms of correct language usage, i.e., language systems such as Standard English, BrE or AmE or even International English. English in use comes in an incredible range of different forms, varieties, dialects and accents which have grown tremendously, comprising New Englishes in Asia and in Africa and English-based pidgins and creoles all around the world. Given the notorious fuzziness of its boundaries, perhaps there is no reason to ask: "Who actually owns English?" (Hayhoe/Parker 1994) and "Is it English?" (Görlach 1996) anymore.

L2 varieties of English are indigenised non-native varieties that challenge much sociolinguistic theory since they cannot simply come under models of second language learning nor under those of first language variation (Kachru 1983). These varieties have emerged in language contact situations and developed their hybrid nature in multilingual regions in which native-like patterns of indigenous transmission and use have progressively entered the superstrate language (Schneider 2007). Yet, anthropological approaches to language contact point to the fact that languages do not come into contact in any meaningful sense, rather *speakers* do, under a wide range of historical and social circumstances such as colonialism, slavery, and, more recently, under new forms of globalisation (Garrett 2004).[13] In such situations, speakers make selections from a pool of linguistic variants available to them and, through such a mixture of features, they

13 For a detailed discussion of the spread of English, models of English in the world, creolised forms of English, and language contact in L2 settings cf. Mesthrie (2017), Schneider (2017, 2007), Trudgill (2017), Winford (2017), Mesthrie/Bhatt (2008), McArthur (1992a) and Kachru ([1986] 1990).

reproduce, recreate and appropriate elements of a selected language (Mufwene 2001).[14] In short, L2 varieties of English are "norm-developing" in the sense that the norms produced by L1 varieties, which are defined as 'norm-providing', are further developed and reproduced in local contexts in order to suit local needs better (Kachru 1985). This process is called 'nativisation' (Schneider 2007) and, according to Kachru ([1986] 1990:21–2):

> [it] must be seen as the result of those productive linguistic innovations which are determined by the localized functions of a second language variety, the 'culture of conversation' and communicative strategies in new situations, and the 'transfer' from local languages.

While L1 varieties and accents of English are generally assumed to reveal the regional origin and the social status of the speakers (McArthur 1992b), L2 varieties and accents of English do not necessarily reveal the social status of the speakers because their English tends to be influenced by other factors, such as their L1 or their ability to produce new sounds (Bettoni 2006). In order to delve into the structure of L2 English accents, it is important to take a step back and shed light on the term 'accent' itself, which has so far been used without further explanation. The present section provides more detailed information on the sociolinguistic dimension of accents. In addition, features of L2 accents of English and issues concerning the perception of accents will be discussed and related to identity construction.

Accents are generally defined according to pronunciation features in contrast to dialects, which also include vocabulary and grammar as distinguishing elements (Chambers/Trudgill 2004; Hughes *et al.* 2005; Trudgill 2000). Therefore, an accent shows specific phonetic realisations which distinguish it from other accents. Most phonologists describe accent development as the result of phonological interference (Chambers/Trudgill 2004). According to McArthur (1992b:9), accents are generally viewed as a "way of speaking that indicates a person's place of origin and/or social class". However, this definition does not fully apply to L2 English accents because through an L2 accent it is not possible to make statements about the speaker's social class although the social status may play a crucial role regarding the accessibility to higher education and the

14 Salikoko Mufwene's (2001) theory of the ecology of language evolution applies directly to contact situations. The 'feature pool' consists of the sum total of all individual forms and variants that each of the speakers involved, with diverse language backgrounds, brings to the contact situation.

quality of language teaching and, in turn, results in a diverse command of the language, both phonologically and syntactically. Thus, a more suitable definition that excludes L2 accents as markers of social status and that takes into account the native language(s) of the speaker and his or her pronunciation skills is required. Bussmann (1996:3) defines accent as an "[i]diosyncratic pronunciation of a foreign language, especially due to the articulatory or phonotactic characteristics of one's native language".

In the case of L2 accents in general and L2 accents of English in particular, attitudes tend to be influenced by national and regional stereotypes which, for instance, may make a Southern Indian accent sound 'sing-song' and 'funny' and a Northern Indian one 'smoother' and 'thick' (Regnoli 2019a, 2016). According to Beinhoff (2013:42), "for NNS-accents [non-native speaker-accents], attitudes regarding the social status of the speaker are likely to be replaced with attitudes towards national stereotypes or personal experiences with people of a specific nationality". Furthermore, attitudes toward L2 accents might be stronger the more they differ from what is perceived as a neutral or standard accent. The idea of a neutral or standard accent seems to be well established in the folk (Niedzielski/Preston 2003), and the remark that somebody speaks 'without an accent' or with 'hardly any accent' is often used to refer to non-regional accents (Beinhoff 2013). In folk theory, these remarks indicate that the folk perceive the accent in question as neutral (cf. Section 5.2.2.2). However, the concept of a neutral or standard accent is not accepted in sociolinguistics since every accent carries some indexical information about the speaker, e.g., whether he or she is an L1, L2 or learner speaker of English and his or her origins. Moreover, according to Sailaja (2009:37) "a standard accent in an individual is not a constant or a perfect set of all the sounds identified as standard", and different contexts require more formal or informal accents.

The literature on English standards and norms reveals considerable disagreement as to what standard English is. The term itself creates some confusion as to whether it refers to written or spoken English. Davis (1999) and Bex (1999) argue that the standardisation of English has been mainly regarded as referring to the written language and, specifically, to a group of influential writers that have contributed to set a specific standard against other varieties. This standardisation has led to certain attitudes and ideologies which have survived until today (cf. below).[15] Yet, according to Trudgill (1999), Standard English is a dialect

15 Here, ideologies are referred to as "sets of beliefs about language articulated by the users as a rationalization or justification of perceived language structure and use" (Silverstein 1979:193)

of English without any related accent, which clearly indicates that the standard is evident in written language more than in speech. Moreover, there seems to be a strong connection between the Standard English dialect and the RP accent. Nevertheless, such a connection is unidirectional since "all RP speakers also speak Standard English, [whereas] the reverse is not the case" (Trudgill 1999:118). Both are purely social concepts which, unlike other dialects and accents, are not related to any particular region but rather to speakers of certain social and educational backgrounds. As Beinhoff (2013:43) puts it:

> [w]hile a standard written language is easy to describe and to identify by looking into a dictionary, the notion of a 'standard' accent is much more difficult to explain since it is not only variable within time and region but also with regard to social restrictions which influence the preference for accents.

Thus, an accent becomes a standard for purely social reasons, and neutral accents do not exist since every accent evokes some sort of attitude in the listener.

RP is the most influential and heavily institutionalised accent of Great Britain and is used in second-language teaching in so-called post-colonial countries such as India or Nigeria. McArthur (1992b: 850–1) argues that RP is

> the accent generally associated with educated BrE and used as the pronunciation model for teaching it to foreign learners [....] [and] it is often informally referred to by the British middle class as a BBC accent or a public-school accent and by the working class as talking proper or talking posh.

This definition reveals both integrative and dissociative attitudes towards RP: while, on the one hand, it seems important from a sociocultural point of view since it confers some sense of correctness, it shows, on the other, some resentment when it is referred to as 'talking posh'. As discussed in Sections 2.4 and 2.5, these statements are based on extralinguistic factors since "any coherent notion of inherent phonetic or phonological superiority" (Carr 1999:134) does not exist.

The notion that RP is correct implicitly points to the existence of incorrect or less correct accents of English. This position is reflected in the 'Deficit Hypothesis' and the 'Difference Hypothesis', which represent two different views on variation in accent and which have influenced World Englishes theories concerning the idea of nativisation (Kachru [1986] 1990, 1983). The 'Deficit Hypothesis' adopts a prescriptive approach to language since it promotes the idea of correctness and regards social success and access to privileges as depending on language habits. The hypothesis was formulated in the context of L1 accents and compared the inferiority of the so-called 'restricted code' of lower classes to the superior 'elaborated code' of the middle class (Bernstein 1971). The 'Deficit Hypothesis' is certainly applicable to L2 accents as well since it may promote stereotypical attitudes of L1 speakers towards L2 speakers or L2 speakers towards other L2 speakers, thus influencing social communication.[16] This mechanism may lead to very frustrating experiences for the speaker to the extent that his or her own identity is threatened, especially in cases where he or she uses a very elaborate code in his or her L1 but has a rather restricted one in English. An appropriate example is that of educated Indian speakers who have attended vernacular-medium schools in the subcontinent or that of first-generation Indian immigrants who have acquired English at later stages of life, often in the host country and who, therefore, do not have an elaborate code in their L2.

Conversely, the 'Difference Hypothesis' adopts a descriptive approach to language and supports the notion that accents simply differ without further value being attached to them (Labov 1972a). In this case, the focus is on differences in language habits and their use within and between speech communities.

However, although scholars seem to be divided into those who support a more prescriptivist approach and those who aim at a more egalitarian view of accents, it is important to bear in mind that research on language attitudes requires both. The present study combines both approaches in what has traditionally been acknowledged as the emic and etic perspectives (cf. Sections 4.1.2 and 4.3). In the words of Beinhoff (2013:46–7), they may be defined as follows:

> a descriptive approach towards all accents [is required] especially when [...] [attitudes] are analysed and discussed, i.e. the more phonetic and phonological side of research on attitudes towards linguistic features. At the same time, it is indispensable to consider the effects that accents have in society and to know about the influence of accents on individuals and their possible ideas about accents and their speakers, i.e. the social psychological and sociolinguistic part of language research. Both aspects are brought together when the phonetic input of the own accent and other accents are transformed into linguistic and attitudinal output.

The social input tends to determine how accents are perceived in terms of attitudinal orientations. Moreover, non-regional accents such as RP tend to be perceived as social standards in post-colonial English societies, where speakers are taught English with respect to this specific norm presented as the pronunciation target. In consequence, many L2 English speakers self-evaluate their accents in comparison to this target and try to adjust their way of speaking accordingly (Regnoli 2016).

16 For a detailed discussion of overt and covert language attitudes of native speakers toward second-language speakers cf. McKenzie (2015).

Moreover, considering that in the Outer Circle, or norm-developing L2 settings, the English language is generally used as a *lingua franca* (hereafter ELF), it has been argued that it should not be the goal of L2 English speakers (and learners) to imitate L1 accents. Instead, they should aim to achieve mutual intelligibility with other speakers of EFL from around the world. The 'Lingua Franca Core' (hereafter LFC) proposed by Jenkins (2000) is an inventory of pronunciation features that are necessary to maintain intelligibility in international communication. For instance, it might not be necessary for L2 English speakers to acquire dental fricative sounds if they cannot master them given that they occur very seldom in many accents of English. Interestingly, these features are placed outside the core along with all other features of pronunciation that occur in L2 varieties of English. In this sense, Jenkins (2007, 2000) argues that, by teaching features outside the core receptively, rather than productively, L2 English speakers can still understand other accents of English and retain some features of their L1 accents. However, the theorisation of the LFC remains controversial in that it does not take into account the different accents developed in post-colonial settings and, although English is here used as a *lingua franca*, the LFC does not apply to such contexts since intelligibility is most generally reached among speakers of different L1s. Moreover, the LFC only considers intelligibility and does not provide insight into the possible role of such features in forming and influencing attitudes.

As mentioned above, L2 speakers of English tend to compare their own accents with a target variety of English, mainly standard BrE or AmE. This comparison is evident in the speakers' meta-linguistic comments about their ways of speaking. In particular, when they are asked to identify specific features of their accents, the folk recur to both segmental and prosodic features (Niedzielski/Preston 2003). As far as phonology is concerned, Uffmann (2017) argues that L1 interference is an interference by constraints and that if, for instance, there is no final devoicing in the L1, one cannot expect a sudden and repeated emergence of final devoicing in nativised varieties. Further research explicitly addressing this issue has highlighted the role of constraints in the comparison between non-native or nativised varieties and the substrate systems of the L1 in question. In his analysis of Vernacular Liberian English, Singler (1996) points out that what is transferred from Loma – the substrate language that he refers to as the 'alpha basilect' – is not phonological processes or rules but rather output constraints. Specifically, Loma does not allow closed syllables, hence coda consonants. When conversing in English, Loma speakers either delete the offending consonant in coda consonants or add a final vowel, thus resyllabifying the consonant into an onset position. Interestingly, both strategies are found in Vernacular Liberian

English, but in different prosodic contexts: if the word is monosyllabic, a vowel is added, if the word is polysyllabic the final consonant is deleted. Considering that there are no processes of insertion, deletion and resyllabification in Loma, what happens in Vernacular Liberian English is that no such rules are transferred, but rather Loma constraints are.

As can be seen, the influence of a person's L1 on his or her accent in an L2 is evident since "articulatory or phonotactic characteristics of one's native language" (Bussmann 1996:3) determine the L2 accent. Moreover, the folk perceive accent variation also in relation to the speaker's L1 (cf. Section 2.4). However, there are a multitude of factors that can influence performance in an L2 and that determine the way L2-sounds are pronounced. For the purpose of the present study, the two most important theories on phonological acquisition and speech perception that need to be examined are Kuhl and Iverson's (1995) 'Native Language Magnet' (hereafter NLM) model and Escudero's (2007) 'Linguistic Perception' (hereafter LP) model. These theories are based on complementing assumptions as to how L2 accents are constituted. According to Kuhl and Iverson (1995), the L1 tends to alter the underlying perceptual mechanisms responsible for the processing of language. In this sense, speakers identify speech sounds in relation to prototypical L1-speech ones and show particular preferences in sound variation when they have difficulties in mastering certain sounds. A prototypical sound functions as a perceptual magnet for similar ones since it "pulls other members of the category toward itself" (Kuhl/Iverson 1995:123). For instance, with respect to /v/, it could be assumed that according to the NLM model, Bengali speakers of English would be less likely to discriminate between /v/ and similar sounds as opposed to L1 speakers of English who have this sound in their repertoire. Since Bengali English speakers usually substitute /v/ with /bh/, the sound /bh/ might be more prototypical that /w/ for them although both sounds are very similar. Thus, the NLM model may account for the preference of /bh/ in substituting /v/ by Bengali speakers of English.

A further model which also considers the influence of the L1 on L2 perception and production is the LP model developed by Escudero (2007). This model is set within the framework of Boersma's (1998) Functional Phonology, which connects cognitive linguistic knowledge with speech perception. Within the LP model (Escudero 2007:125), perception is regarded as:

> a process mediating between (i) the acoustic-phonetic input in the outside world and (ii) the perceptual representation of language sounds, which, in turn, act as the input to (iii) the recognition system, which is responsible for accessing words in the mental lexicon.

According to the model, language-specific knowledge influencing speech perception is based on a perception grammar which enables the categorisation of the acoustic signal on the perceptual input. In this sense, speech sounds are analysed according to their perceptual representations whose recognition would depend on the speaker's familiarity with the input language. In other words, the LP model implies that when listening to the L2 in question for the first time, speakers create a copy of their L1 perception grammar and its categories and use this copy as a separate perceptual system which is then adjusted to the categories of the L2. By suggesting the existence of two separate systems for the L1 grammar and the L2 one, the model may account for the occurrences of foreign accents and the reasons why they show features of the speakers' L1s.

However, with regard to nativised varieties of English, the question is further complicated by the sort of fluidity of norms and cognitive systems that guide the acquisition of English. In Indian varieties of English, for instance, English sounds are not always replaced by regional equivalents. [ʒ] is absent in both Indo-Aryan and Dravidian languages, but still has been acquired by most of them. Conversely, [θ] and [ð] are also absent in Indian languages and are absent even in Indian varieties of English (Sailaja 2009).

The influence of the L1 on the L2-performance is also visible on a more socio-cultural level due to the fundamental role that identity plays in L2-acquisition. The role of language in constructing a person's social identity has already been illustrated (Section 2.4), and the influence of L1 on L2-acquisition is based on the mechanisms and processes described there. As seen above, with regard to L2 accent acquisition, L2 speakers of English might wish to retain some features of their L1s in their L2 accents in order to mark membership or strive for distinctiveness. In this way, "the L1 exerts a socio-cultural influence on the L2-accent and even though certain L2-speech sounds could technically be produced in a native-like manner, they are not" (Beinhoff 2013:65). Moreover, the speaker's preference of a particular target native accent is crucial in shaping the nativised accent as well. This is especially evident in the acquisition of English accents where the two most influential accents, i.e., BrE and AmE, are present, in L2 education (the former) and in popular culture (the latter).

However, identifying a nativised regional accent of English does not seem to be as straightforward as might be expected. Unlike native accents of English, L2 regional English accents have more in common with non-native, norm-dependent accents of English such as Italian English or German English. In such cases, listeners tend to be better at identifying imitated and exaggerated accents than authentic ones since they rely on certain stereotypical phonetic patterns which suggest the existence of a "cognitive prototype of an accent" (Neuhauser/

Simpson 2007:1808). Yet, the ability to identify an accent certainly depends on the listeners' exposure and their familiarity with the accents in question.

In conclusion, a focus on phonetic and phonological variation is crucial to shed light on how an accent is perceived. Moreover, variation in individual features might influence the perceived distinctiveness of an accent and might change the social attributes assigned to the speaker. This means that the perception of the speaker's social identity might, in turn, be affected, as in the case of Indian speakers of English, who are clearly identifiable as Indians through their accents, but seldom recognised through their local IndE ones.

2.7 Indian Accents of English

IndE is an umbrella term used to describe the multiplicity of varieties of English spoken in the Indian subcontinent by speakers of varying fluency, ethnic, linguistic and socio-cultural backgrounds (Kachru 1983). Here, English has been in use for more than four centuries, first as the language of missionaries and early merchants, then as the language of the British colonial power and finally, after Independence in 1947, as the 'associate' official language of the Indian Union and as a second *lingua franca* in addition to Hindi (Sailaja 2009). While almost all L2 varieties of English have reached the third phase of Schneider's (2007) 'Dynamic Model of Post-colonial Englishes', i.e., nativisation (cf. Section 2.6), according to Mukherjee (2007), IndE is currently in the fourth phase of Schneider's model, during which English continues to be widely used in the media, education, the economy, and as a pan-Indian link language (cf. Tab. 2.7.1).

As Fuchs (2016:11) points out: "[t]he question of which standards to use and teach is characterised by paying lip-service to BrE while in practice promoting the emerging Indian standard". General Indian English (hereafter GIE) has traditionally been acknowledged as the ideal target to refer to in primary and secondary education (CIEFL 1972). Yet, there is a continuum of English used by Indians, typically referred to as 'cline of bilingualism', ranging from basilectal to acrolectal varieties which are marked by various degrees of L1 influence and subsequent accentedness (Wiltshire 2005; Gargesh 2004; Kachru [1986] 1990). While at the basilectal level, the influence is quite marked, earlier studies state that there is a substantial degree of uniformity at the acrolectal level as far as discourse organisation, lexis (Lange 2012) and monophthong and diphthong realisations (Maxwell/Fletcher 2010, 2009; Narang *et al.* 2011) are concerned.

Tab. 2.7.1 Development of IndE in Schneider's (2007, 2003) Dynamic Model of Post-colonial Englishes according to Mukherjee (2007)

	Phase	Start date	Event
Phase 1	Foundation	1600	East India Company established
Phase 2	Exonormative stabilisation	1757	Battle of Plassey
Phase 3	Nativisation	1835	Macauley's Minute on Indian Education
Phase 4	Endonormative stabilisation	1968	Three-language formula
Phase 5	Differentiation	Future	?

The Indian subcontinent is a good example of the heteroglossia of many South Asian contexts and of the complexity of multilingualism. Yet, "estimating which languages are spoken by how many people in India is difficult because the only available data-source, the Indian census, is based on self-reported information" (Fuchs 2016:12). The most recent data available are based on the 2001 census. According to the last figures, Hindi is the language spoken the most, closely followed by Bengali, Telugu, Marathi, Tamil, Urdu, Gujarati, Kannada, Malayalam and Oriya, Punjabi and Assamese. In consequence, 790 million Indians stated that their L1 is one belonging to the Indo-Aryan branch of the Indo-European family, 212 million to the Dravidian one, ten million to the Austroasiatic language family and three million to the Tibeto-Burman one (Census of India 2001).

Despite the presence of four different language families, it has been argued that many Indians "share more specific features among themselves than anyone does with an external member of the family" (Montaut 2005:84), such as SOV word order, reduplication, serial verbs and retroflex obstruents. In India, two languages are not enough. As a matter of fact, multilingualism is the norm. Most of the time, children grow up in homes where parents and families speak different L1s. In addition, they acquire different language practices as they move from the family context to that of school. The subsequent fuzziness of language boundaries goes hand in hand with fluidity in language identity (Kachru [1986] 1990; Khubchandani 2001).

As far as scholarly treatments are concerned, Mohanty (2013, 2006) describes the very different multilingual natures of the subcontinent as a widespread bilingualism at the grassroot level. Here, norm maintenance is supported by the non-competing roles of vernacular languages in the society and their complementarities in people's lives. Yet, the substantial division of functional domains positions English "in the driver's seat" (Dasgupta 2002), especially in its use as a medium of instruction where it outranks even Hindi (Mohanty 2006). Although there are 33 languages used in education and 41 languages available for study in school, education in India is not truly bilingual. As Mohanty (2006:279) points out: "education in India is only superficially multilingual, and it remains monolingual at an underlying level. The official three-language formula is more abused and less used". What was an attempt to use an integrative approach to India's language planning turned out to reiterate those hegemonic language practices favouring English.[17] This has much to do with the concept of 'governmentality' as proposed by Foucault (1991). He explains how language practices in school regulate the ways in which language is used and establish language hierarchies in which some languages are valued more highly than others (cf. Section 2.5). Erickson (1987:352) defines those hegemonic practices as follows:

> routine actions and unexamined beliefs that are consonant with the cultural system of meaning and ontology within which it makes sense to take certain actions, entirely without malevolent intent, that nonetheless systematically limit the life chances of members of stigmatized groups.

Such practices ensure that people acquiesce to invisible cultural power and inevitably consider vernacular-medium schools as less prestigious than English-medium ones. English is the language used most as the medium of instruction across Indian states. Urban middle-class Indians consider private English-medium schools as the key to their children's prosperity. According to the National University of Education, Planning and Administration (hereafter NUEPA), the number of children studying in English-medium schools increased by a staggering 274 % to over 20 million students between 2003 and 2011. Of course, this contributes to the creation of strong, and most often dissociative, attitudes towards localised varieties and accents of English. As Bhatt (2017: 307) puts it:

> [...] certain ideological strategies are continually manipulated to legitimize and rationalize the power of 'standard' (English) language. The assumption behind it all is that

17 After post-independence intense language riots concerning Hindi as the national language, in 1968 the National Policy on Education seems to have settled for the so-called 'three language formula' at secondary school level, proposed with the optimistic hope that it would satisfy all three-language pressure groups in the subcontinent: the pro-English one, the pro-Hindi one and the pro-regional-language one. It entails introducing English along with Hindi and a regional language in school education throughout the country so that the children would have an equal language load (Gargesh/Sailaja 2017).

> authority (whether linguistic, political, or cultural) is actually very tentative and is maintained largely by smoke and mirrors – much like the wizard of Oz hiding behind that little curtain. But it is only the ideology critic (Dorothy, Gale's dog, Toto), who thinks to look behind the curtain – everyone else is looking the wrong way!

In spite of such strong (and dissociative) attitudes towards IndE local varieties, the fact that only 23 % of all Indians know some English, but only 4 % are fluent (Crystal 2003; Gradoll 2003; Kachru 2001) show that most of the speakers of IndE may be classified as basilectal. Butler English is an example of this variety of English (Hosali 2005). As mentioned above, at the other end of the cline, there are fluent speakers using an educated variety (Gargesh 2009; Kachru 1983; Sailaja 2009).

Educated speakers of IndE are at the centre of the present study. Choosing acrolectal rather than basilectal speakers as an object of investigation is not an arbitrary choice. Mukherjee's contention that IndE has entered phase four of Schneider's model, i.e., endonormative stabilisation, suggests that the process of perceiving an endocentric standard of IndE has already begun. In fact, sociolinguistic interviews with educated speakers of IndE conducted for the present study suggest that many informants have a mental concept of a standard IndE accent. Masica (1972:2) observed this folk perception more than four decades ago:

> we discovered, in addition to speakers [...] with definite 'Hindi' or 'Malayalam' or 'Bengali' accent [...], a considerable body of speakers from all parts of India whose speech, on the analogy of R.P., did not betray their regional origin, or did so only slightly. Yet, it was not R.P. or any other, although it did share certain characteristics with one or another of them. This generalized Indian English [...] appears to be the *de facto* norm to which the majority of the [...] speakers of English in India aspire. Ought it not to be [...] the *de jure* norm also, for mass-teaching purpose?

For the purpose of the present study, Masica's (1972) work is significant not only because he documents folk perceptions of an emerging standard IndE accent but for his intention to codify a standard IndE accent according to its phonology and pronunciation features. However, although further studies have attempted to codify this new emergent variety (D'Souza 1997; Dasgupta 1993; Mukherjee 2007; Nihalani *et al.* 1979), very little attention has been given to Indian educated accents of English. Most probably, this is also due to the considerable lack of empirical and acoustic research on the phonology of IndE (Fuchs 2016; Sailaja 2012).

IndE is best identified by its phonological characteristics; yet, paradoxically, the variation in the phonology is widespread. According to Sailaja (2009), accent in Indian speech is marked by regional variation although it is possible to talk about a pan-Indian standard accent. In addition, although the L1 exerts some influence on accent, it is important to bear in mind that schooling and peer groups influence accent much more strongly. Acoustic studies of IndE phonology are rare and mainly face issues of generalisability (Sailaja 2012). Early investigations of native language influences on IndE phonology has heightened the need for further studies, as they either documented L1-dependent differences (Nishihara/van de Weijer 2011; Wiltshire/Harnsberger 2006) or IndE similarities across speakers of different native languages (Sirsa/Redford 2013; Wiltshire/Moon 2003). Moreover, most acoustic studies have focused on segmental characteristics, mostly vowels. Little research has investigated the intonation of IndE and its speech rhythm. The following discussion will shed light on studies of both segmental and suprasegmental characteristics of IndE highlighting the need for further investigation in relation to IndE accents.

The vowel inventory of IndE is smaller than in BrE. According to Wells (1982), IndE has ten monophthongs and six diphthongs although some speakers use variable pronunciations (Sailaja 2009). Speakers of standard IndE tend to merge the NURSE, STRUT and COMMa vowels (Bansal 1978; Gargesh 2004; Sailaja 2009). Acoustic evidence has shown that L1 Hindi speakers in particular distinguish between the NURSE and COMMa vowels by duration, but not by quality (Maxwell/Fletcher 2009). Interestingly, L1 speakers of Tamil and Gujarati maintain differences between the NURSE and STRUT vowels (Wiltshire/Harnsberger 2006). There is also some discussion about the realisation of the NORTH and LOT vowels, some suggesting a merger (Bansal 1978; Trudgill/Hannah 2002), others arguing that both are realised as the BrE [ɒ], but with considerable difference in duration, NORTH being longer than LOT (Nihalani *et al.* 1979; Sailaja 2009). In standard IndE, the GOAT and FACE vowels are not realised as diphthongs, but as monophthongs [o] and [e] (Maxwell/Fletcher 2009; Sailaja 2009; Trudgill/Hannah 2002; Wiltshire/Harnsberger 2006). In addition, the START vowel, realised as [ɒ] in BrE, is often pronounced further to the front as [a] in IndE, although acoustic evidence based on data from IndE speakers with Hindi and Punjabi as L1s (Maxwell/Fletcher 2009) and Gujarati and Tamil (Wiltshire/Harnsberger 2006) suggest that an [ɒ] realisation is used as well. Furthermore, IndE does not seem to distinguish between lax and tense vowels, particularly in the case of Bengali speakers of English and L1 Hindi speakers (Bansal/Harrison 1994; Gargesh 2004; Maxwell/Fletcher 2009). Wiltshire and Harnsberger (2006) provide acoustic evidence suggesting that L1 Gujarati and Telugu speakers do not make any length distinctions between the tense vowels FLEECE and FACE and their counterparts KIT and DRESS. However, the difference between the duration of GOOSE – FOOT and START – STRUT is smaller.

In conclusion, Gargesh (2004) reports that the CURE vowel has alternative pronunciations, including a monophthong [u]. However, the general problem with acoustic studies on IndE is that they are usually based on a comparatively small number of speakers, hence it is important not to generalise these findings to the larger population of IndE educated speakers.

While acoustic measurements of the vowel inventory show that there are several sets of vowels that have a tendency to merge, there is only one potential merger in the consonant inventory of standard IndE. This concerns the labio-dental fricative /v/, which is often realised as a labio-dental approximant [ʋ] and at times merged with /w/ (Gargesh 2004; Sailaja 2009). Moreover, the BrE dental fricatives [θ] and [ð] are replaced by the dental plosives [t̪] and [d̪], of which the voiceless phoneme is often aspirated [t̪^{h}] due to the influence of spelling (Bansal 1976; Sailaja 2009). Conversely, the initially aspirated voiceless plosives of BrE [p^{h}], [t^{h}] and [k^{h}] in stressed syllables are always unaspirated in IndE (Bansal 1976; Gargesh 2004; Sailaka 2009). Another allophonic contrast which tends to be neutralised is the difference between syllable-initial clear [l] and syllable-final velarised [ɫ]; only the former is used (Kachru 1994; Gargesh 2004). The plosives [t] and [d] are sometimes not realised as alveolars, but rather as the retroflex sounds [ʈ] and [ɖ] (Kachru 1994; Trudgill/Hannah 2002). Sailaja (2012, 2009) argues that alveolar and retroflex realisation is variable both across and within speakers due to the different phonological inventories of their L1s, with the degree of retroflexion being greater in Southern varieties of IndE (Kachru 1983).

Although the Standard IndE pronunciation (hereafter SIEP) is non-rhotic (Sailaja 2009; Trudgill/Hannah 2002), IndE has often been described as rhotic (Bansal 1978; Gargesh 2004; Wells 1982). More recent empirical investigations show that rhoticity is variable across and within IndE speakers (Chand 2009; Sharma 2005). Moreover, regardless of whether /r/ is pronounced in non-prevocalic position, there are four different phonetic variants: Sharma (2005) mentions approximants and trills, Chand (2009) approximants, trills and flaps, Wiltshire and Harnsberger (2006) fricativised approximants in L1 Tamil speakers of English, Trudgill and Hannah (2002) flaps, and Bansal (1978) approximants and flaps. In short, most differences in the consonant inventory of IndE are phonetic. The only phonological differences are the frequent merger of /w/ and /v/ and the variable rhoticity. For the perception of differences between regional accents of IndE, both phonetic and phonological cues are important since speakers may rely on both kinds of differences when identifying a speaker as Southern or a Northern Indian (to be tested in Chapter 5).

Just as there in unpredictability in the pronunciation of individual words and segments, stress, i.e., the relative prominence with which a syllable is uttered, also tends to be unpredictable. There is a great deal of variation even within one single regional variety of IndE, so much so that generalisation is often difficult (Sailaja 2009). Chaudhary (1989), Gargesh (2004) and Wiltshire and Moon (2003) are among the major works that aim to give a pan-Indian account of stress in IndE, attempting to identify its acoustic correlates. It has been argued that syllabification in particular makes a difference to stress placement with regard to IndEs of the Indo-Aryan group of speakers and the Dravidian one. Although syllable weight plays an equally important role in both language groups, the manner in which a word is syllabified varies. According to Sailaja (2009:30; emphasis in the original): "[t]he different syllable structures assigned take care of the initial stress in "minister of Dravidian speakers who would syllabify the word as *mi.ni.ster* whereas the Indo-Aryan group perceives it as *mi.nis.ter*". Thus, the default stress pattern of IndE speakers tends to follow the stress patterns of their L1s.

As far are IndE intonation is concerned, it has been argued that it differs from BrE with regard to how utterances are divided into intonation phrases, which pitch-accents are commonly used, and the occasional use of a final rising tone (Bansal 1976; Sailaja 2009). Wiltshire and Harnsberger (2006) note that there is considerable difference in the use of pitch-accents between Tamil and Gujarati speakers. While the former tend to use a falling intonation, the latter use a rising one. Similarly, Maxwell and Fletcher (2010) find that L1 speakers of Kannada and Bengali frequently use rising pitch accents.

However, one of the aspects that has so far been neglected in empirical research is speech rhythm. Although suprasegmental features are not standardised in the CIEFL monograph, IndE has most often been characterised as syllable-timed (Gargesh 2004) or more syllable-timed than stress-timed (Fuchs 2016; Sailaja 2012, 2009). Yet, rhythmic variability in local varieties of IndE have, until very recently, been scarcely investigated. Varieties of English have also been described as differing in rhythm. It has been observed that while Inner Circle varieties such as BrE and AmE are more stress-timed, Outer-Circle Varieties such as IndE, Singapore English, and Nigerian English are more syllable-timed (Crystal 1995; Fuchs 2016; Nishihara/van de Weijer 2011).

Traditionally described as syllable-timed (Gargesh 2004), IndE speech rhythm has more recently been evaluated as more syllable-timed than the stress-timed rhythm of BrE (Fuchs 2016, 2014) and AmE (Krivokapić 2013). This tendency towards a more syllable-timed pattern might be related to the absence of weak or reduced vowels in connected speech (Sailaja 2009), stress placement (Chaudhary 1989) and word stress lengthening (Maxwell 2014). Among the few acoustic studies that have so far investigated the speech rhythm of IndE, Krivokapić (2013) examines rhythmic convergence between four speakers of AmE and four speakers of IndE. Focusing her analysis on the duration of stressed syllables and feet, she compares stressed syllable reduction in monosyllabic and multisyllabic feet. Whereas the study finds evidence of stress-timing and syllable-timing in both varieties, the results, however, are consistent with the description of IndE as qualitatively more syllable-timed than AmE.

Sirsa and Redford (2013) investigate whether the sound and timing structures of IndE vary according to the L1 of selected speakers. They measure the rhythmic differences of a text read by seven Hindi English speakers and seven Telugu ones who had attended English-medium schools. Comparing the IndE %V value (46.8 %) with that of BrE (41.1 %; in Grabe and Low 2002), the study provides evidence of a more syllable-timed rhythm in IndE than in BrE.[18] Yet, whether this gradual shift toward syllable-timing is related to the influence of neighbouring and coexisting languages is still underresearched and highly debated. Recent studies have shed new light on IndE target phonology as distinct from that of native Indian languages, suggesting that L1 effects on IndE are minimal and that they may reflect either the incomplete acquisition of the target phonology or the influence of sociolinguistic factors including identity and/or regional variation (Sirsa/Redford 2013; Wiltshire/Moon 2003). Conversely, some other researchers claim that similarities across vernacular languages account for similarities in the IndE produced by speakers with different language backgrounds (Pickering/Wiltshire 2000; Wiltshire/Harnsberger 2006).

Fuchs (2016) addresses the question whether Educated IndE is more syllable-timed than British English from two standpoints: production and perception. While most research has focused on duration, Fuchs proposes a multidimensional approach to the production of speech rhythm by considering diverse acoustic correlates. Moreover, with a total of 20 speakers with different L1 backgrounds, his study provides more systematic results than earlier acoustic studies. The results reveal that the two varieties differ significantly with regard to a number of dimensions, such as duration, sonority, loudness, intensity, pitch and glottal stop insertion. The study also addresses the question whether the difference in speech rhythm between IndE and BrE is perceptively relevant. Applying to his methodology a partially new technique consisting of selective transfer and suppression of segmental and sugrasegmental cues, Fuchs proposes a set of experiments based on intelligibility and dialect discrimination tasks. His findings show that speakers generally find the rhythm of their own variety more

18 %V is a duration-based rhythm metric accounting for the proportion of vocalic intervals in an utterance (Ramus et al. 1999).

intelligible and that listeners are able to identify which variety a speaker is using on the basis of differences in speech rhythm.

The studies above have all provided evidence of a more syllable-timed rhythm in IndE than in BrE and AmE. However, from the perception point of view, not all metrics account for the ease with which listeners are able to discriminate between rhythmic patterns, and more work is required to ascertain how these metrics relate to the subjective experience of linguistic rhythm (White/Mattys 2007). Moreover, with no existing quantitative yardstick, an assessment of the relative adequacy of metrics is clearly not straightforward (Arvaniti 2009), in particular because of the use of different speakers and the variability in speech rate (White/Mattys 2007). The results from Takeyasu and Hattori (2011) reveal that %V is the strongest factor related to listeners' judgements and, together with VtoV, may not only enable listeners to distinguish one rhythmic pattern from another but should also account for the recurrence of audible signal discontinuities (Pettorino *et al.* 2013).[19] On the basis of numerous studies that consider Vowel Onset Points (VOPs) as guiding listeners in the perception of rhythm (Pettorino/Pellegrino 2016) and considering that some prominence instants in the speech signal have been demonstrated to be perceptively more salient than others, %V and VtoV seem to be the cues for speakers' rhythmic identification (Pettorino *et al.* 2013).

Regnoli (forthcoming) addresses this question in relation to the very little research regarding rhythmic contrast in Indian regional varieties of English. In order to ascertain whether rhythmic properties have salience for a first-generation community of Indian university students located in Germany, rhythmic measurements based on two acoustic perceptual parameters (%V and VtoV) were carried out on a one-minute passage read by five speakers each of educated Marathi English and Telugu English. The findings propose that Telugu English is significantly more syllable-timed than Marathi English, as is the case in the speakers' L1s. This result shows that both VtoV and %V capture an important aspect in the rhythmic classification of English varieties. Moreover, it also implies that the Telugu English group exhibits a distinctive pattern at the rhythmic level in relation to Marathi English. This may confirm the folk perception in the community according to which Southern Indians have a distinctive speech pattern although further research is needed (cf. Chapter 5).

19 VtoV intervals correspond to the interval between two consecutive Vowel Onset Points (VOPs). For a more comprehensive account of the %V/VtoV model cf. Pettorino/Pellegrino (2016) and Pettorino et al. (2013)

3 Research Area

Indian migration to Germany is momentous. In 2016, India represented the most important non-EU country of origin for high-skilled migrants and the second most significant sending country for international students (Burkhart *et al.* 2017). Today, Germany represents the country in Europe with the largest number of Indian immigrants after the UK and Italy (Aksakal 2019). From the early 20th century's freedom fighters and students to nurses, engineers as well as contemporary IT-specialists and traders, Indian migrants have been playing a crucial role in the German society. The Indian diaspora in Germany is a fully established and highly influential ethnic group. As a matter of fact, it has become more and more visible through the founding of numerous associations and clubs and through its cultural commitment, political success and the establishment of prominent worship places such as Hindu temples and *gurdwaras*, i.e., places of assembly and worship for Sikhs.

The present chapter provides a full picture of the underresearched topic of Indian speech communities in Germany and, specifically, of the Indian student community of Heidelberg. After an outline of the current state of knowledge about the history of the Indian population in Germany and in Heidelberg, their demographic characteristics and socioeconomic profiles, the chapter will describe their sociocultural and political integration in addition to arguing that the transient aspect of the Heidelberg Indian student community is a valuable sociolinguistic factor in the fostering of network affiliations.

3.1 History

3.1.1 Indian Communities in Germany

Migration from India to Germany began in the 20th century. However, India became a focal point of German intellectual interest and curiosity early despite the lack of colonial connections and major trade relations. Prominent German philosophers such as Georg Wilhelm Friedrich Hegel (1770–1831) and Arthur Schopenhauer (1788–1860), for instance, were fascinated by the rich cultural aspects of India and produced a stunning number of articles and pamphlets on the Indian philosophical thinking (Lütkehaus 2004). Yet, extended visits from Indians to Germany were scarce, and only very few Indians actually stayed for long (Gosalia 2002).

The 20th century was an important turning point in the history of Indo-German relationships. Two groups of Indians gradually started to migrate to Germany. The first one was constituted by nationalists and freedom fighters who sought support for their fight against the British colonial rule. The second, by students who were attracted by the excellent reputation of German universities. During World War I, Indian nationalists saw Germany as a possible ally in their struggle for independence and started to migrate in order to evaluate the opportunities for a combined effort against Great Britain. They had plans to start a joint military campaign against the British in Afghanistan to destabilise the British *Raj* in India. However, all such endeavours failed (Voigt 1999). Yet, with the financial support of the German government, some of the Indian radicals managed to establish a local organisation to coordinate the activities of Indian nationalists abroad. Further socio-political developments in Europe and the eventual defeat of Germany ended these attempts to fight the British colonial rule. Nonetheless, after the end of the Great War, many nationalists found refuge in Germany, where they continued their struggle for independence (Goel 2002; Voigt 1999).

During that time Germany had also become a popular destination among Indian scholars and university students. The city of Munich became the temporary home of many Indians and the first centre of the 'India Institute' in Germany. In addition, three acclaimed visits by the renowned Bengali poet Rabindranath Tagore in 1921, 1926 and 1930 strengthened the reputation of Indian literature and philosophy in Germany and consolidated Indo-German diplomatic relations (Voigt 1999). In 1928, the Indian National Congress opened in Berlin an Indian Student Information Bureau (Goel 2002).

As a matter of fact, students were the ones who contributed to the first major wave of Indian immigration to Germany after World War II. After some cooperation agreements between the two nations, in the 1950s, some one thousand engineering and computer technology students were granted scholarships by several German institutions and thus migrated to Western Germany, i.e., the Federal Republic of Germany (FRG), to further their education. While some of them returned to India after their studies, some stayed and formed the nucleus of today's Indian diaspora in Germany, working as professionals and traders and establishing themselves in the German middle class (Goel 2007; Gosalia 2002; Gottschlich 2013).

In the late 1960s and early 1970s, almost 6.000 Malayali Catholic women were recruited by German Catholic institutions to work as nurses in German hospitals (Goel 2002). Many of these "Indian angels" (Goel 2002:61) intermarried with Germans and contributed towards the hugely disproportional share of Christian

Indians in the diaspora in Germany, at least if compared to religion statistics in India (Schnepel 2004). Overall, the Indian community resulting from this period consisted of professionals (e.g., nurses, doctors, and engineers), academics (e.g., scientists, scholars, and students) and businessmen (Singhvi 2001).[20]

A new migration impetus arrived in 2000 with the launch of the German chancellor Gerhard Schröder's Green Card initiative, which brought a new wave of approximately 20.000 IT professionals and highly qualified technicians to the country (Faist *et al.* 2017; Westerhoff 2007). This initiative was formalised with the implementation of the New Foreigner Law in 2005, allowing preferential entrance for migrants with higher professional backgrounds (Chanda/Mukherjee 2014). According to Gottschlich (2012:2) "[t]his has been so far the last major influx of a specific immigrant group from India to Germany".

However, there are no statistics on the states of origin of the newly arriving migrants from India. With the exception of Indian nurses from Kerala and Punjabi Sikhs, there are hardly any reliable data.[21] Yet, it is worth mentioning that both ethnicities continue to constitute significant minorities within the Indian diaspora in Germany. Other than that, all estimations on the ethnic origin of Indian immigrants are little more than mere guesses.

3.1.2 Indian Communities in Heidelberg

Heidelberg is a university town situated in the Southwestern German federal state of Baden-Württemberg (hereafter BW). According to the Consulate General of India, Munich (hereafter CGI, 2019), the total foreign population of the state is over 1.6 million (11 %), which makes it one of the most immigrant-rich states of the country. Over the past decades, BW has emerged as an important pillar of growing and expanding Indo-German relationships. The leadership in BW considers India as an important partner for trade, investment, technology collaboration, higher education and quality human resources.

Migration from India to BW has been given relatively little attention. It began shortly after World War II and exploded during the 1950s, with students, high-skilled professionals and entrepreneurs being the first wave of Indian migrants

20 Indian engineers were hired by several German Science and Technology companies until 1973, when Germany ceased issuing working visas for guest workers (Gottschlich 2013).

21 In the 1980s, hundreds of Punjabi Sikhs sought political asylum in Western Germany. Many of them found ways to stay in Germany legally even after their asylum requests were denied (Goel 2007).

in the state (Gottschlich 2012; Singh/Rajan 2016). Later in the 1960s particularly Indian nurses migrated from Kerala and, in the early 1980s, it was the turn of humanitarian migrants (Khadria 2014). After 2000, Indian migration was again mainly characterised by high-skilled professionals and student mobility.

As in the rest of Germany, the Indian diasporic community in BW is historically characterised by a heterogeneous group with regard to motivation, Indian states of origin as well as ethnic and religious composition (Butsch 2017). Today, IT professionals and students are the two major components of the Indian diaspora in BW due to (i) the highly advanced services that constitute the core of the state's economy (mechanical, automotive and electrical engineering, information technology, electronics, aerospace, biotechnology and health services) and (ii) its great concentration of universities and its variegated higher education landscape (CGI 2019).

The city of Heidelberg is no exception, a university town, home to around 150.000 people of 160 different nationalities, among them almost 47.000 with a migration background (Stadt Heidelberg 2017). Though small, the Indian local community is quite active and comprises four distinct groups: (i) migrants who settled in the 1960s either for higher education purposes or to work as nurses in local hospitals, got married to German nationals and are now retired; (ii) migrants settling in the late 70s and 80s, currently in the restaurant business; (iii) IT professionals who settled for fixed tenures and (iv) University students (CGI 2019). The first three groups form a stable community which, however, is not to be considered either a speech community or a community of practice in any meaningful sense.[22] Although the present project will not go into this,

22 The original plan of the present study was to work with both the Indian student community and the stable one in order to compare the attitudes of both populations towards regional varieties of Indian English. However, after starting my fieldwork in the stable community, retrieving useful information about its historical background and discussing with older members for three weeks, I realised that the community could not come under either a strict or loose definition of 'speech community' or 'community of practice' since most of its members did not share a common language and were not integrated in the community itself (cf. Section 2.2 for further details on speech communities). In fact, in-group affiliations seemed to be rather loose and discontinuous, and members' identities did not match with a pan-Indian one anymore, let alone with a more ethnic one. Moreover, older members were not familiar with English since English-medium schools had not been institutionalised yet by the time they left India. For this reason, they were proficient either in their first language or German. In conclusion, the above considerations combine to justify excluding these speakers from the present investigation.

it is worth mentioning that the oldest members of the community are female Malayali Catholic nurses who came from India at a very young age (usually, in their early 20s), started to work in hospitals and health institutions, soon got married to locals and became integrated in the German middle-class. Members of the Malayali community gather at church every first Sunday of the month to worship, spend time and eat together. For the overall picture, the stable community is mainly constituted of restaurant and shop owners and high-skilled workers. Similar to the small Malayali community, both groups are integrated locally and play a crucial role in the economic growth of the city and of BW in general (Aksakal 2019; CGI 2019).

The Indian student community is the only community of practice in the city and, today, Indian migration in Heidelberg is mainly characterised by student mobility. The excellent education and research opportunities provided have been attracting undergraduates and graduates from India for years. The European Molecular Biology Laboratory (EMBL), the German Cancer Research Centre (DFKZ), the Max Planck Institutes (MPI), the University of Heidelberg and the SRH Heidelberg University of Applied Sciences are all major educational institutions in which Indian students are registered.[23] Today, the Heidelberg Indian community mainly consists of upper middle-class students who came to Germany in order to further their education and improve their professional skills. Having generally had an English-medium education and having pursued a bachelor's degree in their mother country, these students are enrolled here at different master's and Ph.D. courses covering Physics, International Business and Engineering, Medical Anthropology and Transcultural Studies. The majority plan to get an internship and a post in Germany for a short time and then to return to India financially independent and economically stable. Not only does their transient position provide insight into the sociolinguistic situation of the community, their network allegiances and attitudinal orientations (cf. Chapter 5), but it also contributes to significant changes in the demographic characteristics of the Indian population as a whole (cf. Section 3.2.1) and in their socioeconomic profiles either in Heidelberg, BW or, overall, in Germany (cf. Section 3.2.2).

23 Many universities in Germany, Heidelberg included, offer international students the possibility to enrol at selected courses taught entirely in English. Thus, admission does not require any proof of skills in German.

3.2 Social Situation

3.2.1 Demographic Characteristics

According to the figures of the Ministry of External Affairs, Government of India (hereafter MEA 2018), there were 108.965 non-resident Indians (NRIs) living in Germany at the end of 2018. The German Federal Statistical Office (hereafter DESTATIS 2017) mentions 97.865 NRIs residing in Germany at the end of 2016. After a slight decline between 2003 and 2004, the numbers, which had been around 35.000 for most of the 1990s, have been growing steadily ever since (cf. Fig. 3.2.1). Today, the Indian diaspora is the first minority ethnic population among the two other diasporic communities of subcontinental India, i.e., Pakistan and Sri Lanka, residing in Germany (cf. Fig. 3.2.2). It mainly comprises highly skilled professionals, technocrats, businessmen, traders, nurses, and, in the last decades, there has been an increase in the number of qualified migrants in the fields of IT, banking and finance.

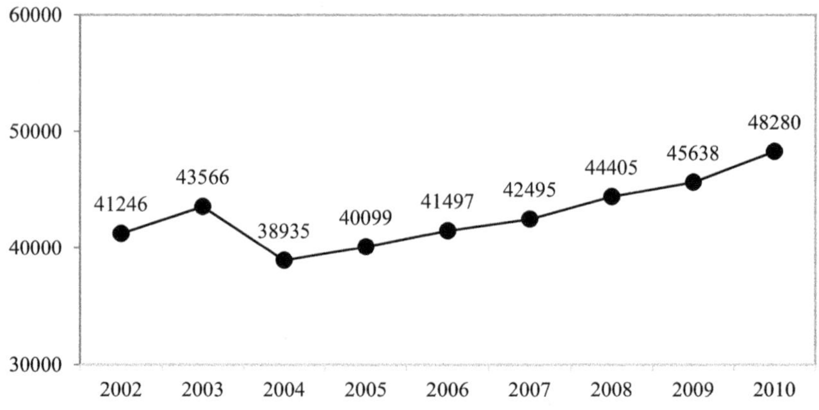

Fig. 3.2.1 NRIs in Germany 2002–2010 (DESTATIS)

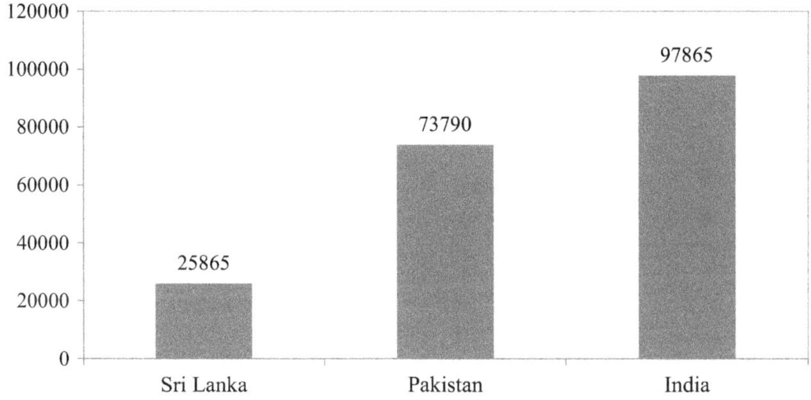

Fig. 3.2.2 Foreign citizens in Germany – South Asia 2016 (DESTATIS)

Data from the DESTATIS (2017) reveal that qualified professionals are the largest group of NRIs living in Germany on a temporary residence permit, followed by Indian students. This is no surprise considering that, according to the German Federal Office for Migration and Refugees (hereafter BAMF 2017), in 2016 India represented the most important non-EU country of origin for highly skilled professionals and the second most significant country sending international university students (Burkhart *et al.* 2017).

Between 1990 and 2015, Indian migrants in Germany increased by more than 114 % (Department of Economic and Social Affairs of the United Nations, hereafter UN DESA 2015). Furthermore, figures from the DESTATIS reveal that some 12.009 Indian citizens came to Germany in 2009, while only 10.374 left the country, thus resulting in a net migration surplus of 13.6 %. In 2008, the surplus was even higher (16.4 %), with 11.403 Indians coming and 9.532 leaving (cf. Fig. 3.2.3). In the words of Aksakal (2019:1), the increasing relevance of Indians in Germany is due to "[...] demographic and macroeconomic trends linked to labour shortages", which push Germany to be "[...] gradually engaged in creating legal channels for the attraction of qualified labour migrants and in parts international students".

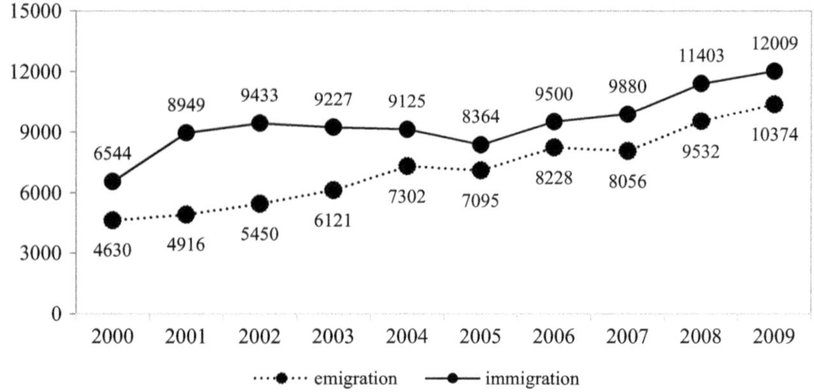

Fig. 3.2.3 Immigration and emigration of Indian citizens to and from Germany 2000–2009 (DESTATIS 2010)

The spatial distribution of Indians in Germany mostly resembles that of the local population (cf. Tab. 3.2.1). Data from the DESTATIS (2010) report that immigrants from India tend to settle in urbanised areas and mainly in the South of the country. Compared to the overall percentage of the Indian population, there is an overrepresentation in three of the main largest cities of Germany (i.e., Hamburg, Frankfurt am Main and Berlin) as well as in the Southern states of BW and Bavaria, which also include major metropolitan areas such as Stuttgart, Heidelberg and Munich. With the spatial distribution being kept constant, as of 2014 there were 13.081 NRIs living in BW. In the last 8 years, there has been an increase of at least 175.8 %. As for the latest data available, there are approximately 20.000 NRIs currently living in BW, making it the 18.3 % of the entire NRIs community living in Germany (Consulate General of India, Munich [hereafter CGI] 2019).

Tab. 3.2.1 Spatial distribution of the Indian diaspora in Germany according to states (DESTATIS 2010)

State	Indian population	German population
North Rhine-Westphalia	10.590	17.849.025
Bavaria	7.633	12.531.925
Baden-Württemberg	7.241	10.754.865
Hesse	6.714	6.067.609
Berlin	2.946	3.450.889
Hamburg	2.902	1.783.975
Lower Saxony	2.323	7.923.536
Saxony	1.821	4.151.011
Rhineland-Palatinate	1.586	4.006.296
Saxony-Anhalt	760	2.339.439
Schleswig-Holstein	732	2.833.747
Bremen	693	659.927
Brandenburg	617	2.506.160
Mecklenburg-West Pomerania	597	1.643.566
Thuringia	574	2.237.434
Saarland	551	1.018.926

The Indian population in Heidelberg has been growing steadily over the last 15 years. According to the figures of Stadt Heidelberg (2019), there has been an increase in both NRIs and PIOs of a staggering 230.7 % between 2003 and 2018, currently making it a combined strength of 1.055 individuals (cf. Fig. 3.2.4).[24]

24 All data from Stadt Heidelberg are the result of help by its Office of Urban Development and Statistics.

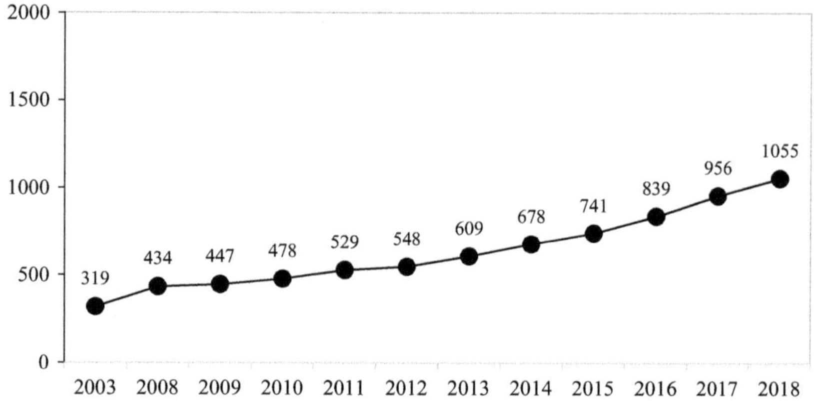

Fig. 3.2.4 NRIs and PIOs in Heidelberg 2003–2018 (Stadt Heidelberg 2019)

The significant imbalance between men and women in the Heidelberg Indian community resembles that of the Indian population in Germany as a whole, whose main sectors are massively male-dominated (cf. Fig. 3.2.5).[25] Despite some early progress made in the years 2010–2011, however, this imbalance has not been overcome yet. While in 2010 women constituted only the 36.1 % of the Indian population in Germany (DESTATIS 2010) – which still is the highest number registered in the country in the last 10 years – the Heidelberg female population amounted to 41.2 % (Stadt Heidelberg 2019). Today, the ratio of women to men in Heidelberg is even more unbalanced, the Indian female population consisting of 39.7 % of the entire community.

Gender disproportion goes hand in hand with age imbalance. Data from the DESTATIS (2011) show that the Indian community in Germany is composed of a rather male young population group. This is no surprise since the Indian diaspora is mainly constituted of male professionals and students.

25 A case in point is the composition of the highly skilled Green Card immigrants from India who came to Germany between 2000 and 2004. According to Venema (2004), only 365 female computer experts found their way to the country, compared to the 4.476 male IT professionals.

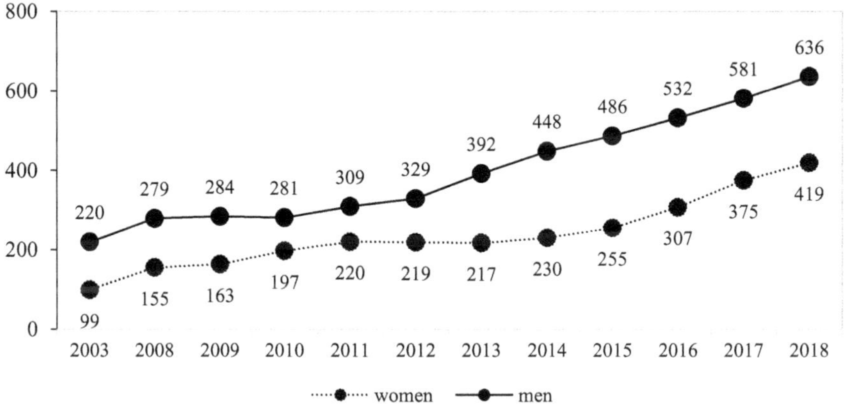

Fig. 3.2.5 Ratio of men and women in the Heidelberg Indian community (Stadt Heidelberg 2019)

Their average age of 32.9 years is more than 10 years younger than that of the local population in spite of an also young student population. Almost two thirds of all NRIs living in Germany are between 25 and 45 years old, compared to a little over a quarter of the local population which falls into that category. In addition, while more than 20 % of all Germans are more than 65 years old, only 2 % of the Indian population in Germany has already reached that threshold, resulting in a ratio of 1:10. This disproportion is mirrored in the Heidelberg Indian community as well. Figures from Stadt Heidelberg (2019) show that the community has always been predominantly male and young (18–44 years old) and that, more recently, the gap has been getting wider (cf. Fig. 3.2.6). Young adults (between 18–29 and 30–44 years old) are the two predominant groups of the community, which mainly consist of high-skilled professionals and students.

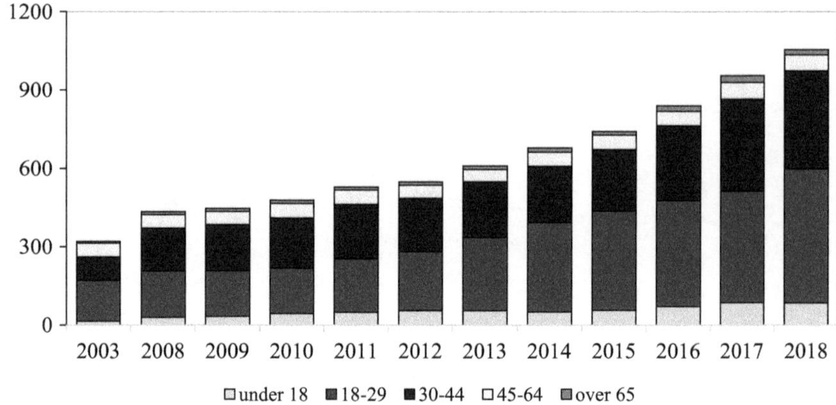

Fig. 3.2.6 Age profile of the Heidelberg Indian community (Stadt Heidelberg 2019)

Indian student mobility both in Germany and in Heidelberg has been growing steadily over the last 10 years and is currently on the rise (CGI 2019). Figure 3.2.7 provides information on the changes in the number of Indian students who were granted a residence permit for educational purposes for 5 years (Mayer *et al.* 2012). Reported data attest that the inflow of Indian students has been increasing by 32.5 % between 2007 and 2011. According to the CGI (2019), "[t]he number of Indian students in Germany has more than doubled in the last five years".

In their study on international students in Germany, Hoffmeyer-Zlotnik and Grote (2019) shed new light on student enrolments at German institutions between the winter terms of 2012/13 and 2017/18. Their data report that Indian student mobility has increased by a massive 138.3 % in 5 years only and that, today, Indians form the second largest group of international students enrolled at German universities (cf. Fig. 3.2.8).

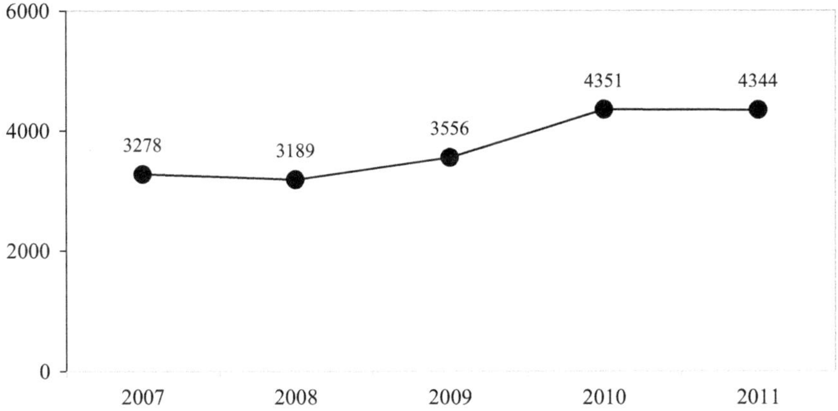

Fig. 3.2.7 Numbers of people with a residence permit for the purposes of studying (section 16 subs. 1 of the Residence Act) (Mayer *et al.* 2012)

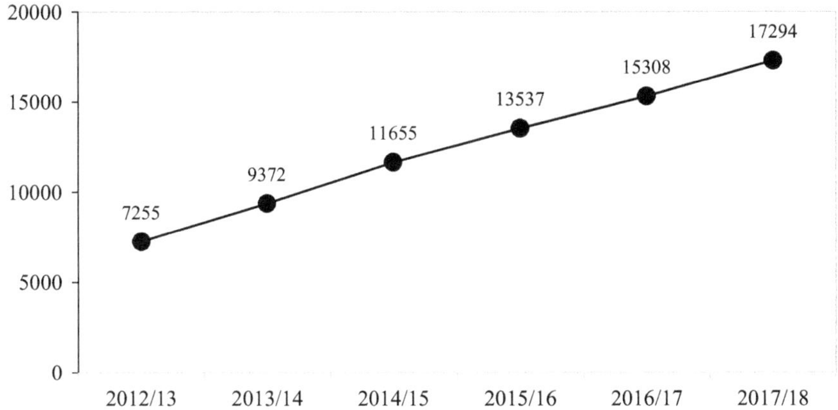

Fig. 3.2.8 Indian mobile foreign students the winter terms of 2012–2018 (Hoffmeyer-Zlotnik/Grote 2019)

Among the 17.294 Indian students currently enrolled at different German institutions, around 4.600 are registered at various universities in BW and Bavaria (CGI 2019). BW has the greatest concentration of universities and the most diverse higher education landscape in Germany, including nine research universities, 15 out of the 83 Max Planck Institutes located in Germany and 14 Fraunhofer Institutes. Moreover, BW boasts a large number of elite German universities such as the Universities of Heidelberg, Konstanz, Tübingen and Stuttgart, not to mention the Karlsruhe Technology Institute (KIT) and the SRH Heidelberg University of Applied Sciences (CGI 2019).

Heidelberg provides excellent education and research opportunities for students and scholars from all over the world and has been attracting undergraduates and graduates from India for years. Indian students in Heidelberg are enrolled at different educational institutions and, particularly, at the German Cancer Research Centre (DFKZ), the University, the European Molecular Biology laboratory (EMBL), the Max Planck Institutes (MPI) and the SRH Heidelberg University of Applied Sciences. According to the CGI (2019) "[t]hese students are involved in frontier areas of S&T research". As for the latest data available from the SRH University Heidelberg (2019), there are 382 Indian students currently registered at different master's courses covering International Business and Engineering, Computer Science and Information Technology.[26] Although there are no data available regarding the total number of Indian students currently enrolled at the University of Heidelberg, figures from the Division of Student Affairs and Teaching (2018, 2017) attest at 128 the total number of Indian students who enrolled during the winter term of 2017/18 and at 137 during the 2018 summer term (cf. Tab. 3.2.2).[27]

Tab. 3.2.2 Indian students enrolled at Heidelberg in winter 2017/2018 and summer 2018 (University of Heidelberg 2018, 2017)

Semester	**Country of origin**	**Total**	**Men**	**Women**	**Bachelor's students**	**Master's students**	**Staatsexamen**	**Ph.D. students**	**International students**	**Other**
Winter 2017/18	India	128	55	73	3	53	3	56	11	2
Summer 2018	India	137	59	78	3	52	3	64	12	3

26 The data have been specifically requested from the International Relations office of the SRH Hochschule Heidelberg. Further information was not disclosed because of the impossibility of the university to create such reports.

27 The University of Heidelberg does not disclose further data to third parties. The data presented here have been specifically requested from the Graduate Academy on the basis of time spent doing fieldwork among the Indian student community.

A compelling aspect of the Indian student diaspora in Germany and, specifically, in Heidelberg, is its temporary migration. A study conducted by the BAMF (2016) analysed the temporality in both Indian high-skilled and student mobility to Germany by reflecting the numbers of those in the same population who left the country 2 years after their arrival. The data indicate that temporary migration is far more significant among professionals than students and that more than a half of high-skilled migrants and almost one fifth of Indian students are temporary migrants living in Germany up to 2 years. The transient aspect of both communities is a crucial factor influencing not only the demography of the Indian diaspora in Germany but also its socioeconomic profile (cf. Section 3.2.2) and its sociolinguistic patterns (cf. Chapter 5).

Although the present research will not go into this, for the overall picture it is fundamental to address the question of how many PIOs are currently living in Germany. Answering the question, however, is not easy since there are hardly any data on Indians after they have obtained the German citizenship (Gottschlich 2013). Yet, figures from the DESTATIS attest at 8.076 the total number of naturalised Indians who became German citizens between 2002 and 2010. Additional figures from the High-Level Committee on the Indian Diaspora estimate the number of PIOs in Germany at 10.000 (Singhvi *et al.* 2001). However, given the further influx of Indian immigrants to Germany in the wake of the Green Card initiative, it seems justified to consider this figure as a mere minimum (Faist *et al.* 2017; Venema 2004). As for the latest data available, there were 37.128 PIOs living in Germany at the end of 2018 (MEA 2018) and 7.600 living in BW at the end of 2014 (CGI 2019).

3.2.2 Socioeconomic Profile

As mentioned above, the overall Indian migration to Germany can be described as high-skilled labour (cf. Section 3.1.1). In response to both demographic and macroeconomic trends linked to labour shortages, Germany gradually engaged in allowing the preferential entrance of migrants with special professional backgrounds (Aksakal 2019; Gottschlich 2013). From the introduction of the Green Card in 2000 to the implementation of the New Foreigner Law in 2005 and the EU Blue Card into the National Residence Act in 2012, Germany managed to reduce bureaucratic barriers and accommodate to migrant societal conditions in order to achieve more tolerant yet selective migration policies (Beine *et al.* 2016; Wogart and Schüller 2011).

Except for the immigrants under family reunification regulations, high-skilled professionals and students comprise the largest group of NRIs living in

Germany on a temporary residence permit under the new legislation of the Aliens Residence Act of 2004 (cf. Tab. 3.2.3). With regard to their occupational profiles, Indians in Germany divert from the general South and Southeast Asian migrant population. The percentage of low or semi-skilled workers tends to be lower in comparison and the proportion of high-skilled or self-employed professionals is significantly higher. As of 2015 about 41.7 % of Indians residing in Germany were professionally qualified, 25 % were semi-skilled, and about 13 % worked in elementary occupations (cf. Tab. 3.2.4) (Palstring 2015).[28] According to Gottschlich (2012), NRIs usually work in middle-class positions, and their average income is among the highest of all migrant groups in Germany. For instance, Indian IT experts who came to Germany through the Green Card regulations had to earn at least € 51.000 per year in order to be eligible for a temporary residence permit (Kolb 2005).

Tab. 3.2.3 NRIs in Germany according to type of temporary residence (DESTATIS 2010)

Type of residence	Indian population		
	Total	Male	Female
Education and Study	5.152	3.948	1.204
Work, mostly high-skilled	8.970	7.507	1.463
Refugees	407	308	99
Family Reunification	11.537	3.959	7.578
Other	3.774	3.019	755
Temporary residence permit (all)	26.638	16.134	10.504

28 It is important to note that about 40.2% of PIOs without a migration experience of their own occupy managerial positions (cf. Table 3.2.6; Palstring 2015).

Tab. 3.2.4 Qualifications of Indian migrants in Germany (Palstring 2015)

Occupation (major groups ISCO-08)	**German population**	**People with Indian migration background**		
		PIOs with no migration experience	**PIOs with migration experience**	**NRIs with migration experience**
Armed Forces Occupations	4.9 %	*	*	0.0 %
Managers	17.4 %	40.2 %	10.3 %	5.1 %
Professionals	19.1 %	11.8 %	20.6 %	41.7 %
Technicians and Associate Professionals	13.5 %	*	11.6 %	12.6 %
Clerical Support Workers	15.5 %	9.6 %	8.7 %	4.4 %
Service and Sales Workers	1.5 %	*	24.1 %	18.1 %
Skilled Agricultural, Forestry and Fishery Workers	12.7 %	*	*	*
Craft and Related Trade Workers	6.6 %	*	6.9 %	2.9 %
Plant and Machine Operators and Assemblers	8.4 %	*	6.0 %	1.8 %
Elementary Occupations	0.5 %	*	10.5 %	12.9 %
Total	100.1 %	61.6 %	98.7 %	99.5 %

The Indian NRI community living in BW is no exception. The state is among the most prosperous and wealthiest regions in Europe, with a generally low unemployment rate and a fast-growing economy. According to the CGI (2019), the composition of the state economy is as follows: services (60.3 %), manufacturing (32.5 %), construction (4.9 %) as well as agriculture and forestry (0.4 %). Moreover (CGI 2009:2):

> [h]ighly advanced mechanical and automotive engineering; electrical engineering; information technology, electronics, aerospace, biotechnology, health services, etc constitute the core of the economy of Baden-Württemberg. The other strong sectors include aerospace, telecommunications, electronics, environment and energy efficient technologies; bio-technology, health sciences, and precision engineering.

Considering that the region's showcase sectors are technology-based and that this knowledge-based economy is driven by the state's continuous investments in higher and technical education, it is no surprise that a high concentration of Indian skilled professionals and students are attracted by working in some of the state's major enterprises. Students are generally granted the opportunity to work as interns for large enterprises and companies including Bosch, Daimler, Festo, Kärcher and particularly ABB and SAP as part of their undergraduate and graduate courses (CGI 2019).

All research institutions located in Heidelberg, offer bachelor and master's students the opportunity to combine theoretical knowledge and practical experiences benefiting from the close cooperation with large local enterprises and industries. In terms of career perspectives, graduating from these universities increase the students' "chances of securing an excellent position in the software and IT industry" by working for "large enterprises such as AIRBUS, ADIDAS, AUDI, BOSCH, BMW, BASF, DEUTSCHE BOERSE, DKFZ, SAP, TRIUMPH, VERIVOX, etc. and many more small-sized and mid-sized companies" (SRH 2019). These job prospects attract many Indian students to pursue their higher education in Heidelberg, and while some members of the Heidelberg Indian student community aim to settle in Germany or somewhere else in Europe after completing their graduate courses, the majority plan to get an internship and a post in Germany for 2 to 5 years and then to return to India, financially independent and economically stable.

3.2.3 Religious Centres and Cultural Associations

High-skilled mobility and the general higher educational levels of NRIs suggest that many Indians migrating to Germany belong to higher caste groups (Punnamparambil 2008). However, the precise configuration of caste in Germany is difficult to assess. According to Gottschlich (2012:5):

> a valuable source can be matrimonial websites such as GermanMatrimonials.com or LifepartnerIndia.com which oftentimes specify caste groups, thereby implying that caste might still play a major role in spouse selection among NRI and PIO in Germany.

Here, most of the potential grooms regard themselves as twice-born Hindus belonging to one of the three higher *varnas*.[29] Among these groups,

29 India's caste system divides Hindus into four rigid hierarchical groups based on their *karma* (work) and *dharma* (religion/work): Brahmins (priests and intellectuals), Kshatriyas (warriors and rulers), Vaishyas (farmers, traders, and merchants) and the Shudras (labourers). Outside of their caste system there are the *achhoots* – the Dalits or the untouchables. Over the centuries, the main castes have been further divided into about 3.000 castes and 25.000 sub-castes, each based on its specific occupation. Although after reaching Independence India's constitution banned discrimination on the basis of caste and the influence of caste has somewhat declined in recent decades,

Brahmins – more specifically, *Lohars* and *Sharmas*, and Kshatriyas – including *Boyars*, *Guptas*, *Agrawals*, *Naidus*, and *Vellalars* – are the most common self-identifications. Some spouses regard themselves as Vaishyas as well. Although they could provide a broad idea of the caste structure in the Indian diaspora in Germany, all of these specifications are hardly representative since they are based on qualitative data collected randomly.

The difficulty in assessing the caste configuration in the Heidelberg Indian community resembles that of the Indian population in Germany. While there are no available data regarding the caste structure of the local communities of PIOs and high-skilled professionals, data from the present database seem to align with data retrieved from the Indo-German matrimonial websites. Members of higher caste groups in general and Brahmins in particular are the major components of the student community (cf. Tab. 3.2.5)

Tab. 3.2.5 Caste configuration in the Heidelberg Indian student community

Caste	N	%
Brahmin	25	42
Vaisya	10	18
Kshatriya	11	17
Unspecified	9	15
No	4	7
Inter-caste	1	2
Total	60	100

In line with the difficulty in retrieving information about the caste configuration, there are no available data regarding the religious structure of the Indian diaspora in Germany. However, considering the considerable heterogeneity of the Indian population in Germany (cf. Section 3.1.1), it is safe to assume that it is mainly constituted of Hindus, Catholics, Muslims and Sikhs.

According to the latest figures from the BAMF (2017), Hinduism is a minority religion in Germany, practiced by the 0.1 % of the total population. Over the years, migrating Hindus have established temples all over the country, thus contributing to the religious and cultural diversity of Germany. The Iskon (International

especially in urban areas, caste identities remain strong. As a result, last names are almost always indications of what caste a person belongs to. For a more comprehensive account of the caste system cf. Bayly (2001).

Society for Krishna Consciousness) temple in Heidelberg is one such example. Established over 20 years ago, it is devoted to the worship of the Hindu god Krishna. Today, the temple attracts devotees from Heidelberg and around with its peaceful ambience, in-depth religious teachings, rituals and festivals.

The Indian Catholic community is among the oldest groups of PIOs residing in Heidelberg and mainly consists of Malayalis (cf. Section 3.1.1). Many Malayali Catholic members of the Indian student community usually join the religious services as well. Overall, the Indian student community consists mainly of Hindus and Christians (cf. Tab. 3.2.6).

Tab. 3.2.6 Religious composition of the Heidelberg Indian student community

Religion	N	%
Hindu	51	85
Christian	5	8
Muslim	2	3
Jahn	1	2
Sikh	1	2
Total	60	100

The Indian diaspora in Germany is a fully established and highly influential ethnic group. Since its very inception, it has been making itself visible through the founding of various associations and organisations aiming to both enhance Indo-German relations and bridge the gap with the mother country. These associations contribute to increasing the visibility of Indian cultural practices – performed in rituals, festivities and art forms – and to reproduce ethnic and national identities. Furthermore, they are essential self-help systems through which members may find support for preventive services (Oberkircher 2006).

In an age of unprecedented international mobility, these associations may play an important role in developing their linguistic and cultural systems and may affect the degree to which distinctive varieties in the new-formed groups emerge and heritage languages are maintained (cf. Chapter 5). While these factors are still under-theorised in sociolinguistic research, in wider social theory and the social sciences they have been attracting interest for some decades now – especially in relation to transnationalism – because "[they have] forced analysis to rethink certain traditional notions of social structure" (Sharma 2014:218).

Indian associations in Germany are active institutions, they are mainly involved in the integration of both NRIs and PIOs in the local environment and in their transnational activities (Saravanan *et al.* 2018). On the whole, there are three types of Indian associations in Germany: (i) Indo-German societies, or, *Deutsch-Indische Geschellschaften* (hereafter DIGs); (ii) Indian associations initiated by Indian diasporic groups; (iii) Indian student associations. Although the distinction between the three is rather clear-cut, the boundaries are somewhat fluid. Few DIGs collaborate with local Indian associations to organise events and obtain grants. In addition to these broad categories, Saravanan *et al.* (2018:8) argue that:

> there are roughly 700 Indian priests and second-generation Indians who are actively involved in promoting development activities. These groups, largely individual or family initiated, function as charities and as non-government organizations (NGOs).

These associations represent diverse ethnic groups and broadly fulfil the functions of every potential migrant organisation as described by Gaitanides (2003), i.e., (i) serving as gateways for the newcomers; (ii) maintaining the group's cultural capital; (iii) supporting individual and collective identities; (iv) offering challenges for individual fulfilment; (v) generating the group's social capital; (vi) activating private self-help; (vii) improving service provision through voluntary engagement; (viii) helping with preventive services; (ix) solving conflicts; (x) exerting social control; (xi) articulating interests; (xii) providing humanitarian aid and support, especially with regard to transnational activities; (xiii) providing knowledge of the home country.

Information on the number of Indian associations in Germany is difficult to obtain since there are no statistics on country-specific associations, and the Indian Embassy only keeps records of registered associations which either approach the Embassy or collaborate with it.[30] Figures from the MEA (2019) attest at 19 the total number of Indian associations in Germany (cf. Tab. 3.2.7). However, the database does not seem to be updated as to include other registered associations (cf. below). Hence, it seems to be justified to hold this measurement as a mere minimum considering that recent data attest at some 122 the total number of Indian associations located in Germany (Saravanan *et al.* 2018).

---

30 In 1953, Deutsch Indische Geschellschaft (DIG), was founded as one of the very first central organisations of the Indian diaspora in Germany. Today, it has 33 chapters and more than 3.500 registered members (Gottschlich 2012).

Tab. 3.2.7 Indian associations in Germany (MEA 2019)

	Association Name	Location
1	Association Indian Students Aachen (AISA)	Aachen
2	Indian Association Bonn e.V. (IAB)	Bonn
3	Sneham e.V South Indian Association Bonn	Bonn
4	Darmstadt Indian Association (DIA).e.V.	Darmstadt
5	Bharat Samiti e. V.	Köln
6	Bharat Verein e.V.	Frankfurt
7	Kerala Samajam e.V.	Frankfurt
8	Telugu Velugu Germany (TVG) e.V.	Frankfurt
9	Rhein-Main Bengali Cultural Association e.V.	Frankfurt
10	Goan Association Germany e.V.	Frankfurt
11	Vishwa Hindu Parishad e.V. of Germany	Frankfurt
12	Frankfurt Tamil Sangam(FTS) e.V.	Frankfurt
13	Rhein Main Kannada Association e.V.	Frankfurt
14	Indian Ladies Club e.V.	Kelkheim
15	Indian International Association of Rhine-Waal University of Applied Sciences	Kleve
16	Sikh Verband Deutschland e.V.	Köln
17	Marathi Mitra Mandal Germany e.V.	Krefeld
18	Indien Forum Frankfurt e.V.	Nauheim
19	Gujarati Samaj Germany e.V.	Neu-Isenburg

Among the 122 registered Indian associations in Germany, about 20 are student associations. They are involved in the dissemination and sharing of information regarding issues including, but not limited to, student visa, job opportunities, cultural events and scholarships. Moreover, they provide suitable emergency contacts and help connect students with potential employers in small and medium-sized Indian/German companies for job and/or internship opportunities. The majority of registered Indian student associations in Germany are partners of a project entitled 'Indian Students in Germany', initiated by the Embassy of India in Berlin with the purpose of mediating among the various student associations spread in the country (cf. Tab. 3.2.8).

Heidelberg is home to one Indian association, i.e., the Heidelberg Indian Students Association (hereafter HISA), a non-profit organisation established in 2003 by a group of Indian students with the intent of bridging the gap between the Indian migrant community and the local one. The organisation "is dedicated towards the welfare of the Indian students and community in and around

Heidelberg" (HISA 2019) and has been proudly working in this direction from the last 16 years. The community is in constant growth and now includes Indian working professionals and International members as well. HISA is driven by an enthusiastic committee which works voluntarily to achieve the aims of the organisation. Along with the posts of President, vice-President and Manager, the HISA committee also includes a treasurer, a cultural secretary, advisors and international volunteers.[31] The association is constantly engaged in the organisation of cultural events (movie nights, flash mobs), festivals (Diwali, Holi, Navratri, Independence Day), Yoga days as well as Business Entrepreneurship and start-up competitions. In addition, sessions for 'returning experts' who "have gained technical or managerial skills through study and work in Germany and who then go on to use their knowledge and expertise in their country of origin" (BAMF 2019) are organised in collaboration with the Centre for International Migration and Development. HISA is currently working on a project dealing with waste segregation management awareness in India, supported by the Centre for International Migration and Development, and collaborating with platforms like DAAD.

31 During the year 2017–18 I held the position of 'International Volunteer' and helped in the organisation of cultural events.

Tab. 3.2.8 Indian student associations in Germany (Indian Students in Germany 2019)

	Association Name	Location
1	Association Indian Students Aachen (AISA)	Aachen
2	Indian Students Association at TU Berlin	Berlin
3	Indians students association Bremen	Bremen
4	Indian Students' Association – Bremerhaven (ISA-BHV)	Bremerhaven
5	Indian Association Chemnitz	Chemnitz
6	BTU Indians Cottbus	Cottbus
7	Darmstadt Indian Association	Darmstadt
8	Indian Association Dresden	Dresden
9	Frankfurt Indian Scholars Association	Frankfurt
10	Nirmiti: Göttingen	Göttingen
11	Indian Students Association at TUHH	Hamburg
12	Indischer Verein Hannover	Hannover
13	Heidelberg Indian Students Association (HISA)	Heidelberg
14	Indisch Deutscher Verein Ingolstadt e.V.	Ingolstadt
15	Indians students association Kaiserlautern	Kaiserslautern
16	Kiel Indians	Kiel
17	Indian International Association of Rhine-Waal University of Applied Sciences	Kleve
18	Magdeburg Indians	Magdeburg
19	Association of Indian Students in University of Paderborn	Paderborn
20	Indian Students Association in Stuttgart	Stuttgart

The association has been officially recognised by the University of Heidelberg as an international student organisation and has been a life-partner of the 'Indian Students in Germany' project, working in collaboration with the Indian Embassy in Germany. At present, HISA has some 300 registered members (with a fairly equal number of men and women) coming from the University of Heidelberg, the European Molecular Biology laboratory (EMBL), the Max Planck Institutes (MPI) and the SRH Hochschule Heidelberg. Although the majority of the community consist of students, it is important to mention that HISA includes members from the PIO and NRI local communities as well. Many of these high-skilled professionals work from companies like SAP, ABB and BASF.

In line with the aims of the organisation and the 'Indian Students in Germany' project, HISA collaborates with different partners, including the TK Health Insurance, i.e., one of the largest public health insurance providers in Germany, Bluebilities GmbH, a recruitment talent acquisition company located in Berlin that assists job seekers to get recruited and Migration Hub Heidelberg, a network providing support to international social projects working with asylum seekers and refugees in Heidelberg.

Among the many aims of the association, HISA is committed to the maintenance of transnational networks and the strengthening of Indo-German relations. In 2017, two Indian regional newspapers, the 'Gujarati Magazine: Global' and the 'Sakal: Pune' dedicated an article on the efforts and successes of HISA and its role in the Indian diaspora in Germany. In 2018, HISA was awarded the 'Sarojini Naidu – Gottfried Wilhelm Leibniz Leadership Award', a distinction conferred by the 'Indian Students in Germany' project in association with the Embassy of India. The award included a citation and cash prize of € 100 and is traditionally awarded "to the association/individual who has contributed to the betterment of situation of Indian students in Germany and assisted in their integration into the German society" (Indian Students in Germany 2019).

4 Methodology

4.1 Research Design

4.1.1 Quantitative and Qualitative Formulae

Experimental linguistic research offers a wide range of methods, approaches and designs to suit a variety of subfields. The distinction between quantitative and qualitative approaches is essential although studies using both are commonly widespread. Researchers adopting the former approach seek to investigate phenomena by collecting numerical data and analysing them statistically while the latter are concerned with establishing categories on the basis of the data themselves and tend to use a more classificatory approach. As seen in Tab. 4.1.1, quantitative approaches are traditionally based on large-scale samples and standardised research tools according to which the analysis of frequencies and probabilities of occurrence allow for generalisations relating to a wider, macro-level population. The qualitative approach, on the other hand, aims at an in-depth understanding of the phenomena studied and tends to focus on individual occurrences, taking both the situation and the context of utterances into account in order to make inductive (and more subjective) claims.

Tab. 4.1.1 Schematic comparison of quantitative and qualitative research formulae (adapted from Lamnek 1995:245 and Schlieben-Lange 1991:121)

Quantitative approach	Qualitative approach
Standardised items	Open items
Macro level	Micro level
Large scale	Individual cases
Deductive	Inductive
Objective	Subjective
Random sampling	Judgement sampling
Static	Dynamic

Dialectologists have been using numerical data to describe language variation and language attitudes for over a century now (Chambers/Trudgill 2004; Francis 1983; Preston 2010:87). Yet, the need for more refined and rigorous methods has become apparent with the first sociolinguistic studies. Accordingly, Labov (1966a) and Trudgill (1974) are considered pioneers due to their adoption of statistical tools and sampling methods from the social sciences – mainly sociology, developmental psychology and (economic) geography – to compare language behaviour between different social groups (Abbuhl *et al.* 2013).

Whereas the introduction of quantitative methods in modern dialectology and sociolinguistics was crucial, a reverse trend in the direction of more qualitative methods – which again came from the social sciences but had been taken over in sociolinguistics – was registered a couple of decades ago (Mayring 1992; Zwickl 2002). According to Löw-Wiebach (2005:33): "qualitative research is a prerequisite for quantitative measuring simply because the categories and items used in quantitative formulae have to be established first by means of a qualitative approach".[32]

Mixed methods are currently a common option for the investigation of complex research questions and have seen a marked increase in recent decades. Mixed-method approaches combine quantitative experimental designs with more qualitative approaches. In many fields of study, even more so in linguistics, a uniquely quantitative or qualitative approach misses out important aspects because it either relies on figures and percentages or on deductive and subjective explanations. Since variation is often not a question of presence versus absence but one of 'how-much when with-whom why-(not)', i.e., of relative frequency (Sankoff 1980:77–8), mixed-methods show that quantitative and qualitative approaches are not incompatible or mutually exclusive, but rather helpful devices in the facilitation of a deeper understanding of complex phenomena (Angouri 2010; Hashemi 2012; Mayring 2014).

The present study uses both quantitative and qualitative methods in what is referred to as the 'convergent parallel design', according to which qualitative and quantitative data are collected independently and concurrently from all members of the population at issue (Creswell/Plano Clark 2011). Yet, as further described in Section 4.2, sequential timing has been preferred during individual tasks, beginning with a quantitative strand. According to this 'explanatory sequential design', the quantitative strand receives the greatest emphasis in the study, and results are followed up by a qualitative phase (Abbuhl *et al.* 2013).[33] The quantitative approach and statistical testing have been used to handle the number of respondents (n = 60) concurrently with the number of extralinguistic variables (n = 3). The qualitative methods have been used to elicit information on accent and dialect variation within the student community (cf. Section 4.2).

32 For further details concerning quantitative and qualitative methods in social research cf. Salkind (2010), Lamnek (1995), Schlieben-Lange (1991) and Fasold (1984:61–146).

33 The pre-investigation of the present study was carried out from March to May 2016. At that time, considering the difficulties in accessing the community due to time

Furthermore, in a community where no previous research has ever been carried out, a quantitative approach alone seemed unrealistic because of the highly complex social situation of the transient student community. Hence, a combination of the two methodologies have proved to be effective and ensured the three desiderata of both qualitative and mainly quantitative research, i.e., validity, reliability and replicability (Punch 1998:101; Schlieben-Lange 1991:119).

4.1.2 Sampling Methods

A crucial and foremost element of empirical linguistic research is to decide *a priori* what kind of data to collect, e.g., naturalistic spoken data, questionnaire data, judgement data and the target group, e.g., small populations or large-scale populations. Ideally, the most reliable method for examining the language use of a specific group would be to gather information from each and every person in the population. Yet, with the exception of small-scale populations, e.g., tribal speech communities, this method is rather impractical. Hence most researchers only focus on "some people in the group in such a way that their responses and characteristics reflect those of the group from which they are drawn [...] This is the principle of *sampling*" (De Vaus 2001:60; emphasis in the original). For instance, De Vaus advocates a quantitative approach in population sampling since it aims at providing a representative sample in order to reflect the population as a whole. Qualitative studies, on the other hand, focus on individuals and thus do not aim at representativeness (Zwickl 2002:32). These non-probability methods cannot be used to make any statistical inference about the population in question and therefore "one must [...] accept that statistically rigorous representativeness is not a primary issue in the research design" (Rice 2010:232).

When it comes to probability (quantitative) methods, most social scientists argue that representativeness can only be assumed if the characteristics of the sampled subgroup match those of the population at large. Hence, representativeness implies the avoidance of biases in the data. However, sampling errors often occur since a sample is hardly ever a perfect replication of the statistical distribution of all subgroups (Buchstaller/Khattab 2013). In empirical linguistics, social representativeness is not achieved easily since "language varies across a wide

---

restrictions and the qualitative/quantitative data imbalance, the explanatory sequential design was reversed. The study placed more emphasis on the qualitative phase (semi-structured recorded interviews collected from eleven participants), which, in turn, informed a quantitative phase (internet-based survey administrated to forty-one participants) used to test and to confirm the findings from the first phase (Regnoli 2016).

range of social dimensions within a population, such as speakers' age, gender, sexuality, ethnic identities, regional background, educational level, and many others" (Buchstaller/Khattab 2013:75). All of this leads to a considerable challenge for linguists when it comes to sampling and avoiding biases in the data at the same time. As Sankoff (1974:21–2) points out, the most important decision a researcher should take is to define *whom* to investigate. As she puts it: "good data is defined as language materials of sufficient type and quantity, as well as materials which take into account the social context in which the language data is gathered".

Linguists have traditionally used sampling probability methods that strive for representativeness. However, the most commonly used ones are 'convenience sampling', 'random sampling', 'stratified sampling', 'ethnographic sampling', and 'network sampling'. 'Convenience sampling' usually strives for convenient accessibility rather than representativeness. In small-scale communities or in hardly accessible ones, for instance, researchers have no other option than sampling volunteers. Although this method restricts the application of statistical analyses as well as possible generalisations, in some cases it is theory-independent and hence justified (Hatch/Lazaraton 1991:42). It is generally used in pre-investigations or pilot studies since it allows researchers to survey the field before setting up a more elaborate sampling design.[34]

In 'random sampling', each individual has the same chance of being selected and will be treated as representative of a given total population. According to De Vaus (2001:60; emphasis in the original): "[this is] the surest way of providing equal probability of selection [...] This involves listing all members of the population (this list is called a *sampling frame*) and then [...] 'pulling their names out of a hat'". However, the method has not proved to be feasible in sociolinguistic studies: "[t]ruly random samples of the type used in opinion polls, marketing research, and other social surveys have proven to be both unmanageable and unnecessary [...]" (Chambers 1995:39).

Group differences and intra-group ones have always been the main interest in sociolinguistic research (Labov 1972a). In such cases, 'stratified random sampling' (also referred to as 'judgement sampling' or 'quota sampling') is used systematically. Building on Sankoff (1974) and Rice's (2010) suggestions that contemporary empirical linguistic research should rely on the principle that a sample needs to be representative for the purpose of the study, this method

34 This was the case in the pre-investigation within the Heidelberg Indian student community, in which volunteers were the only ones I was able to gain access to through the community. In consequence, they were the only ones to be sampled (Regnoli 2016).

allows researchers to identify the type of subgroups they want to investigate first and then to sample these groups systematically.

Intrinsically antithetical to 'random sampling' is 'ethnographic sampling'. Ethnographic data collection entails the discovery of emic categories and of salient social and cultural contrasts within a given community.[35] Hence, individuals are sampled according to ethnographic relevance. Eckert (2000:69) describes this approach as follows: "while survey fieldwork focuses on filling the sample, ethnographic fieldwork focuses on finding out what is worth sampling". As in 'convenience sampling', the ethnographic version is not statistically representative (Eckert 2000; Tagliamonte 2006:27), yet neither merely subjective but rather intersubjective for the convergence of its categorisations with the community's assessment (Buchstaller/Khattab 2013:80).

'Social network (or 'snowball') sampling' is partially similar to the ethnographic method but with a more quantitative assessment. The method was first experimented by Milroy and Milroy (1992), who contacted their participants by being referred from friend to friend in working-class neighbourhoods in Belfast. This 'friend-of-a-friend' approach measures individuals' network status and network flows (Milroy/Gordon 2003).[36] Similarly to 'convenience sampling' methods, 'social network sampling' focuses on voluntary membership. Interestingly, membership in 'network sampling' is not established by the researcher, but rather by the participants themselves (Chambers 2009; Meyerhoff 2002).

The differences and similarities between sampling methods are visualised in Tab. 4.1.2.

Tab. 4.1.2 Sampling methods encoded according to intrinsic similarities. Differences are shown in columns; similarities in rows

Probability methods	**Non-probability methods**	
Random sampling		
Judgement sampling		
Network sampling	Ethnographic sampling	Convenience sampling

35 Cf. Duranti (1997) and Pike (1967) for further details on the emic and etic perspectives. A further discussion of ethnography will be provided in Section 4.3.

36 For a full account of network bonds in the Heidelberg transient community of Indian university students cf. Sections 3.2 and 4.3.

Despite clear-cut distinctions between probability and non-probability methods, linguistics has recently witnessed a tendency towards sampling method triangulation, hence leading to a relaxation of the concept of statistical representativeness. This is mainly the case in dialectology and variationist sociolinguistics.[37] As Tagliamonte (2006:28) points out: "the critical component of this hybrid methodology for variationist analysis is that researchers decide which type of representativeness is sufficient – or attainable – depending on the focus of the study".

The choices generally made when adopting sampling strategies may arguably be motivated by the researchers' theoretical stances about the fabrics of social structure, their testing aims and, finally, their epistemological commitments. In consequence, the present study would have been rather unlikely to use 'random sampling' for the very concept it entails and proved not to be feasible in the usage of 'judgement sampling' since its predetermined categories would have missed crucial local social contrasts within the community in question. Moreover, the pilot study conducted in 2016 clarified that 'convenience sampling' was not justified, in spite of the speech community being so relatively restricted. The network flows and interactions were so dense and worth investigating that a redirection in the research was needed.

Due to the aforementioned reasons, since a deep sense of the locally salient social (intra)-groupings can only be achieved via sustained presence in the community, the present study combines both ethnographic and network sampling methods from an anthropological and folk linguistic perspective. Although I had already been working within the community one and a half year prior to the present investigation, regaining access to the community was crucial for the intrinsic concept of the transiency of the community itself.[38] Accessing the community for the second time changed and re-shaped my positioning and, hence, the direction of the research. Consequently, a 'friend-of-a-friend' situation was recreated from scratch. The advantage of this approach is that it enables not only to have multiple access points to different parts of the community and to "hang [...] out" (Giddens 2006:85) with different internal subgroups, but also to combine ethnographic and network sampling.

The aim was to obtain participants' information for each of the social variables already partially defined in other sociolinguistic studies (*gender*, *ethnicity* and *time spent in Heidelberg*).[39] The approach was not entirely based on probability-methods,

37 For a more comprehensive account cf. Milroy/Gordon (2003), Eckert (2000) and Cheshire *et al.* (1989).

38 For a further discussion on transient speech communities cf. Section 2.2.2.

39 For an account of the extraction and the coding of the extralinguistic variables cf. Section 5.1.1.1.

but as mentioned above, informants were approached as a friend of a friend or through a voluntary student association. As a consequence of what network and ethnography sampling methodologies entail, i.e., community membership is to be established by the participants themselves and not by the researcher, it was not possible to obtain an equal number of informants in each group except for gender (30 male participants and 30 female ones).

The size of the sample is also important for the research design. While social scientists put great emphasis on large numbers, Buchstaller and Khattab (2013:83) argue that sociolinguistic studies tend to be based on smaller samples mainly for reasons of practicality since they require

> the time-intensive linguistic recording and transcription work which explodes data-handling time by subdiscipline-dependent ratio (ten hours of word-for-word transcription per recorded hour; 1:100 for close phonetic transcription [...].

Many linguists argue that a large number of informants is not even necessary for language research. Labov (1966a:180), for instance, posits that a small sample would produce the same linguistic variation as a larger one because "linguistic behavior is far more general and compelling than many social attitudes or survey responses". Similarly, Sankoff (1980:51–2) claims that the very basic assumption that language is based on mutual intelligibility places a limit on the extent of possible variation. In consequence, "even for quite complex communities, samples of more than about 150 individuals tend to be redundant, bringing increasing data-handling problems with diminishing analytical returns". As far as smaller samples are concerned, quantitative analysis requires at least five individuals per cell in order to make statistical sense about the data collected (Gries 2013).

The present study presents data gathered from sixty speakers (39 master's students and 21 Ph.D. ones) aged 21–30, coming from sixteen Indian states, speaking fourteen different languages as L1 (one Germanic language (English), 9 Indo-Aryan ones, 4 Dravidian ones) and the same number of IndE regional dialects.[40] Table 4.1.3 lists social details of each informant.[41] The size of the sample is justified by the relative 'smallness' of the speech community and proves to be sufficient to allow for generalisations about the entire Indian student population of Heidelberg.

---

40 For further details on the characteristics of the sample cf. Section 5.1.1.1.

41 A coding system was developed to give an insight on the social variables of the informants. The first two letters denote their initials, the next letter stands for their gender, i.e., m = male; f = female, and the last ones stand for the locality they are from. When two informants share the same initials, gender and locality, the first letter of their

Speaker	Gender	Age	L1	State	Religion	Caste	Mother Position	Father Position	Education	School	Years in HD	Faculty	Level of German
ABmDe	M	22	Hindi, English	Delhi	Hindu	Kshatriya	Forewoman, skilled. self-employed	Foreman, skilled. self-employed	English-medium	Private	0.1-1	South Asia Institute	B1
AHfKa	F	23	Kannada	Karnataka	Hindu	Brahmin	Unskilled	Semi-skilled. agricultural	English-medium	Both	0.1-1	Physics	A1
APmTN	M	28	Tamil	Tamil Nadu	Catholic	Vaisya	Forewoman, skilled. self-employed	Foreman, skilled. self-employed	English-medium	Private	0.1-1	Physical Chemistry	B2
ARmKe	M	27	Malayalam	Kerala	Hindu	Vaisya	Unskilled	Semi-skilled. agricultural	English-medium	Private	1.1-5	Mathematics and Informatics	B1
ASfKe	F	24	Tamil	Kerala	Hindu	Brahmin	Unskilled	Employer, manager	English-medium	Private	1.1-5	Physics	A1
ASmMP	M	27	Hindi	Madhya Pradesh	Hindu	Kshatriya	Forewoman, skilled. self-employed	Professional worker	English-medium	Both	1.1-5	Biological Sciences	A2
ATmDe	M	22	Oriya	Delhi	Hindu	Brahmin	Unskilled	Foreman, skilled. self-employed	English-medium	Private	0.1-1	Anthropology	A1
AVmDe	M	24	Hindi, Punjabi	Delhi	Hindu	Unspecified	Unskilled	Employer, manager	English-medium	Private	0.1-1	International Business and Engeneering	B1
BJmGu	M	27	Gujarati	Gujarat	Hindu	Brahmin	Forewoman, skilled. self-employed	Professional worker	Gujarati-medium	Private	1.1-5	Physics	A1
BSmGu	M	26	Gujarati	Gujarat	Hindu	Brahmin	Unskilled	Foreman, skilled. self-employed	English-medium	Private	1.1-5	Medical Physics	B1
DLfMan	F	24	Manipuri	Manipur	Hindu	No	Forewoman, skilled. self-employed	Employer, manager	English-medium	Private	0.1-1	Immunology	A1
DSfWB	F	26	Hindi	West Bengal	Hindu	Vaisya	Unskilled	Professional worker	English-medium	Private	0.1-1	South Asia Institute	A1
DTfUt	F	27	Hindi	Uttarakhand	Hindu	Brahmin	Professional worker	Professional worker	English-medium	Private	1.1-5	Biological Sciences	A2
DVfAP	F	27	Telugu	Andhra Pradesh	Hindu	Vaisya	Unskilled	Foreman, skilled. self-employed	English-medium	Private	0.1-1	Computer Science	B2
GSmDe	M	27	Hindi, Punjabi	Delhi	Sikh	No	Employer, manager	Foreman, skilled. self-employed	English-medium	Private	1.1-5	Biological Sciences	A2

Speaker	Gender	Age	L1	State	Religion	Caste	Mother Position	Father Position	Education	School	Years in HD	Faculty	Level of German
SPfBi	F	25	Hindi	Bihar	Hindu	Brahmin	Unskilled	Employer, manager	English-medium	Both	0.1-1	Informatics	A1
SPmKa	M	23	Kannada	Karnataka	Hindu	Kshatriya	Unskilled	Foreman, skilled. self-employed	English-medium	Private	0.1-1	Information Technology	A1
SSfWB	F	23	Bengali	West Bengal	Hindu	No	Unskilled	Professional worker	English-medium	Private	0.1-1	Economics	A2
SSmKa	M	24	Kannada	Karnataka	Hindu	Brahmin	Unskilled	Employer, manager	English-medium	Both	0.1-1	Information Technology	A2
SSmHa	M	30	Hindi	Haryana	Hindu	Kshatriya	Unskilled	Foreman, skilled. self-employed	English-medium	Both	1.1-5	Computer Science	A2
SSmKe	M	23	Malayalam	Kerala	Hindu	Vaisya	Unskilled	Foreman, skilled. self-employed	English-medium	Both	1.1-5	Physics	A1
SSmMa	M	23	Hindi	Maharashtra	Hindu	Unspecified	Professional worker	Employer, manager	Both	Both	0.1-1	Cancer Biology	A1
SSmUt	M	27	Kumaoni Pahadi	Uttarakhand	Hindu	Vaisya	Unskilled	Foreman, skilled. self-employed	English-medium	Private	0.1-1	Information Technology	A1
STfBi	F	23	Hindi	Bihar	Hindu	Unspecified	Employer, manager	Employer, manager	English-medium	Both	0.1-1	Computer Science	A1
SVmKa	M	23	Kannada	Karnataka	Hindu	Brahmin	Unskilled	Foreman, skilled. self-employed	English-medium	Private	0.1-1	Information Technology	A1
TDfMa	F	28	Gujarati	Maharashtra	Hindu	Brahmin	Volounteer	Semi-skilled. agricultural	English-medium	Private	0.1-1	South Asia Institute	A1
TKfMa	F	25	Oriya	Maharashtra	Hindu	Brahmin	Forewoman, skilled. self-employed	Professional worker	English-medium	Public	1.1-5	Physics	A1
URmRa	M	26	Hindi	Rajasthan	Hindu	Vaisya	Unskilled	Foreman, skilled. self-employed	English-medium	Private	1.1-5	Scientific Computing	A2
VJRfKa	F	25	Kannada	Karnataka	Hindu	Brahmin	Employer, manager	Foreman, skilled. self-employed	English-medium	Private	1.1-5	Physical Chemistry	B2
VRmTN	M	26	Konkani	Tamil Nadu	Hindu	Brahmin	Unskilled	Foreman, skilled. self-employed	English-medium	Private	1.1-5	Information Technology	B2

Speaker	Gender	Age	L1	State	Religion	Caste	Mother Position	Father Position	Education	School	Years in HD	Faculty	Level of German
PNmKe	M	26	Malayalam	Kerala	Hindu	Brahmin	Forewoman, skilled. self-employed	Foreman, skilled. self-employed	English-medium	Private	0.1-1	Chemistry and Earth Sciences	A1
PPmKa	M	22	Kannada	Karnataka	Hindu	Kshatriya	Forewoman, skilled. self-employed	Foreman, skilled. self-employed	English-medium	Private	0.1-1	Physics	A1
PVfKa	F	24	Kannada	Karnataka	Hindu	Vaisya	Unskilled	Foreman, skilled. self-employed	English-medium	Private	0.1-1	Computer Science	A1
RDfKa	F	23	Konkani	Karnataka	Catholic	Brahmin	Employer, manager	Employer, manager	English-medium	Both	1.1-5	Information Technology	A1
RFmMa	M	23	Marathi	Maharashtra	Hindu	Brahmin	Housewife	Foreman, skilled. self-employed	English-medium	Private	0.1-1	International Business and Engeneering	A2
RMfMa	F	23	Marathi, English	Maharashtra	Hindu	Inter-caste	Forewoman, skilled. self-employed	Foreman, skilled. self-employed	English-medium	Both	0.1-1	Transcultural Studies	A1
RNmKa	M	23	Telugu	Karnataka	Hindu	Kshatriya	Unskilled	Foreman, skilled. self-employed	English-medium	Private	1.1-5	International Business and Engeneering	B1
SAmKa	M	24	Kannada	Karnataka	Hindu	Brahmin	Forewoman, skilled. self-employed	Professional worker	English-medium	Private	0.1-1	Computer Science	A2
SDfKa	F	21	Konkani, English	Karnataka	Catholic	Brahmin	Professional worker	Foreman, skilled. self-employed	English-medium	Private	0.1-1	English Literary and Cultural Studies	A2
SDfMP	F	26	Hindi	Madhya Pradesh	Hindu	Brahmin	Professional worker	Professional worker	English-medium	Both	0.1-1	Scientific Computing	A1
SHfUP	F	24	Hindi	Uttar Pradesh	Muslim	No	Unskilled	Foreman, skilled. self-employed	English-medium	Private	0.1-1	Physics	B1
SLfUP	F	22	Hindi, English	Uttar Pradesh	Hindu	Unsure	Employer, manager	Employer, manager	English-medium	Private	0.1-1	English Literary and Cultural Studies	A1
SLmKa	M	27	Tamil	Karnataka	Hindu	Kshatriya	Unskilled	Foreman, skilled. self-employed	English-medium	Private	1.1-5	Computer Science	A2
SMfMa	F	26	Marathi	Maharashtra	Hindu	Kshatriya	Professional worker	Foreman, skilled. self-employed	Marathi-medium	Public	0.1-1	South Asia Institute	A1

Speaker	Gender	Age	L1	State	Religion	Caste	Mother Position	Father Position	Education	School	Years in HD	Faculty	Level of German
HTmUP	M	28	Hindi	Uttar Pradesh	Hindu	Brahmin	Unskilled	Foreman, skilled. self-employed	English-medium	Both	1.1-5	Computer Science	A1
JDfMa	F	24	Marathi	Maharashtra	Hindu	Kshatriya	Unskilled	Foreman, skilled. self-employed	English-medium	Private	0.1-1	Information Technology	A1
JGfMa	F	28	Marathi	Maharashtra	Hindu	Kshatriya	Forewoman, skilled. self-employed	Employer, manager	English-medium	Private	1.1-5	Biological Sciences	A1
JGMfKe	F	22	Malayalam	Kerala	Catholic	No	Professional worker	Professional worker	English-medium	Both	0.1-1	Physics	A1
KDmWB	M	25	Bengali	West Bengal	Hindu	Unspecified	Unskilled	Foreman, skilled. self-employed	English-medium	Both	0.1-1	Physics	A1
KGfPu	F	24	Hindi	Punjab (Chandigarh)	Hindu	Vaisya	Unskilled	Employer, manager	English-medium	Private	0.1-1	Biological Sciences	A1
KMmKe	M	29	Malayalam	Kerala	Protestant	No	Unskilled	Employer, manager	English-medium	Private	0.1-1	Computational Linguistics	A1
MGfUt	F	27	Hindi, English	Uttarakhand	Hindu	Brahmin	Forewoman, skilled. self-employed	Foreman, skilled. self-employed	English-medium	Private	0.1-1	Transcultural Studies	B1
MGofUt	F	25	Hindi	Uttarakhand	Hindu	Unspecified	Unskilled	Foreman, skilled. self-employed	English-medium	Public	0.1-1	Information Technology	A2
MMfKa	F	23	Marwari	Karnataka	Jahn	No	Unskilled	Employer, manager	English-medium	Private	0.1-1	Molecular Biosciences	A1
MNmKa	M	24	Kannada	Karnataka	Hindu	Vaisya	Unskilled	Foreman, skilled. self-employed	English-medium	Private	1.1-5	International Business and Engeneering	B1
NKSfTN	F	28	Tamil	Tamil Nadu	Hindu	Brahmin	Unskilled	Employer, manager	English-medium	Private	1.1-5	Biological Sciences	A1
NPfMP	F	23	Hindi	Madhya Pradesh	Hindu	Brahmin	Unskilled	Foreman, skilled. self-employed	English-medium	Private	1.1-5	Scientific Computing	A1
OFmTN	M	23	Tamil	Tamil Nadu	Muslim	Vaisya	Unskilled	Foreman, skilled. self-employed	English-medium	Private	0.1-1	International Business and Engeneering	A2
PGfMa	F	24	Hindi	Maharashtra	Hindu	Unspecified	Unskilled	Semi-skilled. agricultural	English-medium	Public	0.1-1	Cancer Biology	A1

Tab. 4.1.3 The Heidelberg Indian student community sample (n = 60)

4.1.3 Testing Aims

The testing aims of the present study are multiple: exploring the connection between dependent and independent variables, gaining insight into intercorrelations within the community and detecting possible crucial factors resulting from the transient character of the community. Considering that attending to folk awareness as a dimension of ideology (Kroskrity 2004; Silverstein 1979) and perceptual dialectology (Niedzielski/Preston 2003; Preston 2010, 1999) has stressed the importance of speakers' diverse responses to specific varieties of language (cf. Section 2.3), the first aim of the study is to test whether students' folk perceptions regarding accent variation share a common ground with ascertained linguistic beliefs. In other words, the study aims at undertaking an ethnolinguistic reflection upon the elaboration of mental maps and border perceptions regarding regional varieties of IndE. The second aim is to record attitudes towards selected IndE varieties in relation to the participants' self-stated ethnic identities and linguistic consciousness, i.e., to outline the similarities of and differences between these varieties with respect to perceived accent variation. The third aim is to investigate whether network integration plays a role in the attitudes and the identities of the community members, i.e., to provide an account of the intra-group social factors influencing dialectal variation. These testing aims, which have been based on issues raised in the earlier chapters, may be summarised in the following research questions:

1. How are different IndE accents perceived by the members of the speech community?
2. Do differences in L2 phonological characteristics index local and situated ethnic identities?
3. How do different IndE accents affect language consciousness, attitudes and behaviour?

In order to answer these questions, the study will attempt to confirm that methodology triangulation is appropriate for meeting the requirements of the testing aims.

4.2 Oral and Written Questionnaires

After making principled decisions concerning the research design, researchers have to decide which data collection techniques to employ in order to ensure the effectiveness of the three research desiderata mentioned (Punch 1998; Schlieben-Lange 1991). The elicitation of data is a crucial step in the research since it will impact the results of the study. Methods for data elicitation can be divided into direct and indirect ones. Direct ones require informants to answer questions about their opinions and attitudes towards (perceived) language variation. Indirect ones, on the contrary, are based on the simple criterion that informants do not know that they are being researched (Francis 1983:78–103). However, this approach is ethically incorrect and unjustified since "consent is the cornerstone of ethical research practices" (Eckert 2013:14).

In the field of sociolinguistics, folk linguistics and pragmatics, researchers have traditionally relied on direct methods, either in the form of written questionnaires or semi-structured interviews in order to obtain information about language use and behaviour (Kasper 2008). However, direct methods need to be applied carefully in order to overcome Labov's (1972b:113) 'Observer's Paradox': "[t]o obtain the data most important for linguistic theory, we have to observe how people speak when they are not being observed". This means that a considerable effort has to be made in mitigating observer effects on the 'naturalness' of data, favouring techniques that elicit linguistic information completely indirectly.

The present study advocates deductive mixed-method research and dynamic data collection techniques. Considering my personal commitment to the entire community and the new role I had been assigned (cf. Section 4.3), consent was a primary and crucial concern.[42] Although it was a one-time event, consent depended on the effects that the research was having on the community, hence the reason for anonymity.[43] Consent was documented by agreeing to the terms and conditions of the administered questionnaires.[44]

---

initials differentiating them is included in their coding. DSfWB for instance is a female student from West Bengal. For the assignment of the informants into social groups cf. Section 5.1.1.1. For a list of abbreviations of Indian states and union territories cf. p. vi.

42 During fieldwork, I was a board member of HISA, my role being that of the new international volunteer in cultural events. For a comprehensive account of data collection cf. Section 4.3.

43 Going public was not a concern for most informants. However, anonymity was preferred in order to gather more interesting and natural data, hence their initials were used. For further details cf. Section 4.1.2.

44 Both surveys contained the following sentence: "The information you provide will be treated confidentially. Your participation is voluntary". At the beginning of each session, the importance of consent and anonymity was highlighted when informants were asked to provide their personal data, which would be used only by the researcher and in case of additional questions or doubts to be clarified afterwards.

The complete task consisted of two surveys, a semi-structured recorded interview and a recorded reading passage. It lasted about two hours for each participant. The questionnaire, the interview guidelines and the reading of the passage are displayed in Chapter 8. Since no previous linguistic study has been undertaken within the Indian student community in question, I took advantage of the pre-investigation to gather the categories which are relevant for the research area. As part of the pilot study, recordings of the reading passage were collected and partly used for the present one for the elicitation of knowledge and use of regional IndE accents (cf. Section 4.2.4).

4.2.1 Survey I: Language Background and Language Use

The first part of the task is a face-to-face internet-based survey designed to elicit information on attitudes and orientations and to ascertain if such matters correlate with the patterns of language use described in the second survey.[45] Specifically, the task consists of twenty-nine multiple-choice questions and three five-point Likert scales aiming at gathering information about (i) language background and language use in India and in Heidelberg in different domains, (ii) educational background, (iii) personal language-related plans towards L1 and L2 varieties of English and (iv) identity issues regarding specific languages inside and outside the Indian community.[46]

Overall, but particularly in the Likert scale task, the participants are expected to point to their alleged status within the community depending on their in-group allegiances or distance along with their willingness (or not) to shed their regional, ethnic identities in favour of their more 'general' pan-Indian one (Jayaram 2004). Thus, the aim of the first survey is to help participants 'empower' their folk beliefs by influencing the conscious and unconscious reflections on and reactions to dialectal variation, which is the primary concern of Survey II. By activating what the anthropologist Steven Vertovč (1999) defines as 'diaspora consciousness', i.e., a 'multi-locality' (Friesen/Kearns 2008) that involves dual or

---

45 Both surveys are designed on the online platform esurveycreator.com: <http://www.esurveycreator.com>. The free account was upgraded to the 'student' offer, similar to the 'business' one, which allows for the analysis of the results in real time and automatic online evaluations including data cross-tabulations.

46 Likert scales are partially direct and partially indirect methods of elicitation in which participants are given a numerical scale – usually consisting of an odd number of points (either 1–5 or 1–7) – with the endpoints defined as acceptable or unacceptable and then asked to rate each sentence/stimulus along the scale. For further details cf. Schütze/Sprouse (2013:33–4).

multiple identities, the participants are implicitly stimulated to react along an awareness continuum to specific and locally-situated contexts taking place in their community of practice (Niedzielski/Preston 2003).

The choice of turning to the convenience of internet-based surveys administered face-to-face allows for more control over the whole session. It enables asking for clarifications and returning to some earlier questions easily when the informants feel the need to modify some answers.

4.2.2 Survey II, Section I: Accent and identity

Linguistic surveys can be composed of different types of elicitation frames. In order to elicit particular linguistic features, linguists use either direct elicitations or indirect ones. Survey II combines both techniques, including overt self-reports and covert attitudes towards local IndE accents.

The first section is thus devised to measure the extent to which the informants identify with their hometown/state/geographic location in terms of accent perception. Assuming that the concept of regional identity has not been treated here as static, but rather as dynamic – especially in light of the transient character of the community and the continuous mobility of its members – the aim of Survey II is to elicit overt beliefs and attitudes towards self and others' speech productions. This identification questionnaire, modelled and adapted from Llamas (2000), is an attempt to gain insight into how accent and dialect features that are connected with a certain geographical location are used to express solidarity with or distance towards other speakers of those accents and dialects, and whether and to what extent they reverberate within the community in question.[47]

The section consists of fourteen questions (ten open ones; three yes/no ones and one five-point Likert scale) aiming at eliciting the respondents' awareness of their own IndE accents. Expectations regarding the success of the task are based on the assumption of folk theory according to which "[i]f the folk talk about language, they must, of course, know (or at least believe they know) about it" (Niedzielski/Preston 2003:10). Particularly, the task aims at gathering as much

---

47 Llamas (2000) investigates variation and change in the dialect of Middlesbrough. Results from her questionnaire suggest that, as far the glottalisation of /p/, /t/ and /k/ is concerned, the speech of younger women is more glottalised than that of older people and that this might be due to the fact that young speakers from Middlesbrough do not identify with Yorkshire (where Middlesbrough was located until 1968), but rather with the North-east. By glottalising the consonants, young speakers index their Middlesbrough identity over their more general Yorkshire one.

information as possible about the five main conditions which, according to Silverstein (1981), predict, or enhance, folk scrutiny:

1. 'Unavoidable referentiality', e.g., the general awareness of undifferentiated non-native accents and dialect varieties.
2. 'Continuous segmentability', e.g., the awareness of typical pan-Indian accent features.
3. 'Relative presuppositionality', e.g., the awareness of alleged first-language influence on different non-native accents or dialects.
4. 'Decontextualised deducibility', e.g., the capacity of description of (specific features of) a specific dialect or accent.
5. 'Metapragmatic transparency', e.g., the immediate recognition and subsequent imitation of (specific features of) a specific dialect or accent.

It is worth mentioning that the fact "[t]hat [the] speakers involved are well-educated does not [...] deter [...] from describing the data [...] as folk linguistics" (Niedzielski/Preston 2003:13). Moreover, as well as in Survey I, turning to a face-to-face internet-based survey enables exchanging clarifications with the informants and, most importantly, to check the consistency of their answers in real-time and to ask for more accurate descriptions.

4.2.3 Cognitive Maps

The language regard procedure, i.e., speakers' awakening of a response, described in Section 4.2.2 is thus devised in order to account for the speakers' underlying attitudinal cognitorium with regard to popular beliefs about IndE regional varieties. In order to uncover the degree of perceived difference or similarity between the respondents' hometowns/states/geographic locations and other parts of the Indian subcontinent, they are then presented with a map of India in order to visualise the data gathered in the earlier task.

Data have traditionally been presented in the form of maps since the first dialect geographic surveys, i.e., Georg Wenker's (1877) 'Deutscher Sprachatlas' and Jules Gilliéron's (1902–1910) 'Atlas Linguistic de la France'. As Francis (1983:110) explains:

> [s]ince the major, virtually exclusive, interest of traditional surveys has been in the 'horizontal' geographical dimension of linguistic variation rather than in the 'vertical' social dimension, the most logical and effective mode of displaying the distribution has been in maps.[48]

48 For a more comprehensive account of data maps cf. Glauser (1994) and Francis (1983:110–44).

However, it was only in the 1970s that more statistically sophisticated studies of 'dialect images' began to spread (Inoue 1977/8). Adapting techniques from language attitude studies, Inoue (1995) identifies variety descriptors, e.g., snobbish, plain, funny, and then uses them to characterise the speech of different areas. Drawing on such studies, Preston (1981) and Preston and Howe (1987) develop different joint techniques for perceptual dialectology that have later become the cornerstones of folk theory.[49]

The present task partially follows Preston's cognitive map research design and aims at eliciting speakers' overt and covert ideologies and social stereotypes about IndE accents. The respondents were provided with a minimally detailed map of India and asked to hand-draw boundaries around areas where they believe IndE regional speech zones exist. They were then asked to assign adjectives to the marked areas. In doing so, they indicated characteristics both of the speech and the speakers, a well-known technique borrowed from cultural geography (Gould/White 1986). During the task, the participants were strongly encouraged to use their own adjectives. However, some of them preferred to select them from a predefined pool for confidence issues.[50]

Interestingly, during the task, many speakers were willing to be engaged in open-ended conversations about their motivations and perceptions of the marked speech zones. While the latter were usually kept for the final stage of the session, i.e., the semi-structured interview, it is worth mentioning that the present task was usually the 'turning point' of the data collection. The informants were not feeling those 'interviewer versus interviewee' social and conversational asymmetries any longer. As Labov (1984:40–1) would say, this was the exact moment when the interviewer realised that he was not the 'expert' in the field anymore, but rather the 'learner' who must cede his power to their research participants, the true holders of the community's knowledge.

49 For further details cf. Preston (2010, 1999).

50 While the majority of the participants were quite enthusiastic about the task, some felt 'under pressure' for their need to select the 'right' adjective for the 'right' location. Despite continuous encouragements to feel free to write 'whatever they wanted to', some asked whether it was possible to select some adjectives from a predefined pool. Hence, they were presented with Manchester's first accent and dialect map (Carrie/Drummond 2016).

4.2.4 Survey II, Section II: The Accent Recognition Test

The aim of the present section is to obtain information on listener perceptions and, specifically, their attitudes towards specific features and variants as well as towards the speakers who use them. As seen in Sections 4.2.2 and 4.2.3, there are many ways of eliciting language attitudes directly. However, one limitation of such tasks is that they can induce people to over- or under-report linguistic uses on purpose.[51] In order to overcome the problem, language attitudes have been investigated indirectly via their elicitations towards speakers rather than varieties *per se* and then compared with the earlier sets of data.

While the most widely-used method of language attitude elicitation is the 'Matched Guise Technique' devised by Lambert *et al.* (1960), the present study adopts the 'Verbal Guise' one (Campbell-Kibler 2010), which uses more speakers than only one or two.[52] The guise assembled eight stimuli consisting of one passage read in eight different standard regional varieties of IndE. A reading passage was preferred over conversational speech in order to control for content. To minimise the possible 'unnaturalness' of the reading task, the participants were told that the speakers producing the guises were all informants of the pre-investigation. In this way, they were somehow distanced from the idea of knowing the speakers in question due to their awareness of the transient character of the community.[53] While half of the speakers producing the guises were truly subjects of the pilot study, the other half consisted of members of the present community.

51 Trudgill's (1972) work in Norwich, England, is a well-known case of both phenomena. He notices that women are over-reporting their use of Standard English variants in direct elicitations compared with their actual usages in more conversational tasks, while men are under-reporting their use of standard features.

52 The 'Matched Guise Technique' involves assembling a stimulus consisting of a spoken or read passage in different languages or varieties produced by a single speaker. The method is thus partially indirect and concerns a direct elicitation of attitudes towards speakers and an indirect one towards language. For a more comprehensive account cf. Labov (1972a:310) and Lambert *et al.* (1960).

53 Considering the relative 'smallness' of the community, where almost everyone knows anyone, the participants were told that it was unlikely that they knew the speakers since they were subjects of earlier in-depth fieldwork in the same community. The community is not stable but rather dynamic and every year faces drastic changes in its social structure, i.e., new entries and estrangements. For further details cf. Sections 3.1 and 3.2.

The passage in question was taken from 'Clear Light of Day', a novel by Indian author Anita Desai. The passage was, again, chosen carefully. A further method of lowering the 'unnaturalness' of the task is to use a topic the informants could relate to. Hence, the story of a pre- and post-partition Delhi was considered an adequate choice.[54]

As far as recording techniques are concerned, the last decades have witnessed significant advances in the development of recording technology. In recent studies, many technological options including cell phones, CD recorders and laptop computers have all been successfully used in sociolinguistic research (Podesva/Zsiga 2013).[55] Hence, for the present task, audio data have been captured by a solid-state recorder (Sony ICD-PX333) and, at times, by high quality cell phones. Recordings have then been checked with Praat (version 6.0.29) for finer phonological consistency.

Even though similar accent perception tests take advantage of manipulated speech signals (Fuchs 2016), the speech samples in the present study have been left unedited in order to account for variation in natural speech.[56] The recordings have been put in random order to keep the participants focused on accent variation rather than on the guises. At the beginning of each experiment session, the informants were told that 'within-speaker variation' might occur in the recorded passages in order to prevent them from misjudgements.

The choice of the speakers to produce the different guises has also been approached with care. The eight speakers selected, i.e., four female and four male ones, were all highly educated (enrolled in either master's or Ph.D. courses), came from different Indian states and had different L1s. Thus, they cover ideally the state language/ethnic ratio of the entire subcontinent. Considering that the speakers' perceptions of accent variation seem to concern a rather North to South distinction more than a state-to-state one, two female speakers coming from the same Southern Indian state, i.e., Karnataka, but with different L1s, i.e., Konkani, an Indo-Aryan language and Kannada, a Dravidian one, have been selected in order to account for this folk belief.[57] Table 4.2.1 lists the social characteristics of the guises.

---

54 The passage was first selected and used for collecting audio data during the pre-investigation for phonological analysis.

55 De Decker/Nycz (2011) report that recordings made on an iPhone are of sufficient quality to extract the first and second vowel formant reliably.

56 This decision will most probably influence the results and will thus be taken into consideration in Chapter 5.

57 Information gathered during the time of the pre-investigation.

Tab. 4.2.1 Order, gender, first language, ethnicity, duration and character of the guises

N	Gender	L1	Ethnicity	Length	Impressionistic Characterisation
1	f	Bengali	West Bengal	1:50	Very competent, confident and fluent performance. 'Story-telling voice'.
2	m	Tamil	Tamil Nadu	1:17	Competent, confident and fluent; some pronunciation errors.
3	f	Konkani	Karnataka	1:08	Very competent, confident and fluent performance.
4	m	Gujarati	Maharashtra	1:08	Competent and fluent performance; some mispronunciations.
5	f	Kannada	Karnataka	1:29	Competent performance, but somewhat non-fluent; some interruptions and pronunciation errors.
6	m	Punjabi	Punjab	1:02	Very competent, confident and fluent performance; semantically focused delivery.
7	f	Hindi	Uttar Pradesh	0:58	Very competent, confident and fluent performance; somewhat flat.
8	m	Telugu	Andhra Pradesh	1:22	Competent performance; some interruptions and false starts.

Section II has been arranged as follows: the participants had to listen to the different guises reading the same passage and, after each stimulus, were asked to place each voice on the cognitive map (cf. Section 4.2.3) and to rate the speakers on various measures along 12 semantic differential five-point Likert scales. They were free to listen to each stimulus as many times as they wanted to and were asked to base their judgements on the voice alone.

Specifically, the informants were asked to answer questions about the guise's alleged origin, their degree of certainty, the degree of perceived accent difference, the nature of the cue/clue they had used to identify the guise's origin, the alleged post of the guise, and, finally, to rate the voice along two reliability scales, i.e., <degree of certainty> and <degree of perceived difference>, one readiness-for-action trait, i.e., <accent improvement> and nine status-stressing and solidarity-stressing scales, i.e., <pleasantness>, <correctness>, <intelligence>, <friendliness>, <politeness>, <education>, <attractiveness>, <ambition> and <confidence>. The adjectives chosen were partially based on earlier studies (Beinhoff 2013; Giles 1970; Lambert *et al.* 1960) and were adapted to fit the present work in order to both avoid potentially unreliable effects caused by individual items and to maintain internal structural consistency.

However, as Schilling (2013:106) points out, partially indirect elicitation tasks tend to be considered

> [...] unnatural, and there is no guarantee that the results are reflective of listeners' genuine attitudes. [...] This may be because listeners do not have free access to their attitudes or the ability to accurately convey them, or because they do not wish to express negative attitudes they might really hold.

On the brighter side, Preston (1999:xxxv) argues that

> [n]onlinguists are surprisingly good at distinguishing voices along a dialect continuum [in this case, standard IndE], even at sites where traditional dialect geography has not posited as isogloss. Respondents from different areas, however, "hear" boundaries at different places and with different degrees of intensities, more often making more distinctions closer to the local area and fewer in areas farther from the local area.

The participants were fairly well aware of how to convey their attitudes accurately (cf. Section 4.2.3) and did not feel any pressure when it came to expressing negative attitudes towards the guises. This was most probably due to the naturalistic data.

4.2.5 The Sociolinguistic Interview

After the dialect identification task, the respondents were engaged in an open-ended conversation about the task they had just carried out, IndE regional varieties, speakers of those and related topics. Hence, sociolinguistic interview questions had been grouped into three different modules focusing on: (i) Demography; (ii) Accent and Identity; Language Attitudes and Regard and (iii) Heidelberg and Networking.[58] During each session, the modules were arranged as the interview progressed in order to approximate the flow of natural conversation.

The aim of the task was to yield large quantities of speech that was as casual as possible, with the most vernacular, unguarded speech held to occur when the participants focused their attention on the above-mentioned topics rather than on speech itself.[59] Each session lasted approximately 20 minutes, and a total of 21:54 hours was recorded with a solid-state digital recorder (Sony ICD-PX333).

---

58 The sociolinguistic interview is one of the most important tools for collecting data on language in its social setting. For further details cf. Labov (1972a).

59 Cf. Labov's (1972b:112) 'Vernacular Principle', which suggests that: "the style which is most regular in its structure and in its relation to the evolution of language is the vernacular, in which the minimum attention is paid to speech".

Considering the nature of the study, the audio data were not captured in any sound-proof recording booth of some phonetics laboratory but was the result of language documentation in the field.[60] In consequence, while much effort was made to isolate speech signals and overrepresent ambient noise, obtaining high-quality audio recordings was not the primary concern of the task (as it had been for the recording of the reading passage, cf. Section 4.2.6). As seen in Section 4.2, attitude elicitation techniques, whether direct or indirect, prove to be double-edged weapons when it comes to minimising any overt observer effect (Labov 1984). In order to do this, an attempt "to make the recording equipment as inconspicuous as possible and ensure that the act of recording impedes the progression of the observing events as little as possible" (Levon 2013:207) was made.

Section 4.2.3 has briefly mentioned how power asymmetries are always at stake in every data gathering situation. Interviews are no exception. As Wolfson (1976) contends, interviewees expect interviews to be relatively formal. Hence, capturing and pinpointing vernacular speech is a rather difficult task (Labov 1972a). Perhaps, the fact that the interviews registered some stretches of interaction which were either more 'formal' interview-like or more relaxed and conversational suggests that the attempt to avoid the difficult dual role of the investigator implied in Burton's (1978:165) statement that the network method leads to an "empathetic and analytic immersion into a social world" has been partly successful.

4.2.6 The Reading Passage

In addition to questions designed to spark natural speech, the traditional sociolinguistic interview has a series of additional tasks aiming at yielding conscious, monitored, standard-like speech. Reading passages are one such example (Labov 1972a). Researchers interested in connected speech have traditionally used either passages written to fulfil the needs of a specific study or standard reading passages, e.g., Fairbanks' (1960:27) 'Rainbow Passage' or Aesop's 'The North Wind and the Sun'.

However, the passage selected for the present study is the one already discussed in the accent identification task (cf. Section 4.2.4). While the 'social' choice of the passage has been exemplified above, the linguistic one is justified by the very same design of the passage since it exemplifies a wide range of the sounds of English in a different array of phonological contexts. In addition, it allows the recognition of typical IndE features (cf. Section 5.1.3.2).

60 For a more comprehensive account of the data collection cf. Section 4.3.

The task aimed at capturing high-quality connected speech acoustic data for finer phonological analyses. Hence, unlike in the sociolinguistic interview task, maximising the robustness of the linguistic signal was a crucial step. Passages were recorded either in the participants' households or in quiet open spaces in order to achieve as high a signal-to-noise ratio as possible. Hence, the solid-state recorder (Sony ICD-PX333) or, at times, high-quality cell phones, were positioned close to the speakers' mouths to gain an effect as similar to that of a directional microphone.[61] The majority of the recordings are sampled at 44.100 kHz. However, the solid-state recorder sampled the signal at an increasingly higher rate (96.100 kHz).[62] Each session lasted approximately one minute, and a total of 1.12 hours was recorded. Before beginning the recording, the participants were asked to familiarise themselves with the reading passage first and then to read it at their most comfortable speed.

The different methods described in the present section offer a range of alternative techniques, i.e., written data, attitude elicitations and sound recorded data gathering. They all serve different methodological purposes, and, as shown in Fig. 4.2.1, they are grouped and ranged from left to right in terms of increasing 'naturalness'.

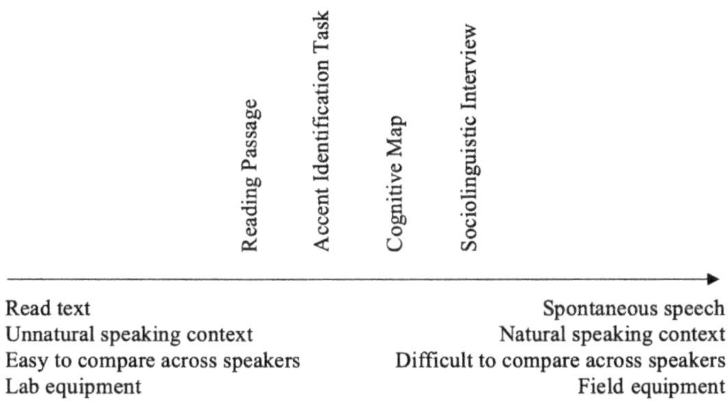

Fig. 4.2.1 Range of data collection designs (adapted from Podesva/Zsiga 2013:180)

61 'Directional microphones', also known as 'cardioid' or 'unidirectional microphones' capture the audio signal only from the direction the microphone is pointing at. For further details cf. Podesva/Zsiga (2013:169–94).

62 The sampling rate value determines the frequency range of the digital signal. The higher the sampling rate, the higher linguistically meaningful frequencies. A sampling rate of 22 kHz is generally sufficient for capturing worthwhile investigating frequencies. 44

4.3 Data Collection

Through the combination of Malinowski's (1922) and Boas' (1917) theories of social behaviour with more traditional sociolinguistic ones, dialectal variation was analysed in relation to the social matrix in which the linguistic patterns detected were embedded. Thus, an insider perspective as well as an outsider one have been adopted in order to interpret the linguistic behaviour of the community members better (Duranti 1997). Developing an emic/insider perspective has helped interpret the participants' linguistic behaviour in light of the social context in which it occurred. Yet, keeping one foot outside of the goings-on of the community has been crucial in order to capture its social structure. The fact that I am Italian has facilitated my task because the respondents did not feel the need to be careful about expressing their views about IndE accents – which is a fairly delicate matter for the community. Being a *quasi*-outsider has proved very helpful since I was not considered biased in any possible way. This led many respondents to make every effort to explain their points of view about accents, which revealed interesting folk comments and a large amount of linguistic sophistication (cf. Section 5.2).

While accessing the community, it was fundamental to be mindful of the cultural and social sensitivities of the group because the way the informants related to me and my social position might have influenced the linguistic data and the information that was provided, hence, the direction of the research (Duranti 1997). Talking about accent variation in the Indian subcontinent is a delicate matter in the community, especially in relation to ethnicity. For this reason, it was originally planned not to tell the participants that the research interest was in their ideas about different accents, but rather about Indian languages, English, and their usage in India and in the host country. Part of the rationale for originally concealing the topic arose from the hope that the respondents would be interested enough in language to discuss it naturally. Fortunately, often no more than a small lead was required to elicit such talk. In order not to dominate the discussion, lengthy stories and authority-status had to be avoided so that the respondents would not conclude that nothing more needed to be said (Niedzielski/Preston 2003). Hence, it has been crucial to constantly reshape the position in the community according to different contextual domains. To borrow Duranti's (1997) terminology, three roles had to be assumed during the fieldwork: that of a researcher, that of the community in question and that of the researcher's disciplinary tradition.

---

kHz is the standard sampling rate. The use of higher sampling rates maximises the range of future uses for recordings. For further details cf. Podesva/Zsiga (2013:169–94).

'Ethnographic grounding' has also been considered during the data collection. Asking the respondents for explanations and interpretations of their own comments about dialect and accent variation has proved a crucial practice for folk scrutiny. The positioning as a 'trusted other' allowed the informants to feel comfortable when revealing beliefs and attitudes which might not always have put them (or the ethnicities they represented) in the best light. In other words, the aim of the ethnographic observations was to attempt to create the situation Milroy (1987:69) describes concerning Labov's Philadelphia neighbourhood studies:

> [t]he intention here was to allow the interviewer to simulate a conversation and over a period move towards a more symmetrical interactive relationship so that the interviewing style came to resemble participant observation.[63]

The present observations of social events are focused on Richards' (2003) four components of interaction: (i) the physical setting of events, (ii) the systems and procedures that are followed, (iii) the people who take part, and (iv) the practices (language included) that are observed. Paying attention to such components allowed the identification of those systematic patterns of behaviour which were socially meaningful within the community. Hence, a mixture of both 'formal' events, i.e., meetings, work activities and more informal ones, i.e., lunch breaks, coffees among friends, bumping into people in the street were attended in order to cover as much as possible all the domains relevant for the community.

Ethnography adopts a more inductive, data-driven, bottom-up approach in which relevant social and linguistic phenomena emerge over the course of participant observation. According to Blommaert and Jie (2010:12): "this is what makes ethnography a demanding approach: it is not enough (not by a very long shot) to follow a clear, pre-set line of inquiry and the researcher cannot come thundering in with pre-established truths". The initial approach to the student community was through friends, and later on, through friend-to-friend recommendations and the WhatsApp HISA group. However, the primary privileged informants did not take part in the study in order to reduce to a minimum any bias in the data.

---

63 'Participant observation' is the primary data collection method of ethnographic research. In participant observation, the twofold goal is to become an active member of the goings-on of a community as well as to observe those activities as they unfold. In sociolinguistics, the tradition to use participant observation stems from the works of John Gumperz (1971) and Dell Hymes (1974), the latter proposing the term 'ethnography of communication' to describe that a community's speech and writing are an "aspect of culture worth of study" (Johnstone 2000:84).

The aim of the fieldwork observations was to create a relaxed and 'natural' atmosphere to make the respondents feel at ease. Thus, they were asked to suggest the location for their interviews, which usually took place in their homes, the university library or university cafés in and around Heidelberg. The male participants usually preferred public spaces, while the female ones suggested either their working places or their households as the research setting.

Several problems are likely to occur during fieldwork. They generally include finding and approaching informants, problems with tape-recordings, etc. (Duranti 1999). While the recording equipment was tested umpteen times prior to the recording sessions, fieldwork in the community posed problems concerning finding female informants. High rates of refusals were registered from the female part of the community, the reason being that they were busy or simply not interested in providing information on such matters. In order to overcome the problem, the network approach had to be started afresh several times (cf. Section 4.1.2).

Because ethnography is a 'thick description' (Geertz 1973) of different activities and events, keeping detailed field notes was an important part of the research process, especially at the early stages. During this time, they were written down on a very regular basis and proved to be very helpful in the progression from confusion to understanding. Field notes have been structured according to a template developed by Sakel and Everett (2012), which provides a list of metadata to be collected for language elicitation tasks:

1. type of event observed (formal/informal);
2. date and time
3. community members involved and their degree of participation;
4. location;
5. languages used;
6. notable linguistic characteristics;
7. notable social characteristics.

The final type of data collected in the field was a record of artefacts of the community's cultural life. Artefacts are "the physical materials, images, broadcasts, and other media products that are relevant to your informants' lives [...] It could also include the cars they drive and the food they eat" (Levon 2013:211). For instance, being invited to many informal dinners, the choice of the food usually reflected the informants' ethnic identities rather than their more general pan-Indian one. Interestingly, these artefacts produced a more comprehensive picture of the social life of the community, including ideologies related to the community itself, and led to interpretations of observed linguistic practice.

Understanding when it was the right time to leave the field was not an easy task. However, several researchers talk about a saturation point, which marks the moment when they no longer seem to be collecting any new information. In the words of the anthropologist Don Kulick, the moment of leaving the field comes when the researcher knows "[...] what your informants will say before you ask them the question" (cited in Levon 2013:212). In spite of initial skepticism that there would ever be enough data to reach such a moment, it eventually came when, during the last four or five interviews, Don Kulick's words sounded like a fulfilled prophecy. However, as was the case with the pre-investigation study, leaving the field did not mean that the ethnography was complete due to the continuous changes and developments of observations' interpretations at later stages of the research.

4.4 Data Preparation

The data collected with the aforementioned methods were analysed following the principles of quantitative and qualitative approaches. As discussed in Section 4.1.1, the present study uses both methods in what has been referred to as the 'convergent parallel design' (Creswell/Plano Clark 2011). Data from the accent and identity survey (cf. Section 4.2.2) and the interviews (cf. Section 4.2.5) were computed qualitatively, while those from the language background and language use survey (cf. Section 4.2.1), the cognitive maps (cf. Section 4.2.3), the accent recognition task (cf. Section 4.2.4) and the recorded reading passage (cf. Section 4.2.6) required advanced statistical testing. The quantitative strand received the foremost emphasis, and the results were followed up by a qualitative analysis phase.

4.4.1 Numerical Data: Statistical Testing

Unlike in the qualitative analysis, in the quantitative one data are analysed statistically. Quantitative analysis allows researchers to discover which phenomena are likely to be genuine reflections of people's behaviour in a language or a variety and which are merely chance occurrences. However, the picture which emerges from the latter type of analysis is less rich than that obtained from the former since it tends to sideline rare occurrences and, in some cases, to 'idealise' the data. For statistical purposes classifications have to be of the so-called 'Aristotelian type', i.e., an item either belongs to a given class or it does not. In order to ensure that certain statistical tests provide reliable results, it is essential that minimum frequencies are obtained, i.e., categories may have to be collapsed, resulting in a loss of data richness. While data richness can be regained and displayed with a more qualitative strand, it is important to note that the strengths of statistical testing methods lie in the concrete possibility of being able to draw conclusions about the population from which the sample was drawn (Johnson 2013). The display of numbers and frequencies is called 'descriptive statistics'; it includes numerical summaries (i.e., mean, median, standard deviation) and visual representations of the data (i.e., histograms, bar charts, scatterplots, cross-tabulations, etc.). Descriptive statistical methods describe samples of data but do not attempt to answer questions (make inferences) about the population from which the samples are drawn. This is what 'inferential statistics' does. Inferential statistical methods can make inferences or predictions about the sample data and establish the probabilities according to which observed relations in the data occur in the population from which the samples are drawn. This is crucial for the testing of hypotheses (Baayen 2013; Gries 2013).

Several problems have to be clarified before any analysis can be started. Statistical computer packages like SPSS or R facilitate the use of statistical tests even without advanced knowledge of probability procedures. However, "[t]his is a dangerous procedure [...] because the requirements of statistical tests are ignored, tests are applied wrongly and interpretations are incorrect" (Zwickl 2002:45). In order to circumvent the problem, statistical guidance was asked for before any statistical tests were done.

A further problem, which is connected with the sampling method and the sample size (cf. Section 4.1.2), concerns the 'normal distribution'.[64] Normal distribution is a prerequisite for a number of statistical tests; it is defined by two parameters, the mean and the standard deviation. It is visually described in a bell-shaped curve diagram in which the resulting scores cluster around a midpoint and the numbers decrease symmetrically on both sides (Johnson 2013:290–5). Normal distribution requires at least 30 informants per variable and does not allow for many extreme scores (Hatch/Lazaraton 1991:164–7). Thus, the sampling methods and the sample size selected for the present study are sufficient to measure the normal distribution of each independent and dependent variable.

64 After setting the types of variables under investigation, one of the first things to do is to examine their distribution. A distribution refers to the frequencies of the values of the variables. Sometimes, the distribution is expected to fit a particular shape, called 'normal' or 'Gaussian distribution'. For a more comprehensive account cf. Johnson (2013).

A further point, which is often ignored in social, psychological and sociolinguistic studies is linearity, which requires interval scale data that are problematic to retrieve and analyse if abstract concepts such as 'attitudes' and 'identity' are to be measured (Zwickl 2002). In order to overcome the problem, the use of 'nominal-' or 'ordinal-scale' variables is preferred in sociolinguistic studies. A nominal (also referred to as categorical) scale variable classifies the data according to categories that have no arithmetic value and are mutually exclusive (e.g., binary variables answering with 'yes' or 'no'). On the other hand, an ordinal variable is one where what matters is the order, but not the difference between the values (e.g., Likert scales, cf. Hatch/Lazaraton 1991:54–9; Johnson 2013:289–90). The present study measures both categorical-scale and ordinal-scale variables. While the former are retrieved from the language background and language use survey (cf. Section 4.2.1) as well as from the accent and identity survey (cf. Section 4.2.2), the latter result from the language background and language use survey (cf. Section 4.2.1) and the accent recognition task (cf. Section 4.2.4).

The issues discussed above influence the kind of tests to be chosen for data analysis (cf. Section 4.4.1.2).

4.4.1.1 Descriptive Statistics

Descriptive statistical methods distill the complexities of the data down to a small and manageable set of numbers in order to describe their basic overall properties. This generally constitutes the second step in quantitative analysis, the first one being the display of the data in a tabular or graphical format (Johnson 2013). Descriptive statistical analysis most commonly entails the measure of central tendency, i.e., the 'best estimate' of the value of a given variable. Different definitions of 'best estimate' result in different measures such as the mean, the median and the mode. Calculating the central tendency is nearly always an essential step in data analysis since it is the principal number that gets reported for a distribution or comparison between groups. The most common measure of central tendency in statistical analysis is the mean, which gives an arithmetic average to all scores. It can only be used for equal-interval-scaled variables; it is sensitive to extreme scores, and it assumes an infinite scale. The calculation of the mean (and the subsequent comparison of means) is described as the "powerhouse" (Johnson 2013:295) of parametric and descriptive statistics.

When the values of a variable are ordered from smallest to largest, the median is the centre of the distribution. It differs from the mean in that it is less sensitive to outliers, i.e., unusually small or large values, and it is suitable for rank-ordered data with a finite number of answers. In addition, when the distribution is skewed, the mean can be misleading. In the present study, both measures of central tendency have been used. Even if the median is more appropriate than the mean for most of the tests, the latter is sometimes displayed for the sake of clarity (Johnson 2013).

The third measure of central tendency is the mode, i.e., the most frequently obtained score in a distribution. However, the mode can distort the data if frequencies are evenly distributed. In such cases, the median is preferred.

While the measure of central tendency describes the average, the central or the most typical value of a variable, the measure of dispersion discloses more information about the extent to which the values vary on either side of the central tendency and how the scores are distributed around the mean. By far the most commonly used measure of dispersion is the standard deviation (s.d.), a quantity derived from the variance.[65] A small standard deviation index means that the scores cluster closely around the mean, indicating a fairly homogeneous answering pattern (Johnson 2013).

There are two situations when descriptive statistics analysis can be sufficient: (i) the dataset is purely 'exploratory', i.e., the research is designed to raise questions rather than answering them. In this case, descriptive statistics can suggest some hypotheses to test, and (ii) the sample data are not gathered from a larger population and the researcher does not plan to compare it to another population.

However, there are some cases, such as the present one, in which the research focus is on intra-population subgroups. When diverse subgroups (cf. in the present data: North Indians and South Indians; males and females, etc.) differ according to some descriptive statistics, not only might the researcher be interested in estimating the size of the effect, i.e., the difference between groups, but also in seeing whether it is a replicable and thus significant effect (cf. Section 4.4.1.2).

4.4.1.2 Inferential Statistics

There are two types of variables in inferential statistics: independent and dependent ones. The dependent variable is the one under analysis, i.e., the one in which the researcher is interested (in the present study: accent and dialect variation; metalinguistic awareness). Independent variables are the ones assumed to influence the dependent one (cf. Section 4.4.1). The relationship between the two is

65 Johnson (2013:299) describes the variance as "[...] the sum of the squared distances between each data point and the mean, divided by the number of observations, N".

the main point of interest in quantitative analysis, and their definitions depend entirely on the formulation of the research questions (cf. Section 4.1.3).

Inferential statistics is used to quantify and study data variability and to test hypotheses as well as separate random and accidental variation from meaningful and systematic one. The notion of hypothesis plays a central role. To borrow Gries's (2013: 316–7) definition:

> [an] hypothesis is a statement that makes a prediction about the distribution of one variable (or about the relation between two or more variables) in a population and that has the implicit structure of a conditional sentence (*if…, then…* or *the more/less…, the more/less…*) (emphasis in the original).

Inferential statistics is used to test the alternative hypothesis (H_1) and the null hypothesis (H_0). While the alternative hypothesis claims that there is a relationship in the data, the null hypothesis negates the former, stating that there are no differences between subgroups of the sample (Hatch/Lazaraton 1991). The ultimate goal of inferential statistics is to reject the null hypothesis and to show (i) that there are significant differences between social groups and (ii) that the independent social variables influence the dependent one(s).

The significance value shows the probability with which to reject H_0 and informs the researcher about the extent to which any particular outcome has been obtained by chance. The traditional practice in most applied linguistic research is not to reject H_0 unless there are fewer than five chances in 100 (probability level $p < 0.05$). However, the current research trend is to mark the level of significance at < 0.01 and < 0.001 (Gries 2013). In the present study, all three levels of significance will be applied.

Significance tests examine whether the observed connection between variables can point to a connection in the population from which the sample was drawn. It is worth mentioning that in case some findings do not prove to be statistically significant, it is still possible to show particular trends in the data and argue for a new hypothesis to be established. If the focus is only on significance, important trends might be lost. In the present study, tendencies in the data will also be reported, particularly for the main independent variables: *gender*, *ethnicity* and *time spent in Heidelberg*.

The decision in favour of specific statistical tests is typically made on the basis of the research aims, the scale of the tested variables, and the size and distribution of the involved datasets (Gries 2013:319–23).

The 'chi-square' test is a non-parametric hypothesis-testing method. It tests the significance of the deviation of observed frequencies from expected ones, i.e., whether the variables tested are distributed as expected from a particular probability distribution. In other words, it tests whether the variables are interrelated. One of the assumptions of the chi-square test is that the sample has to be large enough to obtain an expected cell frequency of five (Gries 2013; Hatch/Lazaraton 1991).[66]

To test whether the averages of a dependent variable in two groups defined by the independent variables differ significantly, 't-tests' are frequently applied in linguistic studies (Fuchs 2016). Specifically, this is the case when the data in question involve a normally distributed ratio/interval-scaled dependent variable and a binary independent one. T-tests compare intra-group variation with inter-group variation, based on a comparison of means. If the grouping variable is expected to be influential, the variation between the two groups should be significantly larger than the variation within the groups. Similar to t-tests, but expanded to more than two social groups, ANOVA (analysis of variance) tests are parametric tests used to analyse the differences among group means in a data sample.

The present study uses all the above-mentioned tests in order to capture the different structural patterns of the variables.

4.4.1.3 Correlation

While significance tests examine whether there is a relationship between an independent variable and a dependent one, correlation methods test the strength of the relationship between variables. The accurate assessment of an association of this type can be complex, especially when there are many variables to be analysed and controlled simultaneously (cf. section below). However, as long as an association is linear, it can be measured with a statistic called the 'Pearson correlation'. It is defined as "the *covariance* of the two variables divided by the product of their standard deviations" (Johnson 2013:305; emphasis in the original). Here, the strength of a relationship is expressed via the correlation coefficient, symbolised by r, and always ranged between -1 and +1. A value near -1 means that all the points fall exactly on a downward-sloping line and denotes a strong negative correlation, whereas one near +1 denotes a strong positive one.

If the datasets deviate from normality and there is a nonlinear relation between the variables, it is better to use a non-parametric measure of correlation

66 In cases in which some cells have frequencies below five, it is suggested to compute the 'Fisher's exact test'. One of the reasons why this test is sometimes preferred to a chi-square one is because of the possibility to calculate exactly the significance of the deviation from a null hypothesis rather than relying on approximations (Gries 2013).

such as the 'Spearman's rho' or 'Kendall's tau'. Spearman's rho is calculated using the same methods as *r*, but the data are transformed into ranks first. In this way, continuous data are converted to an ordinal scale. While this makes the method less powerful (because more data are often required in order to observe an effect), it also makes it more robust against outliers. Pearson's *r* quantifies the linearity of a relationship; Spearman's rho assesses its monotonicity. As Johnson (2013:306) puts it:

> [i]n a monotonic relationship, as one variable increases, the other constantly increases or decreases (but not both). If both variables consistently move in the same direction, we have rho=1, and if they consistently move in opposite directions, rho = -1.

Similar to Spearman's rho, Kendall's tau is another non-parametric rank correlation coefficient used to measure the ordinal association between two measured quantities. Its correlation between two variables will be high when observations have a similar (1) rank between the two variables, low when they have a dissimilar (-1) rank between the two variables (Johnson 2013). According to Zwickl (2002:50):

> [c]orrelational methods were once considered crucial in sociolinguistic studies because they were thought to show the strength of the relationship between linguistic variation as the dependent variable and social group membership as the independent (extralinguistic) variable.

A strong correlation was likely to be interpreted as the result of an influence of the independent variable on the dependent one. However, correlation analysis alone is not a good method to support causal relationships. It has to be corroborated by more suitable testing methods because a correlation between two variables might also be influenced by a third (unknown) one, and thus no direct influence between the two might exist (Johnson 2013).

4.4.1.4 Multivariate Statistics

The statistical methods described above are appropriate only for the description of the interrelation between two variables. However, many linguistic phenomena cannot be understood properly unless a great many *explananda* are considered jointly. Especially in light of a complex society and expected interrelations between different social factors (as in the case of the present study), the need for multivariate methods becomes apparent. Multivariate analysis deals with observations made on many variables simultaneously and, in contrast to hypothesis-testing procedures, it is a model-building process (Baayen 2013).

Multivariate datasets fall into two main classes. On the one hand, there are datasets according to which all variables are equally important. Here, the primary research interest lies in the causal relations between the variables (cf. section above) or in the way in which the variables pattern. On the other hand, interest may focus on how a specific dependent variable (defined as the 'response') is predicted from the other independent variables (defined as the 'predictors').

One multivariate method, i.e., 'cluster analysis', is used in the present study. Cluster analysis (also called 'clustering') is designed to detect underlying structures in the data and is described as a structure-developing procedure. For this method, it is not necessary to separate the dependent variable from the independent ones.[67] It is the task of grouping a set of objects in such a manner that objects in the same group (or cluster) are more similar to each other than to those in other groups/clusters. This multivariate method establishes clusters in the data on the basis of distances between the variables.[68] It is a procedure similar to 'factor analysis', which tends to be applied more frequently.[69] The appropriate clustering algorithm and parameter settings depend on the individual dataset and the intended use of the results. Before applying a clustering technique, the researcher has to decide via logical considerations which objects and variables are relevant for the grouping. However, cluster analysis is an iterative process of knowledge discovery or 'interactive multi-objective optimisation' that involves trial and failure. Thus, it is often necessary to modify data pre-processing and model parameters until the result achieves the desired properties. Clustering techniques work in a hierarchical order, i.e., in each step the two closest findings are combined in one cluster (Zwickl 2002).

In the present study, 'bubble-matrix charts' are used to visualise graphically the different clusterings in order to correlate simultaneously multiple variables

67 As in the case of 'regression analysis', model-building is an iterative process that tests which is the model that best predicts the outcome of the dependent variable. Regression specifies how the observed values of the response can be approximated precisely given the values of the predictors. In other words, it helps to discover and support claims on the probability with which certain independent variables affect a dependent one. Cf. Baayen (2013:339–63) for further details.

68 The measure of distance used most commonly is 'Euclidian distance' (Zwickl 2002:52).

69 'Factor analysis' is a statistical method used to describe variability among variables in terms of a potentially lower number of unobserved components called factors. Its basic purpose is to reduce a larger set of variables to a smaller set of components by identifying correlations among variables and isolating the components associated with those correlations. Cf. Walker (2013:454–5) for further details.

with the obtained clustering results. Bubble matrices are useful to represent the data in two dimensions, each variable (e.g., *ethnicity*) being able to have two specific traits (e.g., North Indian, South Indian) represented by size and colour (cf. Sections 5.1.2.2 and 5.1.3.6).

4.4.2 Qualitative Data: Bottom-up vs. Top-down Approaches

The way in which written and spoken texts are processed (thus understood and analysed) is often described in terms of 'top-down' or 'bottom-up' processing. A top-down approach (also known as 'stepwise design') entails the breaking down of a system to gain insight into its compositional subsystems. Starting from 'higher-level' features (e.g., context, background knowledge, overall meaning), the system is reduced into smaller segments and proceeds through a series of steps 'down' to 'lower-level' features (e.g., semantics, syntax, phonology). This deductive approach contrasts with bottom-up processing where there is a progression from the individual elements to the whole. In other words, a bottom-up (inductive) approach equals the piecing together of a system to give rise to more complex systems, thus making the original systems subsystems of the emergent supersystem. Bottom-up processing is based on incoming data from the environment to form a perception (Hesse-Biber/Leavy 2006).

The present study employs both approaches depending on the 'nature' of the data in question. The qualitative data were prepared and analysed through the application of a revised form of the qualitative content analysis developed by Mayring (2014). This three-step procedure traditionally entails (i) transcript condensation, (ii) eventual consultation of additional material to account for unclear texts, and (iii) structuring of the condensed transcripts according to the aims of the study. However, requoting Blommaert and Jie (2010:12): "[...] it is not enough to follow a clear, pre-set line of inquiry and the researcher cannot come thundering in with pre-established truths". For this reason, the first and the last steps were excluded from the analysis for their top-down data processing and were substituted with the writing of analytical memos (Hesse-Biber/Leavy 2006).

In order to structure and organise the data better, the qualitative data analysis software MAXQDA (version 2018.2) was used. The process of coding ethnographic data is similar to the one used for coding quantitative data (cf. Section 4.4.1), and essentially entails assigning 'codes' or categories to small chunks of data (e.g., portions of transcripts, or of interviews) to allow for further comparison (cf. Section 5.2).

The independent variables (*gender*, *ethnicity* and *time spent in Heidelberg*) were coded following the model of stepwise analysis. Data from the accent and identity survey (cf. Section 4.2.2) and the interviews (cf. Section 4.2.5) were transcribed and coded following a bottom-up approach in order to let the data 'speak for themselves'. Considering the large amount of data collected, the help of few consultants from within the community was crucial throughout the reviewing process since they proved to be invaluable analytic resources, especially in the translation of multilingual instances.

5 Results and Discussion

The results will be presented and discussed in two subchapters (5.1 and 5.2). The first one corresponds to three parts of the questionnaire: language background and language use (cf. Section 4.2.1), the cognitive map task (cf. Section 4.2.3) and the accent recognition test (cf. Section 4.2.4). 5.2 considers the correlation between attitudes and accent variation and corresponds to two parts of the survey: accent and identity (cf. Section 4.2.2) and the qualitative interviews (cf. Section 4.2.5).

5.1 Quantitative Analysis

5.1.1 Characteristics of the Data

5.1.1.1 Extralinguistic Variables

Most of the extralinguistic variables used to categorise the participants and to test the parameters influencing different behavioural components correspond to variables used in other attitudinal studies (Beinhoff 2013; Löw-Wiebach 2005; Zwickl 2002).

A major problem emerging in the testing of the effects of extralinguistic variables is the design of questionnaires since the relevant extralinguistic variables have to be determined beforehand in order not to miss important information (Smit 1996). Although the problem cannot be solved entirely, a pre-study might be helpful in the selection of extralinguistic variables. Accordingly, the main objective of the pre-study for the present work was to obtain information on the community as a whole and on the sociolinguistic practices of its members. Both the administered survey and the sociolinguistic interviews provided a great deal of information on useful extralinguistic variables (Regnoli 2016).

On the basis of the main research questions introduced in Section 4.1.3, the primary extralinguistic variables are *ethnicity*, *gender* and *time spent in Heidelberg*. However, other extralinguistic variables are also deemed important for the context at issue: *medium of instruction*, *type of school*, *faculty* and *occupation*.[70] Although in the design of most studies extralinguistic variables usually include up to five

70 *Age* was not considered a crucial extralinguistic variable since the community includes only students in their twenties. However, 31 informants are between 20 and 25 years old and 29 between 25 and 30.

variants (or levels), all variables adopted in the present work consist of two variants since it is important to have a conspicuous number of informants in each subgroup for statistical analysis (cf. Section 4.4.1). *Medium of instruction*, *type of school*, *faculty* and *occupation* are objective variables and straightforward to classify. Of the 60 informants, with the exception of two who had attended vernacular-medium schools and one who had attended both vernacular- and English-medium schools in India, 57 had completed their education in English-medium ones. Among them, 39 had attended private schools, 5 public schools and 16 both. Moreover, at the time of the fieldwork, of all interviewees, 49 were Science students, 11 were majoring in the humanities; 39 were master's students, 21 were Ph.D. candidates.

Tab. 5.1.1. Variables gender, ethnicity and time spent in Heidelberg

No	Gender	N	%
I	Male	30	50
II	Female	30	50
Total		60	100

No	Ethnicity	N	%
I	North	34	57
II	South	26	43
Total		60	100

No	Time spent in Heidelberg	N	%
I	1 month -1 year	39	65
II	1.1 year – 5 years	21	35
Total		60	100

Gender is the only variable which was controlled in order to both guarantee balance in the data and to portray the homogeneity of the student community (cf. Section 3.2.1). In consequence, 30 men and 30 women were interviewed (cf. Tab. 5.1.1)

Time spent in Heidelberg is an objective variable as well; altogether, 39 informants (65 % of the sample) have been living in Heidelberg for up to one year and 21 (35 %) between 1 to 5 years. Overall, the grouping follows both the age groups of the informants and their occupational status. Those who have been living in Heidelberg for up to one year are generally master's students between 20 and 25 years of age, and the second group mainly consists of Ph.D. students between 25 and 30 years old. Moreover, in the present study, one of the main focal points has been the transient aspect of the Indian community. Being a newcomer in the community may imply different perceptions of accent variation. Depending on the students' personal experiences and network allegiances back home, their degree of knowledge and awareness of Indian English accents may differ considerably. Likewise, a more experienced member of the community is expected to have a higher degree of awareness of language perception and production based on network allegiances and kinship within the community. A communal factor, however, is the degree of internationalisation they had been exposed to during their school years in India. Attendance to convent schools, international schools or government ones is a crucial aspect in the degree of overt accent consciousness, hence a close look at the interrelation between accent identification, *time spent in Heidelberg*, *medium of instruction* and *type of school* might shed new light on the informants' levels of metalinguistic awareness in second language acquisition (cf. Section 5.1.3.3.).

Ethnicity has been classified according to the participants' self-identification. Although they differentiate between speakers' origins and accents quite meticulously in the accent identification task (cf. Section 5.1.3.2) and the cognitive map one (cf. Section 5.1.3.7), they generally divide themselves into Southern and Northern Indians. The initial aim was to cluster speakers according to their states of origin. However, this was not feasible. While many states are overrepresented (Maharashtra, Karnataka), others are not represented at all (Jammu and Kashmir, Himachal Pradesh, Jharkhand, Chhattisgarh, Orissa, as well as the seven sister states – except for Manipur), and states like Punjab, Haryana, Rajasthan and Manipur are represented by one speaker only. Hence, in light of the general aims of the present study, i.e., investigating speakers' metalinguistic awareness regarding accent variation, and in order to have enough individuals in each subgroup for statistical analysis, it was preferred to follow the participants' self-identification. Altogether, 34 informants (57 % of the sample) are from Northern India and 26 (43 %) from Southern India (cf. Tab. 5.1.1).

Extralinguistic variables such as *occupational status of parents*, *religion*, *caste* and *level of German* are not treated as independent variables since they do not provide any meaningful insight into perceived accent variation although the initial aim was to include them as well. However, they help sketch a broader picture of the Indian student community as a whole and are thus treated as potential factors contributing to the structuring of the community. Following Trudgill's (1974:32) contention that "social class stratification is primarily based on differences in wealth and income" and that occupation is the main indicator of social class since it is correlated with education and income, the grouping of *occupational status of parents* sheds light on the participants' family backgrounds and contributes to an index-score of the socioeconomic status of the participants. The grouping of the occupational status of the students' parents is based on the general sociological ranking employed in linguistics (Chambers 2009) and, particularly, on Trudgill's (1974) five-component index used for his Norwich subjects (cf. Tab. 5.1.2). Retired parents are classified according to their former occupation. However, variants such as 'unskilled' have been adapted to and interpreted on the contextual framework of India: housewives are included in this category although they are not necessarily unskilled. Students are grouped according to their fathers' and mothers' occupations, and when the mother is a housewife, they are solely counted on their fathers' occupations.[71]

Tab. 5.1.2. Variable occupational status of parents

Level	Father position	N	%
I	Professional Workers	9	15
II	Employers, Managers	14	23
III	Foremen, skilled, self-emp.	33	55
IV	Semi-skilled, agricultural	4	7
V	Unskilled	0	0
Total		60	100

Level	Mother position	N	%
I	Professional Workers	6	10
II	Employers, Managers	5	8
III	Foremen, skilled, self-emp.	12	20
IV	Semi-skilled, agricultural	0	0
V	Unskilled	37	62
Total		60	100

Although *religion* and *caste* have already been discussed (cf. Section 3.2.3), it is important to mention that several Hindu respondents did not mention their caste or indicated that they did not know their caste identity. However, it could sometimes be easily inferred from external factors such as the surnames of the participants. Catholic informants were among the few who talked spontaneously about their religious upbringing and were therefore included in the respective group.

71 It is important to note that in India just 27 % of women participate in the work force (ILOSTAT 2019).

One of the variables used to measure the participants' integration into the Heidelberg sociocultural environment has been their *level of German*. While few had taken German courses in their mother country before moving to Heidelberg, the majority have attended courses *in situ*, benefiting from local institutions, the Heidelberg University's *Sprachlabor* or from some general e-learning platforms. Their willingness to learn the language principally derives from their desire to get better internships and/or employment soon after graduation. However, since 65 % of the community is constituted by newcomers, it is no surprise that 79 % have a beginner/elementary level of German (cf. Tab. 5.1.3).

Tab. 5.1.3 Variable level of German[a]

No	Level of German	N	%
I	A1	34	57
II	A2	13	22
III	B1	9	15
IV	B2	4	7
Total		60	101

a Rounding adjustments may, in some cases, lead to total percentages above and below 100 %.

The possible interdependency of some variables is problematic for the analysis of the main extralinguistic variables. Results may be distorted if interdependencies are not tested and discussed. The variables in the present study have tested for their interrelationship by applying a chi-square test.[72] *Ethnicity* and *gender* are not interrelated or related to any of the other variables. *Time spent in Heidelberg* and *level of German* are interrelated in so far as the less time participants have spent in Heidelberg, the lower their level of German (cf. Tab. 5.1.4).

Tab. 5.1.4 Interrelation of the variables time spent in Heidelberg and level of German (chi square p = 0.015*)

	0.1–1	**1.1–5**
Beginner (A1/A2)	53 %	25 %
Intermediate (B1/B2)	7 %	15 %

72 Chi-square tests the association between two categorical variables. The null hypothesis asserts the interdependence of the variables under consideration. If differences are statistically significant, the frequencies are not distributed by chance. For a more detailed account cf. Section 4.4.1.2.

Apart from categorical extralinguistic variables, factors such as willingness to learn the language of the host country and use of English in the university environment have to be included as possible influences on sociolinguistic behaviour. Particularly in the context of the present study in which English serves as a *lingua franca*, these factors may shed light on network integration within and outside the Indian student community.

5.1.1.2 The Use of English in the Heidelberg University Environment

The context under investigation is very interesting with respect to the community focus of the present work. Traditionally, Heidelberg is a non-anglophone setting, hence English does not hold any official status. However, the prestigious university environment and its subsequent degree of internationalisation allows for the language to be the second *lingua franca* of the town. Many courses are taught entirely in English, hence admission does not require any proof of German skills (cf. Section 3.2).

This rather favourable situation contributes to the development of an overt consciousness of English accent variation among the Indian student community but, at the same time, it somehow prevents many community members from becoming proficient in German. As shown in Tab. 5.1.4, older members of the community have a better knowledge of German compared to their newly arrived counterparts. As a matter of fact, although the participants generally agree on the importance of acquiring at least a basic competence in German to be better integrated into the town environment, only few of them are resolved on improving their knowledge of the language. For this reason, the initial enthusiasm of newcomers to learn German and enrol in *Sprachlabor* courses gradually reduces when they reach a B1/B2 level. An intuitive explanation might be that the community is mobile, and their transiency does not necessarily increase their willingness to improve their language skills in German. It comes as no surprise that the informants who have been improving their German are the ones who plan to settle down in the host country for at least 10 or 15 years.

English is the language the community members use most frequently in Heidelberg. Figure 5.1.1 shows that the difference in percentages between the participants' usage of English and their mother tongue is massive. 83 % of the sample use English more often that their first language (15 %), which is however still widely used (78 %). Although L1 use in Heidelberg will be treated in connection with language background in Section 5.1.1.3, what is interesting here is that, on a daily basis, English is used much more frequently than the participants' first languages despite their strong network allegiances (cf. Section 5.1.1.4).

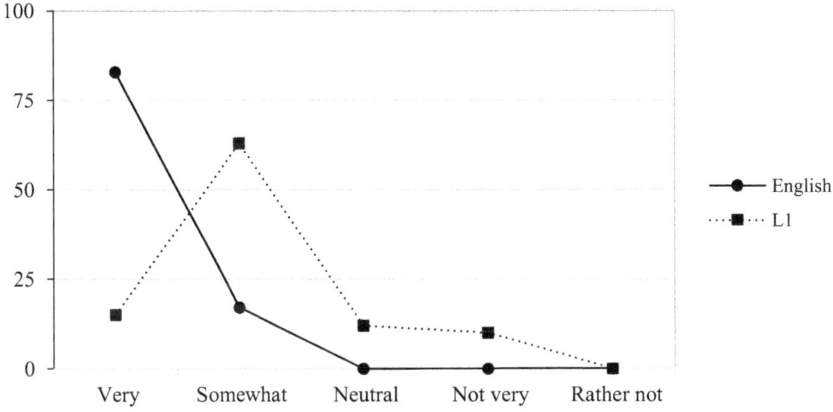

	Very		Somewhat		Neutral		Not very		Rather not		Total	
	N	%	N	%	N	%	N	%	N	%	N	%
English	50	83	10	17	0	0	0	0	0	0	60	100
L1	9	15	38	63	7	12	6	10	0	0	60	100

Fig. 5.1.1 Language use in Heidelberg (in %) *How often do you use your first language now? (I.1.5) How often do you speak English in Heidelberg? (I.3.1).* Rounding adjustments may, in some cases, lead to total percentages above and below 100 %.

These results are in line with those depicted in Fig. 5.1.2, which shows the different domains of language use in Heidelberg and the number of speakers using what language in what situation. 92 % of the sample claim that they frequently speak in English with their German friends and 100 % use English with international people in Heidelberg. Interestingly, the majority of the participants (53 %) prefer to use English with their peers, while 23 % of them are more comfortable talking in their mother tongue or Hindi, the additional *lingua franca* of the student community. In the university setting, 98 % of the informants use English as a means of communication and the same percentage discusses political and technical matters in the same language.

The linguistic scenario slightly changes when the setting shifts from the university setting to the participants' private lives. On a daily basis, 82 % of the sample claim that they use English to speak to office and bank employees. Again, the result was predictable and partially aligns with the former percentages regarding political and technical discussions because of the register and the styles involved. Moreover, 65 % of the informants are more comfortable asking strangers for information in English.

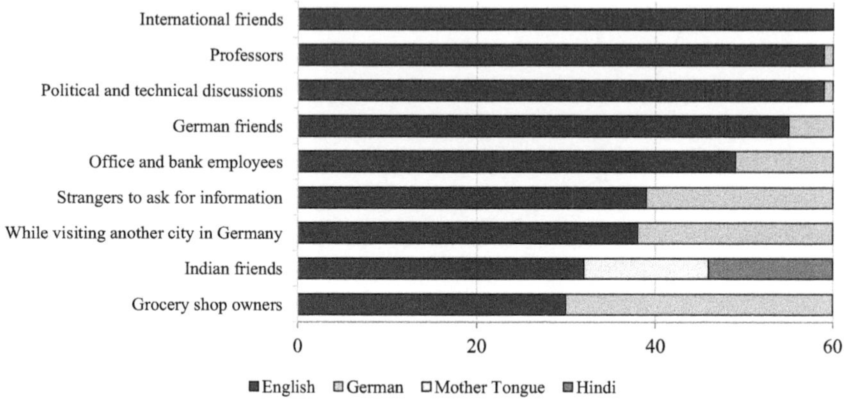

	English		German		Mother Tongue		Hindi		Total	
	N	%	N	%	N	%	N	%	N	%
International friends	60	100	0	0	0	0	0	0	60	100
Professors	59	98	1	2	0	0	0	0	60	100
Political and technical discussions	59	98	1	2	0	0	0	0	60	100
German friends	55	92	5	8	0	0	0	0	60	100
Office and bank employees	49	82	11	18	0	0	0	0	60	100
Strangers to ask for information	39	65	21	35	0	0	0	0	60	100
While visiting another city in Germany	38	63	22	37	0	0	0	0	60	100
Indian friends	32	53	0	0	14	23	14	23	60	100
Grocery shop owners	30	50	30	50	0	0	0	0	60	100

Fig. 5.1.2 Language use in Heidelberg (n = 60) *How do you usually interact in Heidelberg?* (I.3.2) (Kruskal-Wallis p = 0.00003****)

The percentage of community members using English decreases in their journeys outside Heidelberg (63 %) and in their interactions with grocery shop owners (50 %). Here, again, the results are consistent with the idea that the use of English in the university setting is inversely proportional to its use in the local setting.

The Kruskal-Wallis test has been applied to test whether English stochastically dominates German, Hindi and the speakers' mother tongues in everyday interactions in the community.[73] The results reveal significant differences between the subgroups (p = 0.00003****).

5.1.1.3 Language Background and Language Use in Heidelberg

In order to gain insight into the general interactions of the community members in Heidelberg in different domains, four questions are included in Survey I (cf. Section 4.2.1):

- *How often do you use your first language now? (I.1.5)*
- *Use of English in personal interactions (I.2.1)*
- *Use of English in reading general literature (I.2.11)*
- *Interactions with native English speakers (I.2.6)*

The participants generally agree on English being the language they are most likely to adopt on a daily basis (cf. Fig. 5.1.1). Figure 5.1.3 sheds light on their use of English in personal interactions on a five-point Likert scale. The data substantiate earlier findings according to which English is the language spoken most frequently in the university domain (cf. Fig. 5.1.2). 92 % of the sample always use the language in their interactions with professors and university staff, while 73 % are active solely in English on social media. With respect to friends and family, the percentage drop of English usage is massive: 2 % of the informants interact only in English with their family and 27 % with their friends. This finding confirms earlier claims according to which English is seldom used in more private spheres (cf. Fig. 5.1.2).

73 The Kruskal-Wallis test (also known as Kruskal–Wallis H test or one-way ANOVA on ranks) is a non-parametric method for independent measures that relies on the rank-ordering of data rather than calculations involving means and variances (such as the one-way ANOVA test) and allows for the evaluation of the differences between three or more independent samples (treatments). The null hypothesis is that the average orders between all groups are the same (Hatch/Lazaraton 1991:332–5).

The pattern for the use of English in interactions with friends is most distinctive since it shares a similar trend with that for the use of the participants' first language in Heidelberg (cf. Fig. 5.1.3). Together, they show a peak indicating that the informants have a fairly high average of contacts both in English and in their mother tongues, thus suggesting that they spend an almost equal amount of time interacting in both languages in Heidelberg. The somewhat strong use of their mother tongue is a clear example of language maintenance since the participants continue to use their L1s in many domains despite the competition with the two more dominant or majority languages used in Heidelberg (cf. Fig. 5.1.2). This shows their strong network allegiances with the local Indian student community (cf. Section 5.1.1.4) as well as their tight transnational ties with their mother country (cf. Section 5.2.2.3). However, whether they interact more with international people than with their peers is hard to tell since many of the informants prefer to speak English within their community as well (cf. Fig. 5.1.2).

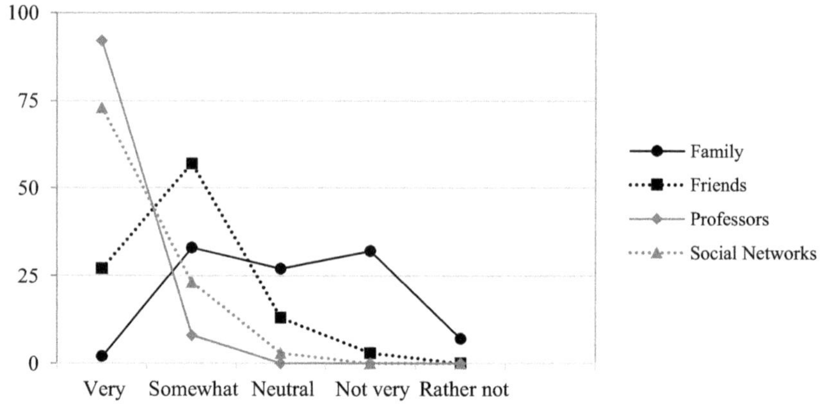

	Very		Somewhat		Neutral		Not very		Rather not		Total	
	N	%	N	%	N	%	N	%	N	%	N	%
Family	1	2	20	33	16	27	19	32	4	7	60	101
Friends	16	27	34	57	8	13	2	3	0	0	60	100
Professors	55	92	5	8	0	0	0	0	0	0	60	100
Social networks	44	73	14	23	2	3	0	0	0	0	60	99

Fig. 5.1.3 *Use of English in personal interactions* (in %) (I.2.1)

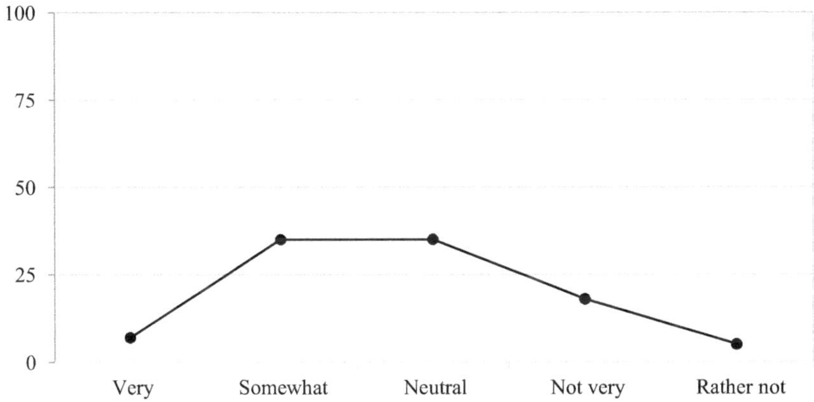

	Very		Somewhat		Neutral		Not very		Rather not		Total	
	N	%	N	%	N	%	N	%	N	%	N	%
L1 interactions	4	7	21	35	21	35	11	18	3	5	60	100

Fig. 5.1.4 *Interactions with native English speakers* (in %) (I.2.6)

While interactions with international people are an everyday matter for the community members, contacts with native speakers of English in Heidelberg are fairly sporadic, yet somewhat constant (cf. Fig. 5.1.4). 77 % of the sample interact regularly with L1 English speakers. However, only 7 % of all the informants have constant interactions with them. With the exception of SLfUP, a female speaker who had lived in Heidelberg for six months and who was enrolled at the Department of English of the University at the time of the fieldwork – hence, who was facilitated in meeting native speakers – the rest of the sample consists of male informants who have been living in Heidelberg long enough to meet with native speakers even outside the university environment. 23 % of the sample claim that they seldom have interactions with native English speakers. Interestingly, the majority of the participants are not questioning their affinity with the category of *native* speakers of English during the compilation of the questionnaires.

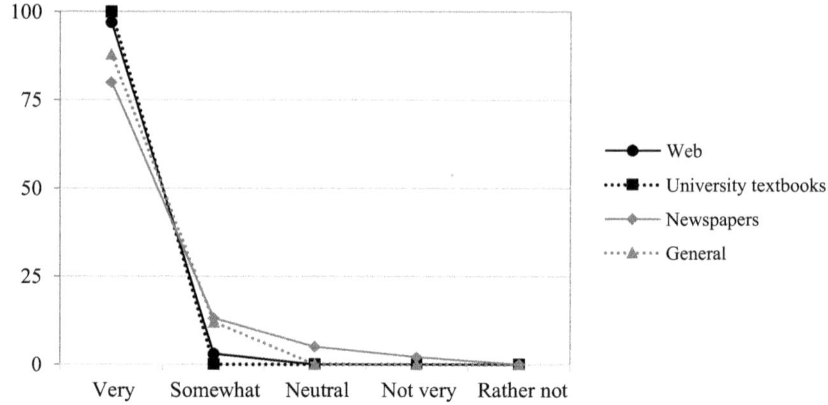

	Very		Somewhat		Neutral		Not very		Rather not		Total	
	N	%	N	%	N	%	N	%	N	%	N	%
Web	58	97	2	3	0	0	0	0	0	0	60	100
University textbooks	60	100	0	0	0	0	0	0	0	0	60	100
Newspapers	48	80	8	13	3	5	1	2	0	0	60	100
General	53	88	7	12	0	0	0	0	0	0	60	100

Fig. 5.1.5 *Use of English in reading general literature* (in %) (I.2.11)

The overt connection they are drawing between specific local language practices and more global assessments of nativeness reflects and fosters what Shuck (2004) postulates as 'the ideology of nativeness', which constructs the categories of 'native English' speaker as contiguous with British or Americans, and 'non-native' with foreigners (cf. Section 5.2.2.2).

Figure 5.1.5 shows that English is dominant in all domains surrounding the reading of general literature and substantiates earlier claims and earlier findings from the pilot study (Regnoli 2016). Interestingly, there are no significant differences among any of the subgroups of the extralinguistic variables selected. This indicates that the community is fairly homogeneous in its language practices despite gender, ethnicity and the amount of time spent in Heidelberg.

5.1.1.4 Network Bonds and Network Integration: Implicational Scaling

The effects of interpersonal relationships on language variation and language perception have long been investigated in sociolinguistics (Cheshire 1982; Gumperz 1982; Lippi-Green 1989; Milroy 1987). Sometimes, they have more impact on the language choices of the speakers than most categorical extralinguistic variables. Although consistent, categories such as ethnicity and gender "may relate indirectly to the procedures of participants in constructing and categorizing social worlds that reflect their analysis of locally meaningful social groupings" (Milroy/Gordon 2003: 116).

The present study aims to shed new light on the closely related concepts of social network and community of practice in relation to language variation and perception. Hence, in order to understand and grasp the specifics of those local practices which are sensitive for the Indian student community in question, it is important to delve into the locally contracted ties that the speakers construct in their everyday lives. At the time of the fieldwork, a network approach was considered suitable since it provides a set of procedures which enable a study of a small community where speakers cannot not be discriminated in terms of any kind of social class index (cf. Sections 4.1.2 and 3.2.2). Moreover, a network analysis offers the possibility to deal with variation between *individual* speakers rather than between groups, which is ideal for the ethnographic perspective of the study (cf. Section 4.3).

A major challenge has been to devise a procedure for characterising differences in the network structure of the community which are indexical of local social practices. A network-strength scale has been devised (maximum score, 4) according to four criteria which assess speakers' network characteristics with reference to those different relationships within their community of practice that have emerged during the fieldwork as significant to the participants. Informants score one point for each of the following conditions they satisfy:

- same faculty as at least two more Indian students;
- proximity to more than five Indian students;
- free time spent with other Indian students;
- regular participation in Indian associations in Germany, particularly in HISA.

Network density has been measured on a five-point Likert scale ranging from (0) highly unintegrated to (4) highly integrated. Network integration indices have then been compared with their rankings in a sociometric diagram. Table 5.1.5 shows the ranking of the 60 participants according to the four criteria mentioned and lists speakers' sociometric rankings in the rightmost column.

The four criteria, identified by the numbers in the sentence above, form an implicational scale such that a positive score for one criterion implies a positive one on all the criteria to its left (but not vice versa). The five discrepancies are indicated by parenthesising the offending coefficient in the scores of the following participants: VJRfKa, PGfMa, APmTN, DLfMan and KGfPu.

In order to assess the development of the set of data in question and to test the fit of the implicational scale, two calculations have been computed: the Guttman Coefficient of Reproducibility and the Rasch Scalability Coefficient. Data from both calculations result statistically significant, i.e., they show less than 10 % error cells (Guttman Reproducibility Coefficient = 0.97*; Rasch Scalability Coefficient = 0.75*).[74]

Network relationships in the community are relatively dense and multiplex. Following the principle of 'anchorage', which entails considering the network from the point of view of the individuals, it is possible to make some general claims about the informal relationships the community members are embedded in (Milroy 1980). Each person may be viewed as a focus from which lines radiate to points, i.e., the other people they are in contact with, in forming the so-called 'first-order network zone'. Intuitively, the more distantly connected people form a second, a third- or a fourth-order zone. According to Boissevain (1974), the first two order zones appear to be most important since individuals generally use second-order contacts to attain different goals: it is the 'friend of a friend' who helps attain such goals.

---

74 The coefficient of reproducibility measures the predictability of responses according to their position within the table. More specifically, Guttman Scales are ones in which the items constitute a unidimensional series such that an answer to a given item predicts the answers to all previous items in the series. The formula of the Coefficient of Reproducibility is 1– Errors/(Total Responses). By arbitrary convention, the coefficient of reproducibility should be higher than 0.9. The Rasch coefficient of scalability is defined as 1 minus the sum of the observed number of errors according to the Guttman scale model over the sum of the expected number of errors. The level of acceptance of the coefficient of scalability should be higher than 0.6. For a more detailed account of the measurements of categorical data and on data scalability cf. Hatch/Lazaraton (1991) and Jobling/Snell (1961).

Tab. 5.1.5 Network Strength Scale (n = 60) (Guttman Reproducibility Coefficient = 0.97*; Rasch Scalability Coefficient = 0.75*)

	1	2	3	4	Tot	Status	Ethnicity	Gender	Years in HD
SDfKa	+	+	+	+	4	highly integrated	s	f	0.1–1
JGMfKe	+	+	+	+	4	highly integrated	s	f	0.1–1
MMfKa	+	+	+	+	4	highly integrated	s	f	0.1–1
AHfKa	+	+	+	+	4	highly integrated	s	f	0.1–1
MGofUt	+	+	+	+	4	highly integrated	n	f	0.1–1
STfBi	+	+	+	+	4	highly integrated	n	f	0.1–1
DSfWB	+	+	+	+	4	highly integrated	n	f	0.1–1
SMfMa	+	+	+	+	4	highly integrated	n	f	0.1–1
AVmDe	+	+	+	+	4	highly integrated	n	m	0.1–1
SVmKa	+	+	+	+	4	highly integrated	s	m	0.1–1
VSmTN	+	+	+	+	4	highly integrated	s	m	0.1–1
MNmKa	+	+	+	+	4	highly integrated	s	m	0.1–1
PPmKa	+	+	+	+	4	highly integrated	s	m	0.1–1
ARmKe	+	+	+	+	4	highly integrated	s	m	1.1–5
SSmKe	+	+	+	+	4	highly integrated	s	m	1.1–5
BJmGu	+	+	+	+	4	highly integrated	n	m	1.1–5
ABmDe	+	+	+	+	4	highly integrated	n	m	1.1–5
ASmMP	+	+	+	+	4	highly integrated	n	m	1.1–5
BSmGu	+	+	+	+	4	highly integrated	n	m	1.1–5
URmRa	+	+	+	+	4	highly integrated	n	m	1.1–5
DTfUt	+	+	+	+	4	highly integrated	n	f	1.1–5
TKfMa	+	+	+	+	4	highly integrated	n	f	1.1–5
JGfMa	+	+	+	+	4	highly integrated	n	f	1.1–5
VJRfKa	(-)	+	+	+	3	integrated	s	f	1.1–5
PGfMa	+	(-)	+	+	3	integrated	n	f	0.1–1
APmTN	(-)	(-)	+	+	2	somewhat integrated	s	m	0.1–1
DLfMan	(-)	+	(-)	+	2	somewhat integrated	n	f	0.1–1
RFmMa	+	+	+	-	3	integrated	n	m	0.1–1
ATmDe	+	+	+	-	3	integrated	n	m	0.1–1
SSmUt	+	+	+	-	3	integrated	n	m	0.1–1
KDmWB	+	+	+	-	3	integrated	n	m	0.1–1
OFmTN	+	+	+	-	3	integrated	s	m	0.1–1
SPmKa	+	+	+	-	3	integrated	s	m	0.1–1
SSmKa	+	+	+	-	3	integrated	s	m	0.1–1
PNmKe	+	+	+	-	3	integrated	s	m	0.1–1

(*continued on next page*)

Tab. 5.1.5 Continued

	1	2	3	4	Tot	Status	Ethnicity	Gender	Years in HD
SAmKa	+	+	+	-	3	integrated	s	m	0.1–1
PVfKa	+	+	+	-	3	integrated	s	f	0.1–1
DVfAP	+	+	+	-	3	integrated	s	f	0.1–1
JDfMa	+	+	+	-	3	integrated	n	f	0.1–1
SPfBi	+	+	+	-	3	integrated	n	f	0.1–1
NKSfTN	+	+	+	-	3	integrated	s	f	1.1–5
ASfKe	+	+	+	-	3	integrated	s	f	1.1–5
VRmTN	+	+	+	-	3	integrated	s	m	1.1–5
SSmHa	+	+	+	-	3	integrated	n	m	1.1–5
SSmMa	+	+	-	-	2	somewhat integrated	n	m	0.1–1
MGfUt	+	+	-	-	2	somewhat integrated	n	f	0.1–1
TDfMa	+	+	-	-	2	somewhat integrated	n	f	0.1–1
RMfMa	+	+	-	-	2	somewhat integrated	n	f	0.1–1
NPfMP	+	+	-	-	2	somewhat integrated	n	f	1.1–5
RDfKa	+	+	-	-	2	somewhat integrated	s	f	1.1–5
GSmDe	+	+	-	-	2	somewhat integrated	n	m	1.1–5
HTmUP	+	+	-	-	2	somewhat integrated	n	m	1.1–5
RNmKa	+	+	-	-	2	somewhat integrated	s	m	1.1–5
SLmKa	+	+	-	-	2	somewhat integrated	s	m	1.1–5
SHfUP	+	-	-	-	1	unintegrated	n	f	0.1–1
SLfUP	+	-	-	-	1	unintegrated	n	f	0.1–1
SDfMP	+	-	-	-	1	unintegrated	n	f	0.1–1
KGfPu	+	-	(+)	-	2	somewhat integrated	n	f	0.1–1
SSfWB	-	-	-	-	0	highly unintegrated	n	f	0.1–1
KMmKe	-	-	-	-	0	highly unintegrated	s	m	0.1–1

The high density of the network may be considered to "function effectively as [a] norm-enforcement mechanism" (Milroy 1980:52) since its interactional (or content) characteristics exert influence on behaviour. In order to avoid the inadequacy of specifying a link without considering its content, the sociometric status of the participants has been compared to their integration indices which, in turn, align with the network multiplexity. The sociometric status shows an interesting correspondence for the highly integrated members since they top the scale for integration just as they do for status. Table 5.1.5 reveals that the volume of exchanges and, therefore, of shared knowledge within the network is great. Highly integrated speakers (n = 23) constitute the "ego" (Milroy 1980:46) or the core of the first-order network zone, and integrated ones (n = 19) form the ego's second-order zone. Well-integrated participants are socially positioned to access multiple sub-communities of practice such as HISA or other Indian communities in Germany. Moreover, the content of the links between the ego and the mediating first-order contact is very tenuous. Highly integrated members and integrated ones usually constitute the linguistically influential peer groups of the community. On the contrary, somewhat integrated (n = 13), unintegrated (n = 3) and highly unintegrated (n = 2) members occupy the more peripheral zones of the network. As described in other network studies (Cheshire 1982), peripheral members (and, particularly, those unintegrated and highly unintegrated) are not generally known by the core members, but only by integrated or secondary ones.

Extreme density generally produces homogeneity of norms and values. According to Milroy (1980:61):

> [s]ince this homogeneity of norms might be expected to extend to interactional and specifically linguistic norms, the density of these networks may partly account for the great consistency with which speakers characteristically show loyalty to vernacular speech norms, despite the social stigma attached to it.

This seems to justify the norm-supporting and norm-constructing network ties and the homogeneity of norms and values that guide the participants' language use within the community (cf. Sections 5.1.1.2 and 5.1.1.3). Besides, the density and the multiplexity of the network support the speakers' first languages resisting institutional pressures to language shift. The close-knit affiliations of the community go hand in hand with network structures as identified in other multilingual communities since, as Giddens (2006) points out, distinctive ethnic communities involving strong personal ties tend to gravitate to form bonds with other networks which have similar cultural and linguistic norms. The Malayali community of Heidelberg constitutes one such example (cf. Section 3.2.3).

Religious communities appear to be important focal points for many diasporas since their networks may account either for the phenomenon of language maintenance or the social trajectory of language shift (Li Wei 1995; Shin 1998). In the community in question, similar triggers have been identified. As a result, it comes as no surprise that 60 % of the Catholic sample have multiplex networks with members of the Malayali Catholic community. Their monthly gatherings not only help foster inter-network allegiances but also shed new light on the sociometric rankings of the social network structure since 40 % of them are highly integrated.

Unlike in stable communities, network ties very seldom weaken in transient multilingual ones. In these contexts, minority languages usually resist institutional pressures to language shift because the close-knit, dense and multiplex affiliations of the community are supported by its transiency. As seen in Fig. 5.1.1, these relatively short-lived contexts promote language maintenance practices – manifest in the stable and continuous use of the speakers' L1s – which, in turn, structure internal network subgroups based on ethnicity (cf. Section 5.2.1.2).

5.1.2 Identity and Diasporic Views

5.1.2.1 Ethnic Identities

Sections 5.1.1.2 and 5.1.1.3 draw attention to speakers' moderate use of their L1s in Heidelberg and on the importance of network structure in resisting sociocultural and institutional pressures to language shift. As a matter of fact, different local identities in connection with language maintenance and language use seem to be rooted in the Indian student community. According to the participants, there are at least two competing ethnic identities in their network: Northern and Southern. However, the sociolinguistic situation is rather complex since some speakers coming from different states hold different opinions regarding their identity affiliation.

5.1.2.2 Identity Development: Cluster Analysis and Bubble Matrices

The first part of the questionnaire, corresponding to Survey I: Language Background and Language Use (cf. Section 4.2.1) aims to shed new light on those mechanisms related to identity development and on what the anthropologist Steven Vertovec (1999) defines as 'diaspora consciousness'. A key feature that distinguishes diasporas from individual migrants is their awareness of their origins and roots. While this is usually heightened by transnational activities and retained in memories, food and other artefacts of the community's cultural life

(Levon 2013), it is generally also mirrored in specific attitudes towards observed linguistic practice.

To gain insight into identity development in Heidelberg, the following questions were asked either in the form of open questions or of five-point Likert scales ranging from strongly agree to strongly disagree:

- *Which language do you most strongly identify with? (I.1.9)*
- *Keeping my Indian languages strong in Heidelberg is important to me (I.3.3)*
- *It is important for Indians living here to pass their language knowledge to future generations (I.3.4)*
- *The use of my background languages is a strong part of my identity in Heidelberg as well as among other Indians (I.3.5)*

In line with the moderate density of the student network, a rather homogeneous set of answers was registered among the extralinguistic variables' subgroups. The analysis of the data in question relies on a multidimensional approach which has been chosen in order to group the questionnaire's responses according to underlying factors in the data and to let them 'speak for themselves'. Hierarchical/agglomerative cluster analysis has been combined with a bubble matrix chart. Both procedures are similar to the more frequently applied factor analysis, with the main difference that the data requirements are not as difficult to meet.[75]

Fig. 5.1.6 shows the tree diagram and bubble matrix chart for seven variables related to identity developing, corresponding to the above-mentioned questions. The variables *L1 interactions* and *English in HD* are discussed in Sections 5.1.1.2 and 5.1.1.3. The metric used to calculate the distance is Euclidean, and the method employed is the Farthest Point algorithm, also known as the Voorhees algorithm (Jones *et al.* 2001).

The tree diagram on the x axis shows the hierarchical and agglomerative ordering of selected variables based on similarities between the clusters starting at the bottom of the tree. The further down the clusters join, the more similar the data are. At a first glance, the tree diagram on the x axis indicates four levels of clustering which join at a rather low linking distance.

75 For an account of cluster analysis and bubble matrices cf. Section 4.4.1.4.

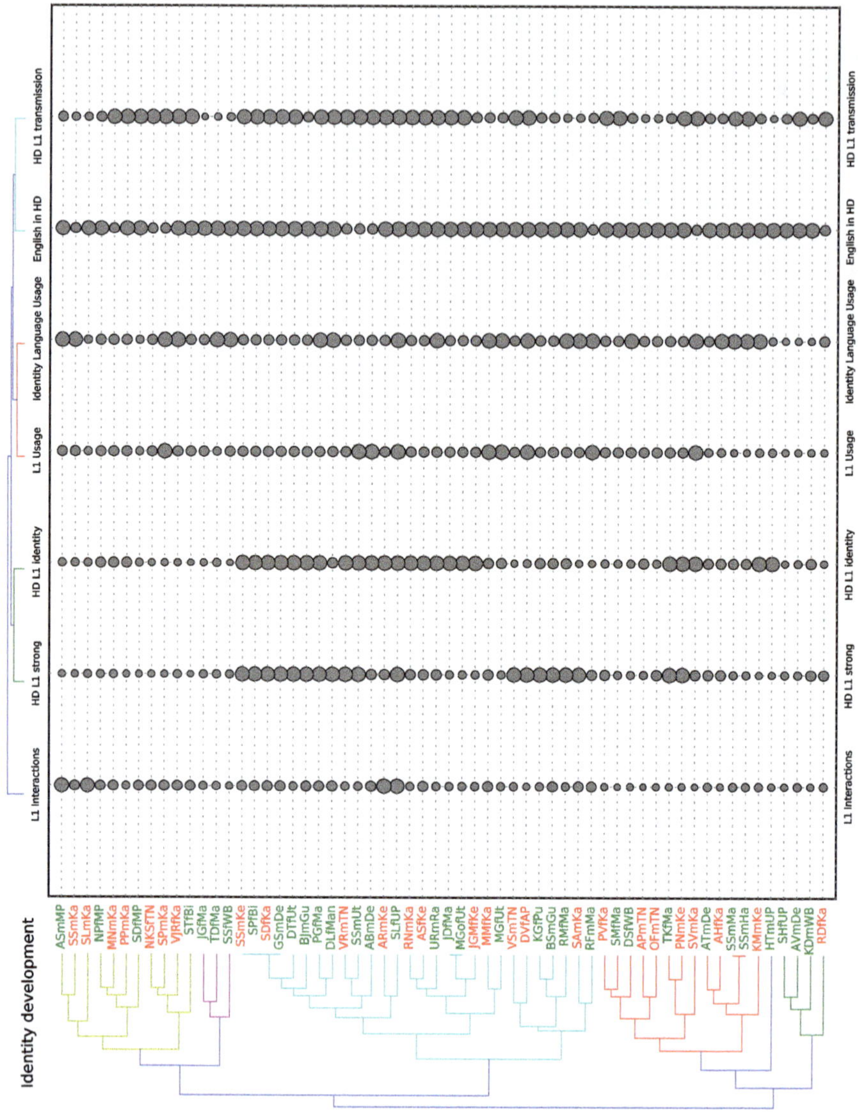

Fig. 5.1.6 Cluster analysis and bubble matrix for identity development. Voorhees' algorithm, Euclidean distances.

A close look reveals that the following variables are related: (i) willingness to use the L1 in Heidelberg frequently (*HD L1 strong*; I.3.3) and use of the L1 as a strong part of the speakers' identities in Heidelberg as well as among other Indians (*HD L1 identity*; I.3.5); (ii) actual use of the L1 (*L1 usage*; I.I.5) and actual use of the language they most strongly identify with (*Identity language usage*; I.1.9); (iii) use of English in Heidelberg (English in HD; I.3.1) and importance to pass their language knowledge to future generations in diasporic settings (*HD L1 transmission*; I.3.4). The correlation between the variables willingness to use the L1 in Heidelberg frequently (*HD L1 strong*; I.3.3) and use of the L1 as a strong part of the speakers' identities in Heidelberg as well as among other Indians (*HD L1 identity*; I.3.5) emphasises the dense network ties of the community resisting language shift processes. Moreover, it sheds light on the ethnic identities of the participants, with 67 % considering their mother tongue the language they most strongly identify with.

The bubble matrix chart on the x axis shows the relation between variables and five-point Likert scales. The radius of every bubble is proportional to the Likert-scale score, i.e., the bigger the bubble, the closer to 1 (strongly agree) the score. From left to right, there is a steady progression towards strongly agreeing with the survey questions, which points to the development of diasporic identity and consciousness.

Both the tree diagram and the bubble matrix chart on the y axis show interesting similarities and differences between the clusters. The tree diagram suggests the hierarchical ordering of the speakers, who have been pre-categorised according to their ethnicities. Northern Indians are portrayed in green, Southern Indians in red. Here, again, the further down the clusters join, the lower the linkage distance and the more similarity between the items. The tree diagram shows the presence of two rather dissimilar clusters, which are subdivided further into three more clusters. However, all the clusters are somewhat homogeneous. This confirms the participants' dense network multiplexity with respect to norms and values surrounding identity development and diaspora consciousness (cf. Section 5.1.1.4). The bubble matrix indicates the value the informants have assigned on a five-point Likert scale to the variables shown on the x axis. Bubble radiuses are proportional to the answer given. In the second sub-cluster of the tree diagram, the correlated variables *HD L1 strong* and *HD L1 identity* show an interesting similarity which is exemplified by the congruence of the Likert-scale values. The latter reveal a concentration of high scores indexing a high level of identity and language consciousness and go hand in hand with the speakers' overt attitudes towards accent and belonging and indexicality (cf. Section 5.2.1).

The above data clustering procedure precedes the analysis of the singular variables for identity development and allows for a more comprehensive interpretation of the results. Subsequently, all variables will be discussed individually.

67 % of the sample agree on their native language being the one they most strongly identify with. The remaining 33 % consider English their identity language. While there is no significant difference in *gender* and *time spent in Heidelberg*, *ethnicity* is an interesting extralinguistic variable to account for. 40 % of the respondents who associate their identity with English come from the South of India and, with the exception of one student from Kerala, they were all born and raised in Bangalore, Karnataka. This comes as no surprise since this state is among the major industrial poles of the subcontinent. Since the 1980s Karnataka has emerged as the pan-Indian leader in the field of Information Technology and is home to India's largest bio cluster. This, of course, brings a high degree of internationalisation into the locals' everyday lives and, as many informants mentioned during the interview session, growing up in Karnataka means being exposed to (different) English(es) since early childhood (cf. Section 5.2.1.1). Northern participants who identify with English come from different states. The majority, however, are either from Maharashtra (15 %) or Uttarakhand (10 %).

The similarities pointed out by the clustering procedure described above between the variables *HD L1 strong* and *HD L1 identity* are in line with this result. In answering the questions *Keeping my Indian languages strong in Heidelberg is important to me* (I.3.3) and *The use of my background languages is a strong part of my identity in Heidelberg as well as among other Indians* (I.3.5), the participants emphasise the pivotal role that their mother tongues play in their everyday lives in Heidelberg. In fact, the two variables show a weak positive correlation ($r = 0.4237$). Although positive (i.e., both variables move in tandem), the correlation may be weak because a quarter of the sample does not associate their native language with their identity. Figure 5.1.7 shows the correlation between the two variables in relation to identity development in Heidelberg. While 32 % of the sample agree on the importance of keeping their background languages strong in Heidelberg, only 2 % do not agree. *HD L1 identity* shows a downward trend ranging from a maximum of 38 % – corresponding to those participants who consider the use of their L1s a strong part of their identity in Heidelberg as well as among their Indian peers – to a minimum of 3 % – corresponding to two female Northern speakers (SSfWB and STfBi) who have been living in Heidelberg for less than six months and who do not associate their identity with their native language. As expected, SSfWB is a highly unintegrated member of the Indian student community (cf. Fig. 5.1.6). Surprisingly, STfBi is a highly integrated member, part of the 'ego' of the network. However, despite her core membership status, she does not associate her identity with her mother tongue, nor does she agree on keeping her L1 strong in Heidelberg. In this sense, her reaction towards questions I.3.3 justifies the one towards I.3.5 in that the use of her first language does not undermine her involvement in the community's network.

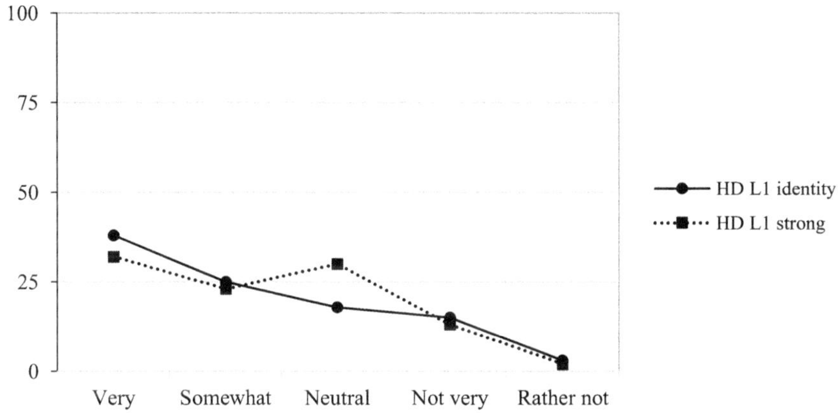

	Very		Somewhat		Neutral		Not very		Rather not		Total	
	N	%	N	%	N	%	N	%	N	%	N	%
HD L1 identity	23	38	15	25	11	18	9	15	2	3	60	99
HD L1 strong	19	32	14	23	18	30	8	13	1	2	60	100

Fig. 5.1.7 Identity development I (in %) *Keeping my Indian languages strong in Heidelberg is important to me (I.3.3) The use of my background languages is a strong part of my identity in Heidelberg as well as among other Indians (I.3.5)* (Pearson Correlation Coefficient r = 0.4237). Rounding adjustments may, in some cases, lead to total percentages above and below 100 %.

It is important for Indians living here to pass their language knowledge to future generations (I.3.4) is the last question aiming to reveal the identity development of the participants. The primary focus of the question is to retrieve information regarding their thoughts about transnationalism and the diaspora, which were discussed during the subsequent interview to check for consistency. Figure 5.1.8 shows that the majority of the sample (57 %) deem it important to transmit their language knowledge to future generations. This result substantiates earlier findings since it points to the dense network structure of the community as being influenced by (and exerting influence on) the members' linguistic behaviour. In addition, it highlights how sociolinguistic practices (such as language transmission) and social relationships (such as in-group network ties and affiliations) affect the processes of language maintenance and shift in transient multilingual communities.

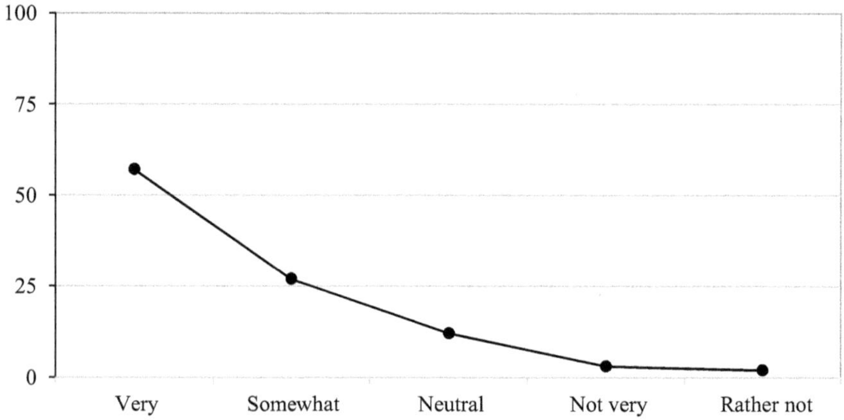

	Very		Somewhat		Neutral		Not very		Rather not		Total	
	N	%	N	%	N	%	N	%	N	%	N	%
L1 transmission	34	57	16	27	7	12	2	3	1	2	60	101

Fig. 5.1.8 Identity development II (in %) *It is important for Indians living here to pass their language knowledge to future generations (I.3.4)*

5.1.3 Language Attitudes and Accent Variation

5.1.3.1 Indian Accents: Evaluation and Stereotyping from a Folk Perspective

Grammaticality and communicative effectiveness are independent issues. Although they often tend to be confused by laypeople, the former refers to what constitutes the rules of a grammar (and the violation of those rules), the latter does so to the inherent value, content and purpose of a specific message (Lippi-Green 1997). The idea or, better still, the abstraction of a standard language and its corollary, non-accent, immediately follows the above-mentioned issues. According to Milroy and Milroy (1991:22–3), the concept of standard language need not be understood as any actual language, but as "an idea in the mind rather than a reality – a set of abstract norms to which actual usage may conform to a greater or lesser extent". In consequence, non-accent may be interpreted as "a collectively held ideal, which brings with it a series of social and regional associations" (Lippi-Green 1997:41). Non-accent is a major issue for many members of the Heidelberg Indian student community. In order to explore the sociocultural mechanisms that guide speakers in their willingness to acquire a non-accent or a neutral accent (cf. Section 5.2.2.2), its counterpart, accent, needs to be addressed first.

As far as linguistics is concerned, the term 'accent' is inherently fuzzy (cf. Section 2.6). Yet, it is widely used by laypeople and, often, in rather interesting and creative ways. The central distinction addressed in Sections 2.6 and 2.7 between L1 and L2 accents is at the core of the present study since the members of the Heidelberg Indian student community seemingly construct their diasporic ethnic identities around their IndE accents. In this specific context, one of the most intriguing and complicated questions of sociolinguistics arises: since L2 varieties of English differ at all linguistic levels and accents are here used to refer to the breakthrough of native language phonology into the target language, where does accent end and dialect begin?

There is a commonly held folk belief in the student community that Southern Indians speak English with a distinctive accent. Their English is often termed 'funny', 'stereotypical' and 'highly influenced by their L1', in contrast to the English of the Northerners, which is commonly described as 'smoother' and 'thick' (Regnoli 2016). What has emerged from the pre-study is that speakers' perceptions of accent variation seem to concern a North to South distinction rather than a state-to-state one. Thus, Survey II, part II is structured in such a way that participants have to listen to a one-minute recording of eight Indian speakers from different states (four from Northern India and four from the South). In order to test the folk belief mentioned above, two female speakers coming from the same Southern Indian state (Karnataka), but with different L1s (Konkani – Indo Aryan and Kannada – Dravidian language) are included (cf. Section 4.2.4).

The results will be presented and discussed from two perspectives. The first one corresponds to the ratings of the eight stimuli for the reliability, intellectuality, amiability and readiness-for-action scales. The second one will account for the participants' evaluations of the Northern and Southern stimuli combined and will consider the informants' ratings in relation to the main extralinguistic variables (*gender*, *ethnicity*, *time spent in Heidelberg*).

Figures 5.1.9–5.1.16 show the ratings of status and solidarity traits of the eight stimuli on a five-point Likert scale. At a first glance, the figures show that the Northern stimuli are rated more or less the same – with the exception of Speakers Four, a Marathi male student with Gujarati origins (cf. Fig. 5.1.12) and Six, a Punjabi male student (cf. Fig. 5.1.14). Although the community has rather similar reactions towards different status and solidarity traits, there are some significant differences among the subgroups of the extralinguistic variables selected.

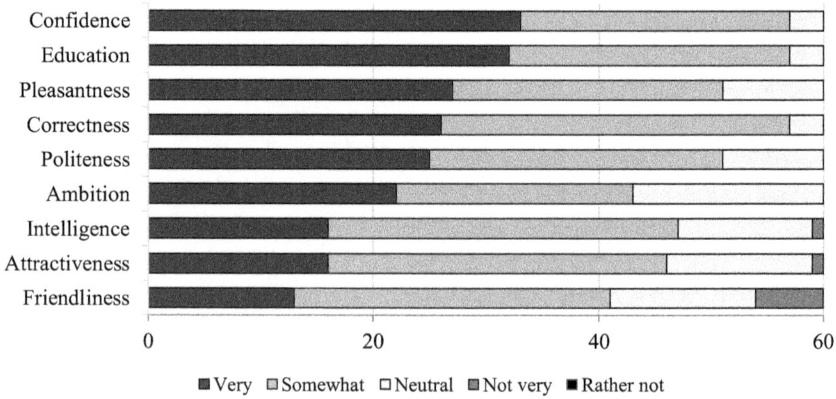

	Very		Somewhat		Neutral		Not very		Rather not		Total	
	N	%	N	%	N	%	N	%	N	%	N	%
Confidence	33	55	24	40	3	5	0	0	0	0	60	100
Education	32	53	25	42	3	5	0	0	0	0	60	100
Pleasantness	27	45	24	40	9	15	0	0	0	0	60	100
Correctness	26	43	31	52	3	5	0	0	0	0	60	100
Politeness	25	42	26	43	9	15	0	0	0	0	60	100
Ambition	22	37	21	35	17	28	0	0	0	0	60	100
Intelligence	16	27	31	52	12	20	1	2	0	0	60	101
Attractiveness	16	27	30	50	13	22	1	2	0	0	60	101
Friendliness	13	22	28	47	13	22	6	10	0	0	60	101

Fig. 5.1.9 Ratings for intellectuality and amiability categories; Speaker One (female): West Bengal (n = 60)

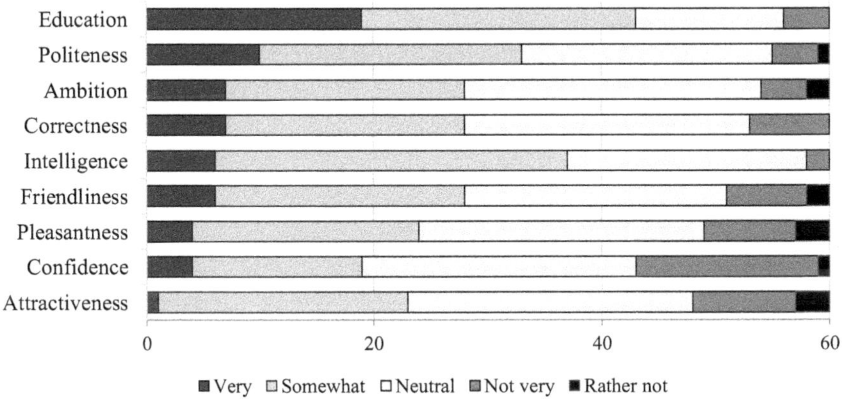

	Very		Somewhat		Neutral		Not very		Rather not		Total	
	N	%	N	%	N	%	N	%	N	%	N	%
Education	19	32	24	40	13	22	4	7	0	0	60	101
Politeness	10	17	23	38	22	37	4	7	1	2	60	101
Ambition	7	12	21	35	26	43	4	7	2	3	60	100
Correctness	7	12	21	35	25	42	7	12	0	0	60	101
Intelligence	6	10	31	52	21	35	2	3	0	0	60	100
Friendliness	6	10	22	37	23	38	7	12	2	3	60	100
Pleasantness	4	7	20	33	25	42	8	13	3	5	60	100
Confidence	4	7	15	25	24	40	16	27	1	2	60	101
Attractiveness	1	2	22	37	25	42	9	15	3	5	60	101

Fig. 5.1.10 Ratings for intellectuality and amiability categories; Speaker Two (male): Tamil Nadu (n = 60)

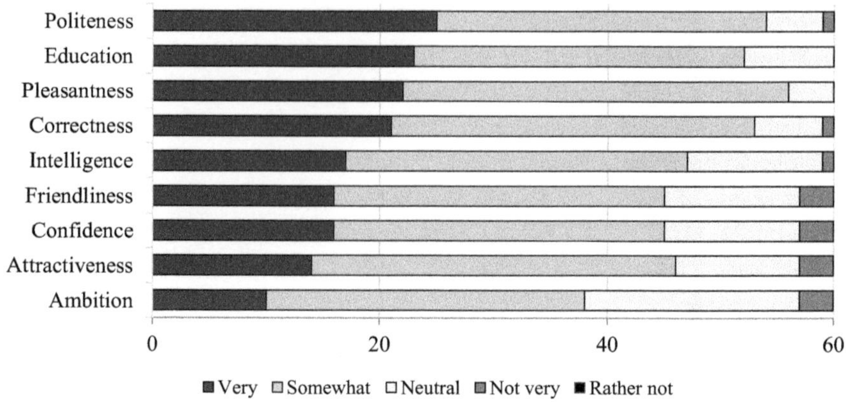

	Very		Somewhat		Neutral		Not very		Rather not		Total	
	N	%	N	%	N	%	N	%	N	%	N	%
Politeness	25	42	29	48	5	8	1	2	0	0	60	100
Education	23	38	29	48	8	13	0	0	0	0	60	99
Pleasantness	22	37	34	57	4	7	0	0	0	0	60	101
Correctness	21	35	32	53	6	10	1	2	0	0	60	101
Intelligence	17	28	30	50	12	20	1	2	0	0	60	100
Friendliness	16	27	29	48	12	20	3	5	0	0	60	100
Confidence	16	27	29	48	12	20	3	5	0	0	60	100
Attractiveness	14	23	32	53	11	18	3	5	0	0	60	99
Ambition	10	17	28	47	19	32	3	5	0	0	60	101

Fig. 5.1.11 Ratings for intellectuality and amiability categories; Speaker Three (female): Karnataka, L1: Konkani (n = 60)

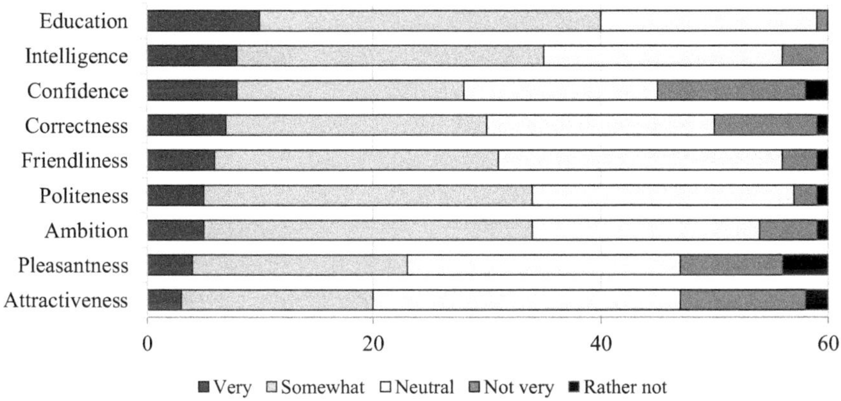

	Very		Somewhat		Neutral		Not very		Rather not		Total	
	N	%	N	%	N	%	N	%	N	%	N	%
Education	10	17	30	50	19	32	1	2	0	0	60	101
Intelligence	8	13	27	45	21	35	4	7	0	0	60	100
Confidence	8	13	20	33	17	28	13	22	2	3	60	99
Correctness	7	12	23	38	20	33	9	15	1	2	60	100
Friendliness	6	10	25	42	25	42	3	5	1	2	60	101
Politeness	5	8	29	48	23	38	2	3	1	2	60	99
Ambition	5	8	29	48	20	33	5	8	1	2	60	99
Pleasantness	4	7	19	32	24	40	9	15	4	7	60	101
Attractiveness	3	5	17	28	27	45	11	18	2	3	60	99

Fig. 5.1.12 Ratings for intellectuality and amiability categories; Speaker Four (male): Maharashtra (n = 60)

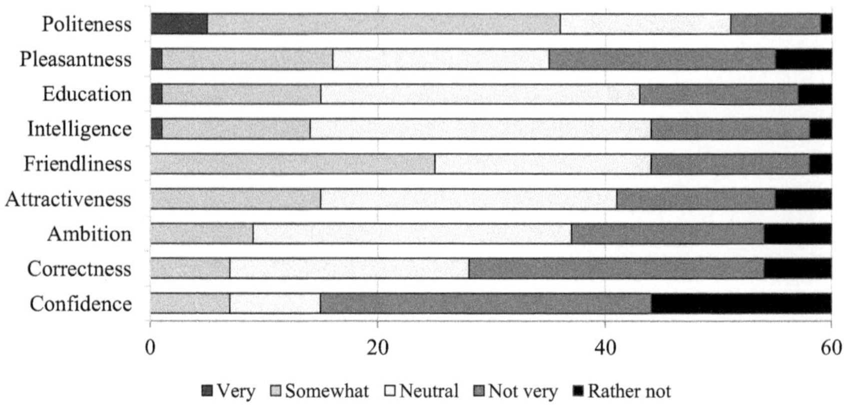

	Very		Somewhat		Neutral		Not very		Rather not		Total	
	N	%	N	%	N	%	N	%	N	%	N	%
Politeness	5	8	31	52	15	25	8	13	1	2	60	100
Pleasantness	1	2	15	25	19	32	20	33	5	8	60	100
Education	1	2	14	23	28	47	14	23	3	5	60	100
Intelligence	1	2	13	22	30	50	14	23	2	3	60	100
Friendliness	0	0	25	42	19	32	14	23	2	3	60	100
Attractiveness	0	0	15	25	26	43	14	23	5	8	60	99
Ambition	0	0	9	15	28	47	17	28	6	10	60	100
Correctness	0	0	7	12	21	35	26	43	6	10	60	100
Confidence	0	0	7	12	8	13	29	48	16	27	60	100

Fig. 5.1.13 Ratings for intellectuality and amiability categories; Speaker Five (female): Karnataka, L1: Kannada (n = 60)

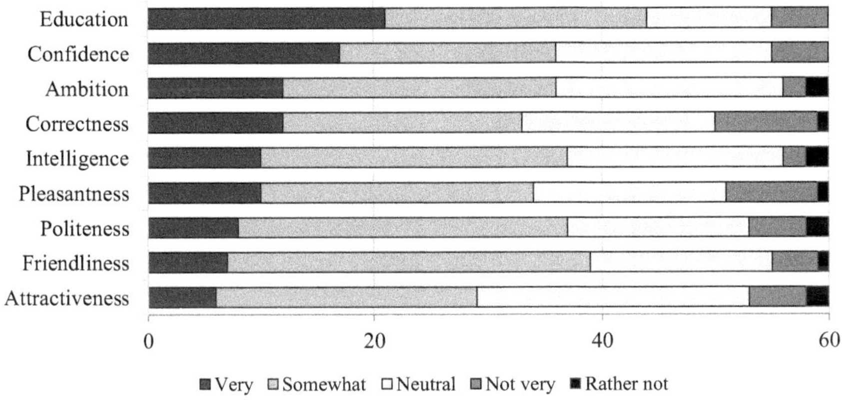

	Very		Somewhat		Neutral		Not very		Rather not		Total	
	N	%	N	%	N	%	N	%	N	%	N	%
Education	21	35	23	38	11	18	5	8	0	0	60	99
Confidence	17	28	19	32	19	32	5	8	0	0	60	100
Ambition	12	20	24	40	20	33	2	3	2	3	60	99
Correctness	12	20	21	35	17	28	9	15	1	2	60	100
Intelligence	10	17	27	45	19	32	2	3	2	3	60	101
Pleasantness	10	17	24	40	17	28	8	13	1	2	60	100
Politeness	8	13	29	48	16	27	5	8	2	3	60	99
Friendliness	7	12	32	53	16	27	4	7	1	2	60	101
Attractiveness	6	10	23	38	24	40	5	8	2	3	60	99

Fig. 5.1.14 Ratings for intellectuality and amiability categories; Speaker Six (male): Punjab (n = 60)

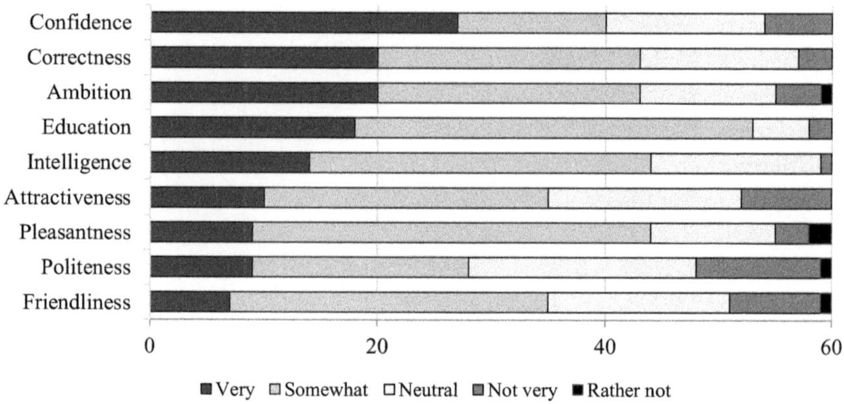

	Very		Somewhat		Neutral		Not very		Rather not		Total	
	N	%	N	%	N	%	N	%	N	%	N	%
Confidence	27	45	13	22	14	23	6	10	0	0	60	100
Correctness	20	33	23	38	14	23	3	5	0	0	60	99
Ambition	20	33	23	38	12	20	4	7	1	2	60	100
Education	18	30	35	58	5	8	2	3	0	0	60	99
Intelligence	14	23	30	50	15	25	1	2	0	0	60	100
Attractiveness	10	17	25	42	17	28	8	13	0	0	60	100
Pleasantness	9	15	35	58	11	18	3	5	2	3	60	99
Politeness	9	15	19	32	20	33	11	18	1	2	60	100
Friendliness	7	12	28	47	16	27	8	13	1	2	60	101

Fig. 5.1.15 Ratings for intellectuality and amiability categories; Speaker Seven (female): Uttar Pradesh (n = 60)

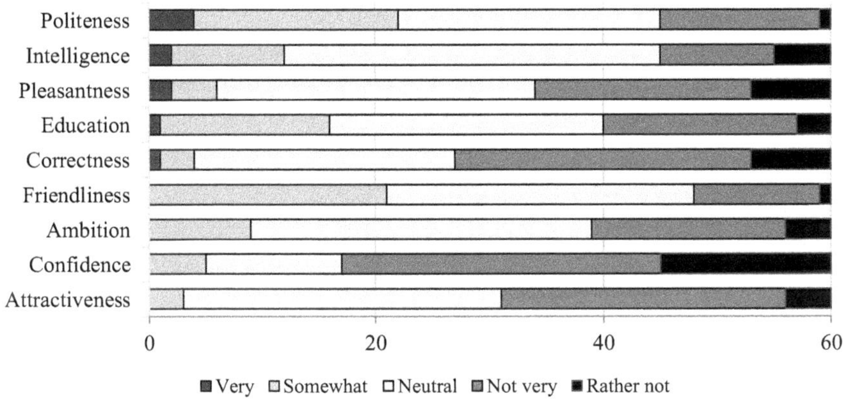

	Very		Somewhat		Neutral		Not very		Rather not		Total	
	N	%	N	%	N	%	N	%	N	%	N	%
Politeness	4	7	18	30	23	38	14	23	1	2	60	100
Intelligence	2	3	10	17	33	55	10	17	5	8	60	100
Pleasantness	2	3	4	7	28	47	19	32	7	12	60	101
Education	1	2	15	25	24	40	17	28	3	5	60	100
Correctness	1	2	3	5	23	38	26	43	7	12	60	100
Friendliness	0	0	21	35	27	45	11	18	1	2	60	100
Ambition	0	0	9	15	30	50	17	28	4	7	60	100
Confidence	0	0	5	8	12	20	28	47	15	25	60	100
Attractiveness	0	0	3	5	28	47	25	42	4	7	60	101

Fig. 5.1.16 Ratings for intellectuality and amiability categories; Speaker Eight (male): Andhra Pradesh (n = 60)

Table 5.1.6 shows that *gender*, *ethnicity* and *time spent in Heidelberg* reveal statistically significant differences between the subgroups with respect to five stimuli. Interestingly, with the exception of Speaker Seven, the stimuli are Southern speakers. The results seem to justify the considerable homogeneity of perception of the Northern guises discussed above. *Time spent in Heidelberg* is the most revealing variable in that, among all the guises and traits, the longer the community members have been living in Heidelberg, the more positively they evaluate the guises (cf. Section 5.1.3.4). With respect to *gender*, there is no univocal behaviour since Speaker Two – a male student from Tamil Nadu – is perceived as more educated by the male informants than the female ones. Conversely, the female part of the sample is significantly surer about the ethnicity of Speaker Eight – a male student from Andhra Pradesh. Finally, with respect to *ethnicity*, Speaker Seven is rated more positively by her Northern peers.

Tab. 5.1.6 p-values of attitude traits for different guises according to the community (Wilcoxon rank-sum)

Speaker 2		
Education	Gender	0.04*
Speaker 3		
Attractiveness	Time spent in HD	0.04*
Ambition	Time spent in HD	0.01**
Speaker 5		
Pleasantness	Time spent in HD	0.04*
Speaker 7		
Politeness	Ethnicity	0.03*
Attractiveness	Time spent in HD	0.01**
Ambition	Time spent in HD	0.03*
Confidence	Time spent in HD	0.006***
Speaker 8		
Degree of certainty	Gender	0.02*

Despite their gender, ethnicity or time spent in Heidelberg, the respondents have a tendency to agree better and have a more unified view about Northern speakers than about Southern ones. The Southern stimuli show no apparent linear patterns in the ratings of reliability, amiability and intellectuality categories – with the significant exception of Speaker Three (cf. Fig. 5.1.11), a female student from Karnataka whose native language is Konkani, a (Northern) Indo-Aryan language. Her ratings are in fact similar to those of Speaker One, a female student from West Bengal (cf. Fig. 5.1.9). The fact that her first language does not coincide with her ethnicity may be the reason that her ratings are very positive and aligned with those of the Northern stimuli (cf. Section 5.2.1.1.2).

In addition, the reported results indicate fine-grained differences in the ratings of Northern and Southern IndE accents in a wide range of traits, with Northern IndE guises having better ratings than the Southern ones. Hence, the respondents' norm-orientation is unidimensional since Northern IndE varieties seem to serve as a superordinate norm in the migrant community. The lack of significance in the reactions of the Northern and the Southern participants towards those attitude traits characterising the Northern and the Southern stimuli is somewhat disappointing since it indexes the linguistic power of the majority, i.e., the Northern Indians, whose views have gradually been accepted and copied by the minorities, i.e., the Southern part of the community. As expected from the pilot study, the Northern Indian participants seemingly have stereotypical views about themselves and the South. Unexpectedly, students coming from the South have by and large taken over the stereotypes of the Northerners about themselves. Anisfeld and Lambert (1964) have already pointed out one such attitude in their studies on bilingualism in Canada with respect to Anglos and Quebecers. The Anglos consider themselves superior with regard to status traits, and the Quebecers agree with them, with the exception that they consider themselves more agreeable in solidarity categories. The latter is the only difference between the results of the present study since the Southern participants do not compensate the perceived lack of their intellectual qualities by judging themselves more polite, friendly, etc.

Interestingly, although the community members react fairly similarly to intellectuality and amiability traits, their perceptions are aligned with the ethnicity of the guises. Their reactions towards Northern and Southern stimuli reach significance for all the status and solidarity scales with the exception of <politeness> (cf. Fig. 5.1.23). Reliability categories do not reach significance with the Bonferroni correction test (cf. Figs. 5.1.17 and 5.1.18). The only readiness-for-action trait, <accent improvement>, is significant (cf. Fig. 5.1.28). Figures 5.1.17–5.1.28 show the attitudes of the Indian students towards South IndE accents and North IndE ones.

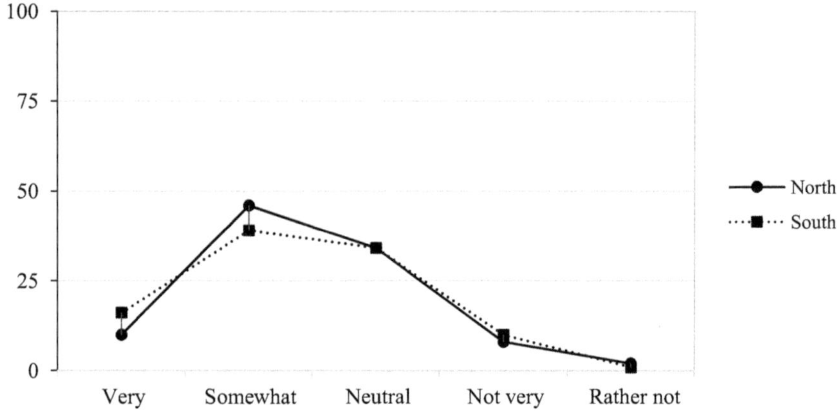

	Very		Somewhat		Neutral		Not very		Rather not		Total	
	N	%	N	%	N	%	N	%	N	%	N[a]	%
North	24	10	111	46	82	34	18	8	5	2	240	100
South	39	16	94	39	81	34	24	10	2	1	240	100

Fig. 5.1.17 Ratings for ethnicity-clustered guises according to the community; Degree of certainty (in %) (Wilcoxon signed-rank p = 0.55 ns; Bonferroni p = 0.06 ns)
a The sum total has been calculated by taking into account the entries for all the ethnicity-clustered guises, i.e., 4 Northern IndE speakers and 4 Southern IndE ones, according to the 60 informants of the sample, i.e., 60x4 = 240. Percentages have been rounded.

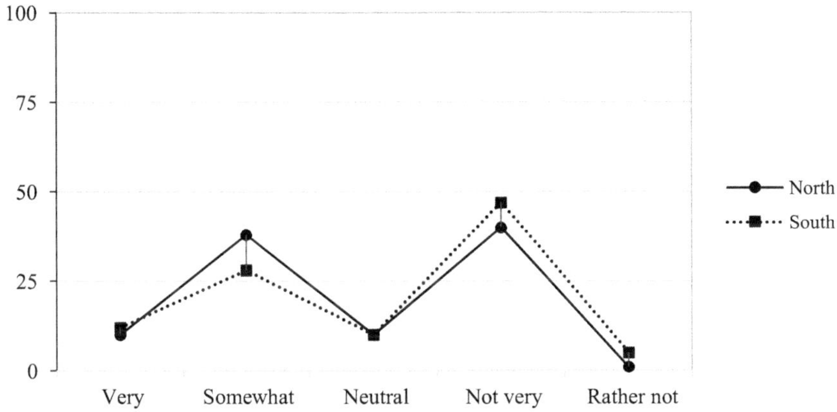

	Very		Somewhat		Neutral		Not very		Rather not		Total	
	N	**%**	**N**	**%**	**N**	**%**	**N**	**%**	**N**	**%**	**N**	**%**
North	24	10	92	38	24	10	97	40	3	1	240	99
South	28	12	66	28	23	10	112	47	11	5	240	102

Fig. 5.1.18 Ratings for ethnicity-clustered guises according to the community; Degree of perceived difference (in %) (Wilcoxon signed-rank $p = 0.01^{**}$; Bonferroni $p = 0.06$ ns)

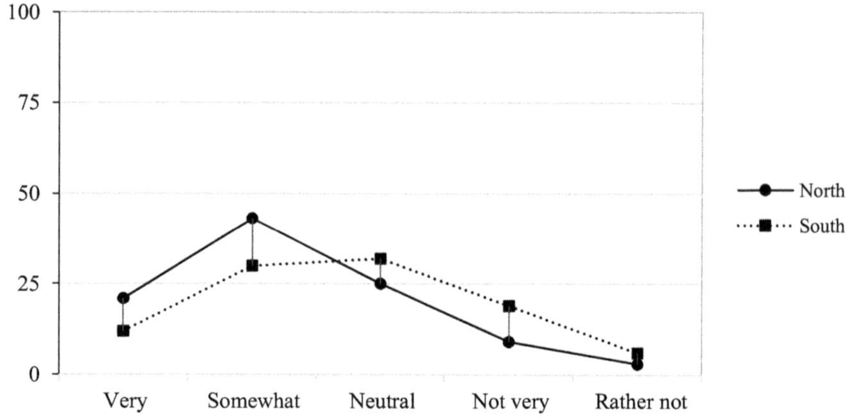

	Very		Somewhat		Neutral		Not very		Rather not		Total	
	N	%	N	%	N	%	N	%	N	%	N	%
North	50	21	102	43	61	25	21	9	6	3	240	101
South	29	12	73	30	77	32	46	19	15	6	240	99

Fig. 5.1.19 Ratings for ethnicity-clustered guises according to the community; Pleasantness (in %) (Wilcoxon signed-rank p < 0.00001****; Bonferroni p = 0.00012***)

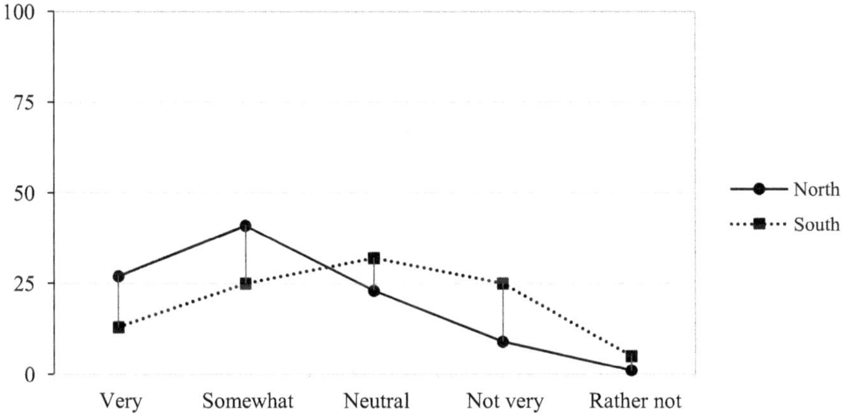

	Very		Somewhat		Neutral		Not very		Rather not		Total	
	N	%	N	%	N	%	N	%	N	%	N	%
North	64	27	99	41	54	23	21	9	2	1	240	101
South	30	13	61	25	76	32	60	25	13	5	240	100

Fig. 5.1.20 Ratings for ethnicity-clustered guises according to the community; Correctness (in %) (Wilcoxon signed-rank p < 0.00001****; Bonferroni p = 0.00012***)

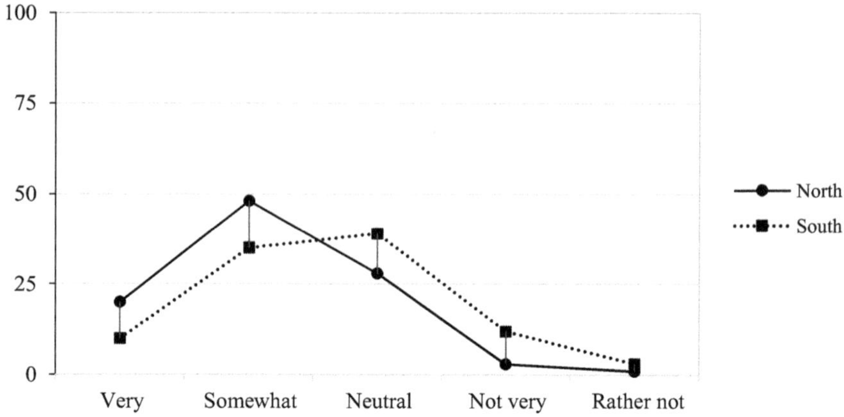

	Very		Somewhat		Neutral		Not very		Rather not		Total	
	N	%	N	%	N	%	N	%	N	%	N	%
North	48	20	115	48	67	28	8	3	2	1	240	100
South	25	10	85	35	94	39	29	12	7	3	240	99

Fig. 5.1.21 Ratings for ethnicity-clustered guises according to the community; Intelligence (in %) (Wilcoxon signed-rank $p < 0.00001$****; Bonferroni $p = 0.00012$***)

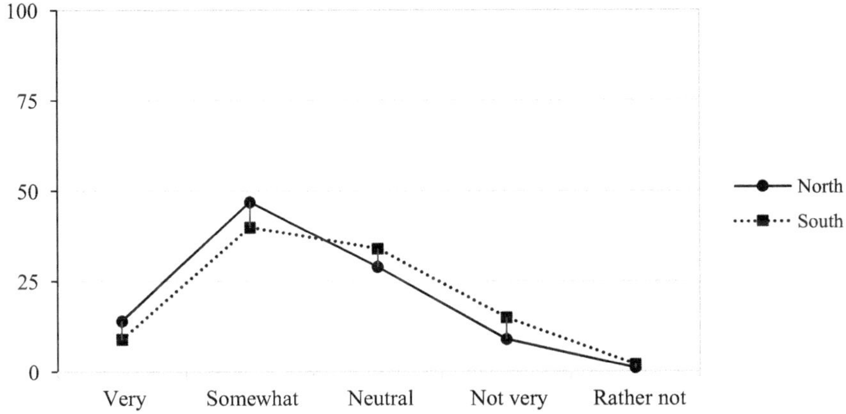

	Very		Somewhat		Neutral		Not very		Rather not		Total	
	N	%	N	%	N	%	N	%	N	%	N	%
North	33	14	113	47	69	29	22	9	3	1	240	100
South	22	9	96	40	81	34	36	15	5	2	240	100

Fig. 5.1.22 Ratings for ethnicity-clustered guises according to the community; Friendliness (in %) (Wilcoxon signed-rank p = 0.005**; Bonferroni p = 0.06 ns)

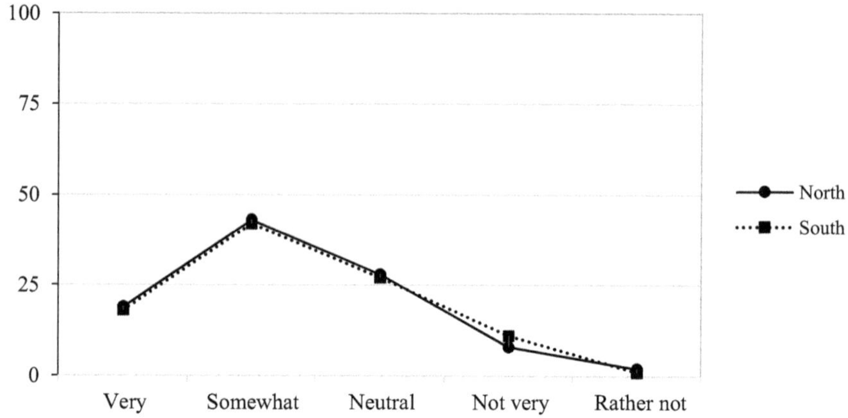

	Very		Somewhat		Neutral		Not very		Rather not		Total	
	N	%	N	%	N	%	N	%	N	%	N	%
North	46	19	104	43	68	28	18	8	4	2	240	100
South	44	18	101	42	65	27	27	11	3	1	240	99

Fig. 5.1.23 Ratings for ethnicity-clustered guises according to the community; Politeness (in %) (Wilcoxon signed-rank $p = 0.49$ ns; Bonferroni $p = 1$ ns)

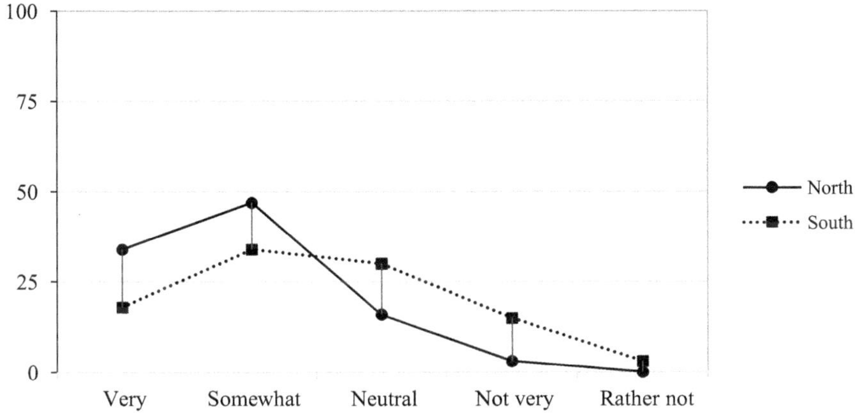

	Very		Somewhat		Neutral		Not very		Rather not		Total	
	N	%	N	%	N	%	N	%	N	%	N	%
North	81	34	112	47	39	16	8	3	0	0	240	100
South	44	18	82	34	73	30	35	15	6	3	240	100

Fig. 5.1.24 Ratings for ethnicity-clustered guises according to the community; Education (in %) (Wilcoxon signed-rank p < 0.00001****; Bonferroni p = 0.00012***)

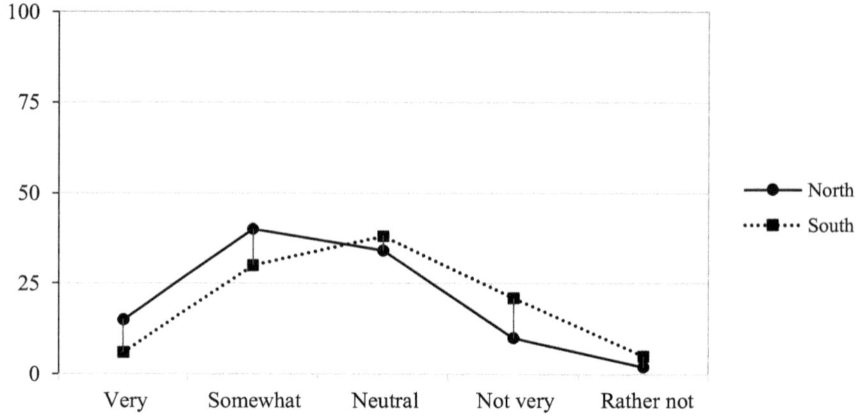

	Very		Somewhat		Neutral		Not very		Rather not		Total	
	N	%	N	%	N	%	N	%	N	%	N	%
North	35	15	95	40	81	34	25	10	4	2	240	101
South	15	6	72	30	91	38	51	21	11	5	240	100

Fig. 5.1.25 Ratings for ethnicity-clustered guises according to the community; Attractiveness (in %) (Wilcoxon signed-rank $p < 0.00001$****; Bonferroni $p = 0.00012$***)

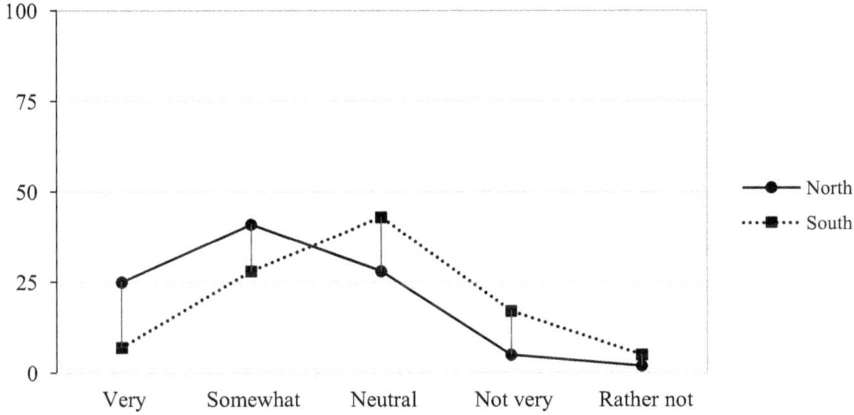

	Very		Somewhat		Neutral		Not very		Rather not		Total	
	N	%	N	%	N	%	N	%	N	%	N	%
North	59	25	98	41	68	28	11	5	4	2	240	101
South	17	7	67	28	103	43	41	17	12	5	240	100

Fig. 5.1.26 Ratings for ethnicity-clustered guises according to the community; Ambition (in %) (Wilcoxon signed-rank $p < 0.00001$****; Bonferroni $p = 0.00012$***)

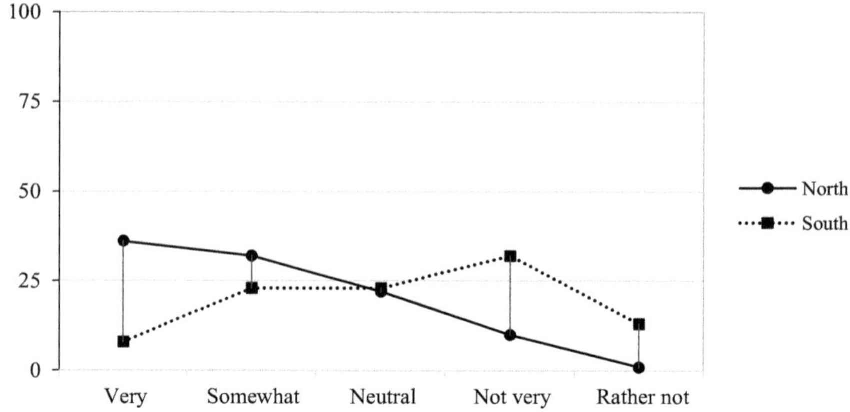

	Very		Somewhat		Neutral		Not very		Rather not		Total	
	N	%	N	%	N	%	N	%	N	%	N	%
North	86	36	77	32	52	22	23	10	2	1	240	101
South	20	8	56	23	56	23	76	32	32	13	240	99

Fig. 5.1.27 Ratings for ethnicity-clustered guises according to the community; Confidence (in %) (Wilcoxon signed-rank $p < 0.00001$****; Bonferroni $p = 0.00012$***)

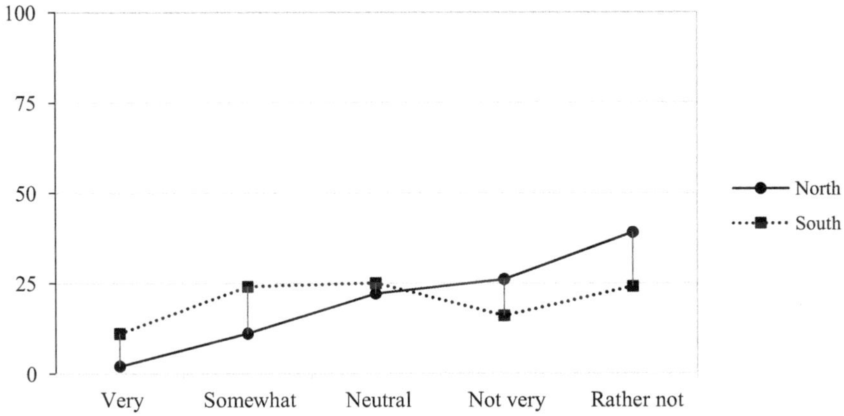

	Very		Somewhat		Neutral		Not very		Rather not		Total	
	N	%	N	%	N	%	N	%	N	%	N	%
North	5	2	26	11	53	22	63	26	93	39	240	100
South	26	11	57	24	61	25	38	16	58	24	240	100

Fig. 5.1.28 Ratings for ethnicity-clustered guises according to the community; Accent Improvement (in %) (Wilcoxon signed-rank $p < 0.00001$****; Bonferroni $p = 0.00012$***)

Northern IndE accents are generally rated more positively than Southern IndE ones for all traits. With some interesting exceptions, the respondents' attitudes towards the majority of the categories are quite uniform, indicating Northern IndE accents as 'somewhat positive' and Southern IndE ones as 'neutral'. <Politeness> is the only amiability trait that does not confirm the trend; in fact, it is not a significant variable in accent discrimination (cf. Fig. 5.1.23). All intellectuality traits, i.e., <correctness>, <intelligence> (cf. Figs. 5.1.20 and 5.1.21), <education> (cf. Fig. 5.1.24) and <ambition> (cf. Fig. 5.1.26) show major discrepancies between Northern and Southern IndE accents. Conversely, with the exception of <confidence> (cf. Fig. 5.1.27), amiability traits diverge less. This may lend credence to the results analysed earlier, which point to Northern IndE accents as somewhat 'superior' with respect to status traits and Southern IndE ones as generally agreeable but still 'inferior' to Northern ones with regard to solidarity categories. The readiness-for-action trait, <accent improvement> (cf. Fig. 5.1.28) shows a rather clear-cut inclination towards rating Southern IndE accents as in need of improvement. This justifies earlier findings from the pilot-study which suggest that South Indians are perceived to have a higher competence in and better command of English in syntactic constructions in spite of their perceived heavily-accented English. According to the community members, a strong accent does not mean syntactic inaccuracy. In this sense, "syntax appears to be a potentially more important domain of norm-maintenance within the community in order to cultivate and maintain the status of a proficient speaker while phonology may be recruited more readily for a construction of a local Indian identity" (Regnoli 2019a:453).[76]

The reactions of the community's subgroups towards ethnicity-clustered stimuli are significant as well. Mean values and standard deviations for readiness-for-action, reliability, amiability and intellectuality categories have been calculated. To assess the statistical significance of the differences in mean ratings of the informants, non-parametric Wilcoxon signed-rank tests (and follow-up Bonferroni post-hoc comparison tests) have subsequently been undertaken for the main extralinguistic variables.

Table 5.1.7 shows the p-values of attitude traits according to *gender*. With the exception of the reliability traits <friendliness>and <politeness>, both the male and the female in-group differentiate between Northern and Southern IndE accents. Although both subgroups react similarly to the categories, their perceptions of ethnicity-clustered stimuli in relation to intellectuality traits diverge significantly, even more so with <confidence> and <education>.

Tab. 5.1.7 Bonferroni-corrected p-values of attitude traits for ethnicity-clustered guises according to gender

Trait	**Male**	**Female**
Pleasantness	p = 0.00528**	p = 0.0288*
Correctness	p = 0.00024***	p = 0.00024***
Intelligence	p = 0.01008*	p = 0.00336**
Education	p = 0.00024***	p = 0.00024***
Attractiveness	p = 0.00192**	p = 0.03072*
Ambition	p = 0.00024***	p = 0.00024***
Confidence	p = 0.00024***	p = 0.00024***
Accent Improvement	p = 0.00024***	p = 0.00024***
Degree of certainty	p = 1 ns	p = 1 ns
Degree of perceived difference	p = 1 ns	p = 0.92 ns
Friendliness	p = 0.37 ns	p = 1 ns
Politeness	p = 1 ns	p = 1 ns

76 Accent improvement will be discussed further in Section 5.2.2.2, where ideologies of nativeness and the neutral or non-accent will be dealt with.

Table 5.1.8 indicates the Bonferroni-corrected p-values for readiness-for-action, reliability, amiability and intellectuality categories for ethnicity-clustered stimuli according to *ethnicity*. As with *gender*, <friendliness>, <politeness>, <degree of certainty> and <degree of perceived difference> do not reach significance.

Tab. 5.1.8 Bonferroni-corrected p-values of attitude traits for ethnicity-clustered guises according to ethnicity

Trait	North	South
Pleasantness	p = 0.01536*	p = 0.00528**
Correctness	p = 0.00024***	p = 0.0024**
Intelligence	p = 0.00576**	p = 0.00432**
Education	p = 0.00024***	p = 0.00024***
Attractiveness	p = 0.00192**	p = 0.03408*
Ambition	p = 0.00024***	p = 0.00288**
Confidence	p = 0.00024***	p = 0.00024***
Accent Improvement	p = 0.00024***	p = 0.00024***
Degree of certainty	p = 1 ns	p = 1 ns
Degree of perceived difference	p = 0.1992 ns	p = 1 ns
Friendliness	p = 1 ns	p = 1 ns
Politeness	p = 1 ns	p = 1 ns

Both the Northern informants and the Southern ones differentiate between Northern and Southern IndE accents and attribute better ratings to the Northern stimuli. <Correctness> and <accent improvement> are one such example. Southern ratings are massively lower than Northern ones and even more so with regard to the Southern informants. This finding supports earlier claims according to which the linguistic practices of the majority, i.e., the Northern participants, tend to be gradually accepted and copied by the minorities, i.e., the Southerners.

The reactions towards ethnicity-clustered stimuli of those participants who have been living in Heidelberg for less than a year and from 1.1 to 5 years are significant as well. Table 5.1.9 shows the p-values of attitude traits according to the subgroups. As with *gender* and *ethnicity*, *time spent in Heidelberg* does not reach significance for both reliability categories, <friendliness> and <politeness>. The clear-cut difference between Northern and Southern IndE accents is visible in all categories, especially in <education> and <confidence>. With respect to the latter, people who have been staying in Heidelberg longer seemingly perceive the North/South difference as more substantial (cf. Section 5.1.3.4).

Tab. 5.1.9 Bonferroni-corrected p-values of attitude traits for ethnicity-clustered guises according to time spent in Heidelberg

Trait	0.1–1	1.1–5
Pleasantness	p = 0.00024***	p = 0.09552*
Correctness	p = 0.00024***	p = 0.01056*
Intelligence	p = 0.00024***	p = 0.07392 ns
Education	p = 0.00024***	p = 0.00816**
Attractiveness	p = 0.00192**	p = 0.02304*
Ambition	p = 0.00024***	p = 0.0288*
Confidence	p = 0.00024***	p = 0.0024**
Accent Improvement	p = 0.00024***	p = 0.00336**
Degree of certainty	p = 1 ns	p = 1 ns
Degree of perceived difference	p = 0.1992 ns	p = 1 ns
Friendliness	p = 1 ns	p = 1 ns
Politeness	p = 1 ns	p = 1 ns

5.1.3.2 Ethnolinguistic Differences: Origins and Clues

The accent recognition task aims at showing the participants' unconscious perceptions of different IndE accents. A further objective is to associate their covert attitudes towards the alleged origin of the stimuli and elicit the participants' metalinguistic awareness in second language acquisition. As a result, the following open questions are included for each guise in Survey II, part II (cf. Section 4.2.4):

- *Identify the ethnicity of the following speakers and assign each voice to the site it belongs on the map provided (II.II.1)*
- *What cues/clues did you consider to identify the speaker's origin? (II.II.3)*

The discussion of II.II.1 will be expanded with respect to the map assignment in Section 5.1.3.7.1. The identification of the guises matches the informants' ratings of readiness-for-action, reliability, amiability and intellectuality attitude traits (cf. Section 5.1.3.1). The 'fuzziness' of ratings of specific guises aligns with their perceived origins. During the task, the participants were first asked to identify the ethnicity of the guises, to describe the cues/clues they had considered for their identification and then to rate them on the scales described above. A possible reason for this 'fuzziness' or 'origin uncertainty' might be related to the specific phonological cues they did (or did not) find, which subsequently did (or did not) hint at the alleged ethnicity of the speaker.

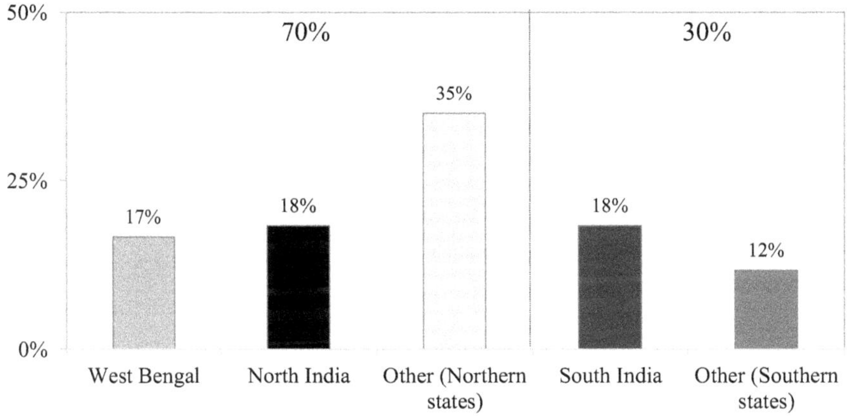

Location	N	%
West Bengal	10	17
North India	11	18
Other (Northern states)	21	35
South India	11	18
Other (Southern states)	7	12
Total	60	100

Fig. 5.1.29 Perceived ethnicity of the guises; Speaker One (female): West Bengal (in %)[a]. Rounding adjustments may, in some cases, lead to total percentages above and below 100 %.

Figure 5.1.29 shows that the majority of the community (35 %) locate Speaker One as belonging to different states of Northern India (most commonly, Delhi).[77] An even percentage thinks that she comes from a rather general Northern or

77 The distinction between 'North India' and 'Other (Northern States)' as well as 'South India' and 'Other (Southern States)' follows the descriptors of the participants as pointed out in the answers provided in II.II.1. The captions 'Other (Northern States)' and 'Other (Southern States)' are umbrella terms used to cluster all the states that the participants enlist in II.II.1 as belonging to either area. The clustering follows the binary ethnicity self-identification process as described by the community members (North Indian/South Indian). For further details cf. Section 5.1.1.1.

Southern area (18 % each), while 12 % agree that she is from some Southern state (most commonly, Karnataka). However, 17 % of the sample indicate that the guise is from the North Eastern state of West Bengal, her actual state of origin. This result is interesting in that it points to the fact that, overall, the student community tends to differentiate speakers on a North vs South basis, rather than a state-to-state one. Interestingly, Speaker One is among the few guises whose precise ethnicity is guessed correctly. This indicates that, according to the community members, the Bengali English accent is among the most easily identifiable IndE ones.

Tab. 5.1.10 Common recognised clues; Speaker One (female): West Bengal

Clue	Frequencies
Tone	15
L1 influence	4
/r/	4
'baba'	4
Total	27

Table 5.1.10 enlists the main salient features the participants mention in accent discrimination. Tone is most frequent (15 of 27). As to the other three clues stated overtly, Bengali English receives remarks in relation to the realisation of the /r/ sound in prevocalic positions in the pronunciation of 'baba' (Bengali for 'dad') and general L1 influence. Considering that most differences in the consonant inventory of IndE are phonetic and that the only phonological ones are the frequent merger of [w] and [v] and rhoticity, it is interesting to note that the perception of Bengali English is mainly phonological.[78]

Figure 5.1.30 shows that the origin of Speaker Two is recognised by 13 % of the sample. However, while 22 % of the community guess that he is from Southern India, another 28 % point to his alleged Northern origin. Considering the large number of responses referring to the Northern states, it is interesting to mention that 28 % locate the speaker as belonging to the less educated and poorest states of the subcontinent (predominantly Bihar). This result seems to

78 A more detailed account of the speakers' perceptions of accent variation and their definitions of key terms such as 'tone' will be provided in section 5.2.1.

support earlier findings indicating that the Southern guises are perceived as significantly less educated than the Northern ones (cf. Section 5.1.3.1).

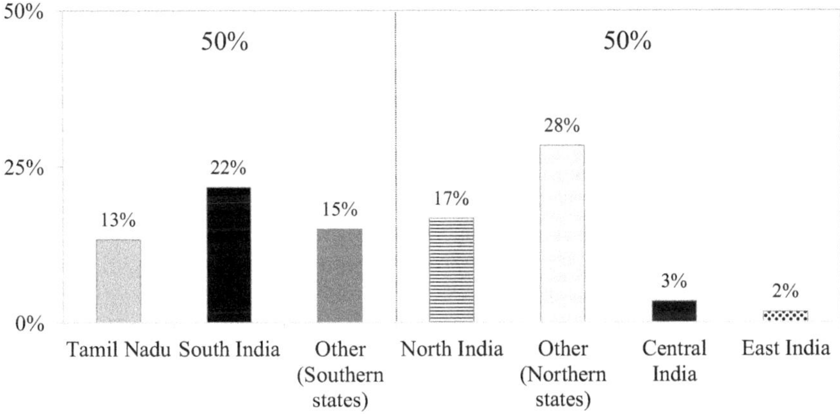

Location	N	%
Tamil Nadu	8	13
South India	13	22
Other (Southern states)	9	15
North India	10	17
Other (Northern states, predominantly Bihar)	17	28
Central India	2	3
East India	1	2
Total	60	100

Fig. 5.1.30 Perceived ethnicity of the guises; Speaker Two (male): Tamil Nadu (in %)

Tab. 5.1.11 Common recognised clues; Speaker Two (male): Tamil Nadu

Clue	Frequencies
Tone	11
'where'	8
'only'	6
Speech rate	5
Total	30

With respect to the clues used for his identification, as with Speaker One, tone is the feature mentioned most. The w/v merger is another common clue as represented in the pronunciation of /where/ as [ˈvɛəɽ], hinting, in addition, at the realisation of /r/ as a flap in non-prevocalic position (cf. Tab. 5.1.11). The pronunciation of /only/ as [ˈɒnli] sheds light on a common phenomenon occurring in many IndE varieties: monophthongisation (Sailaja 2009:25–6). In this case, [əʊ] is realised as the one back rounded vowel [ɒ]. Slow speech rate is the last clue to be identified.

Considering the interesting correlation between the ethnicity of Speaker Three, i.e., South, and her native language, i.e., Konkani, an Indo-Aryan language predominantly spoken in North Western India, it comes as no surprise that many community members are rather uncertain about her place of origin. Thus, many locations are suggested (cf. Fig. 5.1.31).

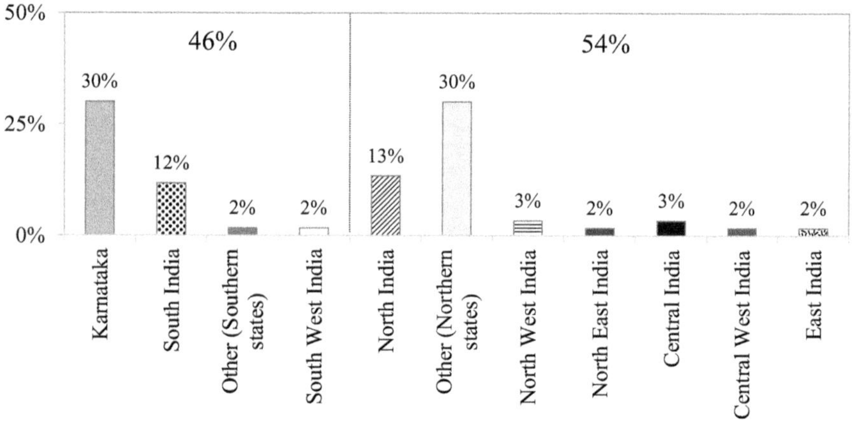

Location	N	%
Karnataka	18	30
South India	7	12
Other (Southern states)	1	2
South West India	1	2
North India	8	13
Other (Northern states)	18	30
North West India	2	3

Location	N	%
North East India	1	2
Central India	2	3
Central West India	1	2
East India	1	2
Total	60	101

Fig. 5.1.31 Perceived ethnicity of the guises; Speaker Three (female): Karnataka, L1: Konkani (in %)

While 30 % of the sample correctly guess her ethnicity, another 30 % locate her in some Northern state (where Konkani is spoken as well). Interestingly, 10 % of the participants attribute her to some further places where Konkani is spoken (i.e., Central India, Central West India, North West India, South West India), whereas a very small percentage (2 %) place her in other Southern states. This may lend credence to an alleged Konkani influence in the phonetic inventory of the guise's English despite her being bilingual in Kannada as well. Table 5.1.12 sheds light on the clues mentioned most frequently. While tone is always widely used for accent discrimination, the realisation of the voiceless alveolar stop /t/ as a voiceless retroflex stop [ʈ] serves as a crucial clue in the identification of Speaker Three.

Tab. 5.1.12 Common recognised clues; Speaker Three (female): Karnataka, L1: Konkani

Clue	Frequencies
Tone	9
/t/	6
Speech rate	4
Total	19

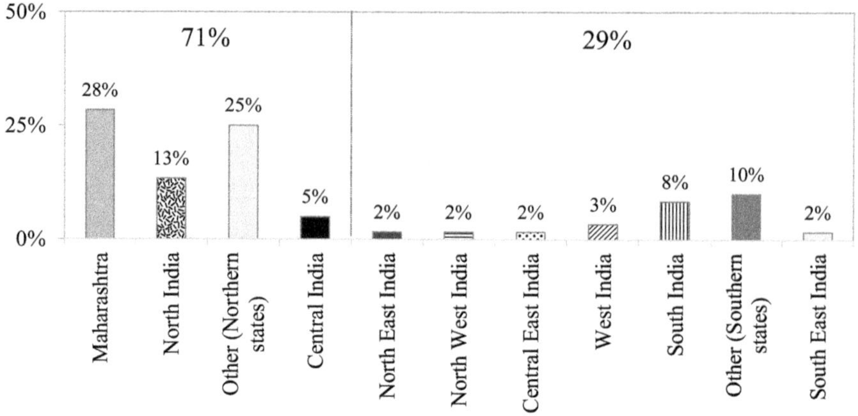

Location	**N**	**%**
Maharashtra	17	28
North India	8	13
Other (Northern states)	15	25
North West India	1	2
North East India	1	2
South India	5	8
Other (Southern states)	6	10
South East India	1	2
Central India	3	5
Central East India	1	2
West India	2	3
Total	60	100

Fig. 5.1.32 Perceived ethnicity of the guises; Speaker Four (male): Maharashtra (in %)

Figure 5.1.32 shows that 28 % of the participants guess the ethnicity of Speaker Four correctly. The percentages related to his identification as a North Indian (13 %) and as coming from some specific Northern Indian states (25 %) indicate that the guesses are fairly accurate. Yet, other estimates locating him in Central India (5 %), West India (3 %) and North West India (2 %) might be considered valid as well since the speaker has Gujarati origins. With respect to the cues used for his identification, tone is, again, the most salient one. However, unlike for the guises described above, no concrete clues or phonetic realisations are mentioned, which leaves rather general features (cf. Tab. 5.1.13).

Tab. 5.1.13 Common recognised clues; Speaker Four (male): Maharashtra

Clue	**Frequencies**
Tone	11
L1 influence	10
Speech rate	7
Total	28

Figure 5.1.33 shows the reactions towards Speaker Five, a female student from the Southern state of Karnataka whose first language is Kannada. Unlike Speaker Three who is easily recognised on the basis of her ethnicity despite her first language not matching with her place of origin (cf. Fig. 5.1.31), Speaker Five is not recognised at all. As is the case with Speaker Two, the guise is perceived to be from North India (30 %) or from other specific Northern states (25 %) because of the more or less explicit connection the participants make with less developed Indian states. Bihar is amongst the states of origin selected most. Interestingly, one in four participants locates her in South India. These 25 % are responsible for the clue for her identification recognised most: the mispronunciation of *Sultanate*, *Tughlaqs* and *Khiljis*, i.e., words of Hindi origin that, according to many community members, are immediate hints for North/South accent discrimination (cf. Tab. 5.1.14).[79]

79 The *Tughlaq* and *Khilji* (or *Khaliji*) dynasties were Muslim dynasties that ruled over the Delhi sultanate in medieval India. For a more detailed account of the history of the Delhi Sultanate cf. Eraly (2015).

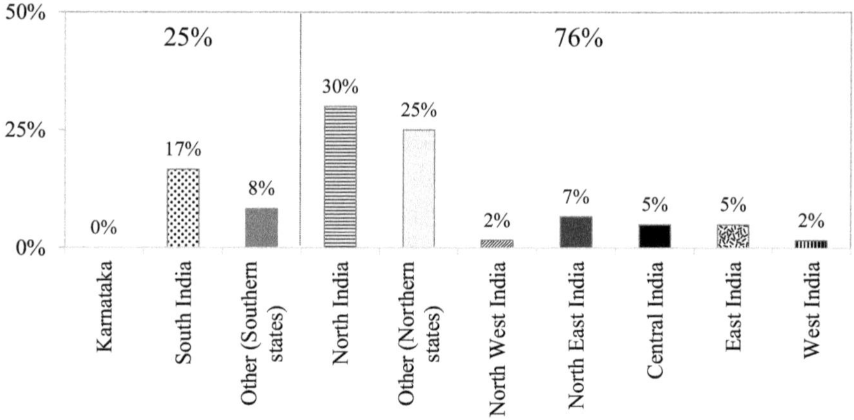

Location	N	%
Karnataka	0	0
South India	10	17
Other (Southern states)	5	8
North India	18	30
Other (Northern states)	15	25
North West India	1	2
North East India	4	7
Central India	3	5
East India	3	5
West India	1	2
Total	60	101

Fig. 5.1.33 Perceived ethnicity of the guises; Speaker Five (female): Karnataka, L1: Kannada (in %)

Tab. 5.1.14 Common recognised clues; Speaker Five (female): Karnataka, L1: Kannada

Clue	Frequencies
Mispronunciation of 'Sultanate', 'Tughlaqs' and 'Khiljis'	11
Tone	6
L1 influence	5
Total	22

Only 7 % of the informants recognise Speaker Six as Punjabi (cf. Fig. 5.1.34). However, his accent is identified as Northern Indian by the majority of the sample (60 %). A few speakers locate him in West India (3 %) because of his 'melodious' English. Interestingly, many community members attribute the same adjective to Punjab as well as Rajasthan/Gujarat (cf. Section 5.1.3.7.2). As with Speaker Four, no explicit clues are pinpointed with respect to the recognition of Speaker Six. Table 5.1.15 shows a list of general recognised features.

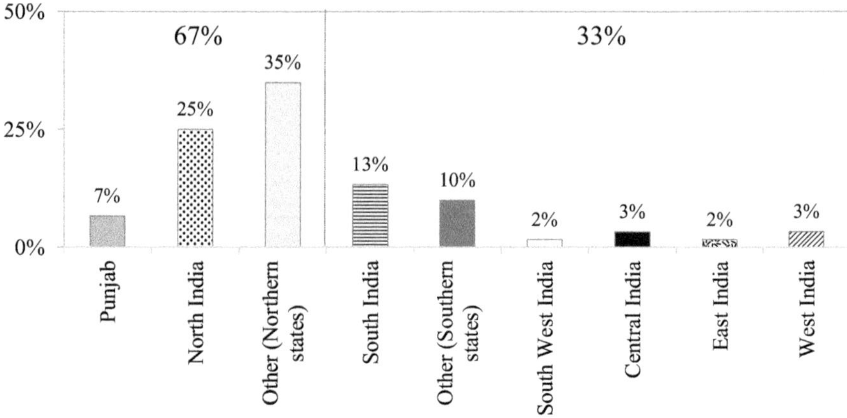

Location	N	%
Punjab	4	7
North India	15	25
Other (Northern states)	21	35
South India	8	13
Other (Southern states)	6	10
South West India	1	2
Central India	2	3
East India	1	2
West India	2	3
Total	60	100

Fig. 5.1.34 Perceived ethnicity of the guises; Speaker Six (male): Punjab (in %)

Tab. 5.1.15 Common recognised clues according to the community; Speaker Six (male): Punjab

Clue	Frequencies
L1 influence	10
Speech rate	9
Tone	8
Total	27

As for Speaker Six, only 7 % of the sample recognise the place of origin of Speaker Seven (cf. Fig. 5.1.35). However, 67 % guess her ethnicity correctly. Interestingly, a third of the community members locate the guise in Southern India, and, specifically, in the main capital cities, i.e., Bangalore, Chennai, because of their relatively high literacy rates. This result sheds light on the delicate relationship between having a (strong) accent and having received a 'proper' education in English. A comprehensive account of these language ideologies and attitudes will be given in Section 5.2.1.1. The relative scarcity of accuracy regarding the clues for the guise's discrimination despite the high percentages of correct identification is interesting, however (cf. Tab. 5.1.16).

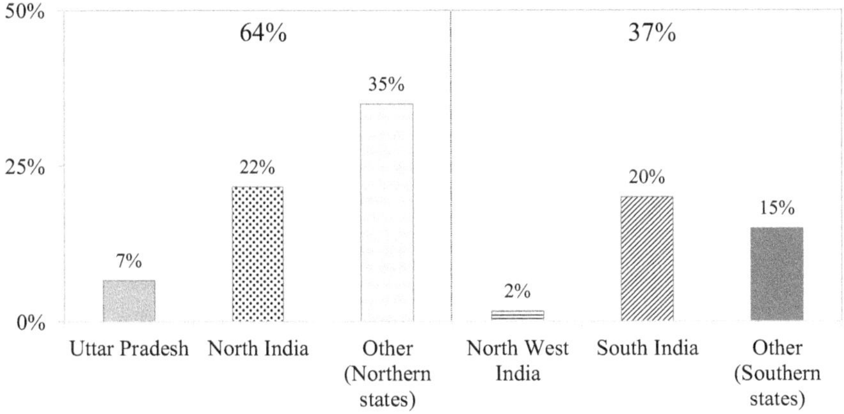

Location	**N**	**%**
Uttar Pradesh	4	7
North India	13	22
Other (Northern states)	21	35
North West India	1	2
South India	12	20
Other (Southern states)	9	15
Total	60	101

Fig. 5.1.35 Perceived ethnicity of the guises; Speaker Seven (female): Uttar Pradesh (in %)

Tab. 5.1.16 Common recognised clues; Speaker Seven (female): Uttar Pradesh

Clue	Frequencies
Speech rate	10
Tone	10
Total	20

The origin of Speaker Eight is recognised by 12 % of the sample (cf. Figure 5.1.36). As is the case with Speakers Two and Five, his ethnicity is generally linked to a Northern one (64 %) for educational reasons (cf. above). This result supports earlier findings which show a significant correlation between Southern accents and a perceived lower level of education (cf. Section 5.1.3.1).

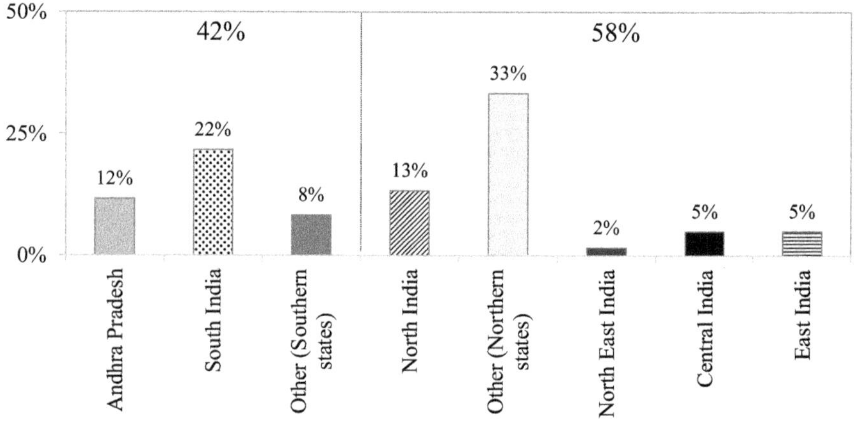

Location	N	%
Andhra Pradesh	7	12
South India	13	22
Other (Southern states)	5	8
North India	8	13
Other (Northern states)	20	33
North East India	1	2
Central India	3	5
East India	3	5
Total	60	100

Fig. 5.1.36 Perceived ethnicity of the guises; Speaker Eight (male): Andhra Pradesh (in %)

Table 5.1.17 sheds light on a new clue that the community use to identify the guise: the realisation of the voiceless alveolar fricative /s/ produced in the post-alveolar region as a voiceless palato-alveolar fricative [ʃ]. Both sounds are homophones for Speaker Eight.

Tab. 5.1.17 Common recognised clues; Speaker Eight (male): Andhra Pradesh

Clue	**Frequencies**
L1 influence	7
Tone	5
[ʃ]	4
Total	16

The results above show that Kannada English (Speaker Three) is the most frequently identified IndE accent according to the community members, soon followed by Marathi English (Speaker Four) and Bengali English (Speaker One). Interestingly, despite the commonly held folk belief of the community, i.e., South Indians have a peculiar and distinctive English accent, Northern IndE accents are detected more easily. These perceived differences, in addition to supporting results analysed earlier (cf. Section 5.1.3.1), indicate that speakers tend to differentiate on a binary level (North vs. South) rather than on a state-to state one. Yet, the reported results shed light on a higher awareness of perception with respect to Southern IndE accents. Although their location is partly recognised or, at times, not recognised at all, Southern stimuli are identified more easily according to precise phonetic realisations which seemingly index specific accents of Southern IndE.

The reactions of the community's subgroups towards the origin of the stimuli and the clues for accent discrimination support earlier findings. Table 5.1.18 shows the accent recognition indices of the male and the female subgroups.

		1 f West Bengal		4 m Maharashtra		6 m Punjab		7 f Uttar Pradesh		2 m Tamil Nadu		3 f Karnataka L1: Konkani		5 f Karnataka L1: Kannada		8 m Andhra Pradesh	
		male	female	male	female	male	female	male	female	male	female	male	female	male	female	male	female
Home State	N	6	4	9	8	3	1	1	3	6	2	11	7			6	1
	%	20	13	30	27	10	3	3	10	20	7	37	23			20	3
North India	N	3	8	5	3	7	8	5	8	5	5	2	6	7	11	2	6
	%	10	27	17	10	23	27	17	27	17	17	7	20	23	37	7	20
Other (Northern states)	N	11	10	6	9	8	13	10	11	6	11	7	11	8	7	10	10
	%	37	33	20	30	27	43	33	37	20	37	23	37	27	23	33	33
North West India	N			0	1			1	0			2	0	0	1		
	%			0	3			3	0			7	0	0	3		
North East India	N			1	0							0	1	3	1	1	0
	%			3	0							0	3	10	3	3	0
West India	N			0	2	1	1							1	0		
	%			0	7	3	3							3	0		
East India	N					1	0			0	1	1	0	1	2	1	2
	%					3	0			0	3	3	0	3	7	3	7
Central India	N			2	1	0	2			0	2	1	1	1	2	1	2
	%			7	3	0	7			0	7	3	3	3	7	3	7
Central West India	N											0	1				
	%											0	3				
Central East India	N			0	1												
	%			0	3												
South India	N	6	5	2	3	6	2	7	5	8	5	5	2	6	4	6	7
	%	20	17	7	10	20	7	23	17	27	17	17	7	20	13	20	23
Other (Southern states)	N	4	3	5	1	3	3	6	3	5	4	1	0	3	2	3	2
	%	13	10	17	3	10	10	20	10	17	13	3	0	10	7	10	7
South West India	N					1	0					0	1				
	%					3	0					0	3				
South East India	N			0	1												
	%			0	3												
total	N	30	30	30	30	30	30	30	30	30	30	30	30	30	30	30	30
	%	100	100	101	99	99	100	99	101	101	101	100	99	99	100	99	100

Tab. 5.1.18 Perceived ethnicity of the guises according to gender

The results suggest that, overall, the male speakers are clearly more accurate in discriminating the guises. However, an interesting division surfaces among the two subgroups: the male speakers are better at recognising the Southern stimuli – with the exception of Speaker Four (female: 70 %, male: 74 %) – while the female speakers tend to be more accurate in the discrimination of the Northern guises. Specifically, the male informants are more accurate in the identification of Speaker Two (64 % as against 37 % of the female subgroup), Speaker Three (male: 57 %, female: 33 %), Speaker Four (male:74 %, female: 70 %), Speaker Five (male: 30 %, female: 20 %) and Speaker Eight (male 50 %, female: 33 %).[80] Their female counterparts are more accurate in discriminating the following guises: Speaker One (female: 73 %, male: 67 %), Speaker Six (female: 73 %, male: 60 %) and Speaker Seven (female: 74 %, male: 53 %). While the results suggest that the male informants are generally better at recognising IndE guises according to both their home states and their ethnicity, it is worth taking into consideration the accuracy of discrimination of the female sample. Their recognition of Northern

80 The total percentages are obtained by adding the respective values of the correct ethnicity locations of each guise.

guises over Southern ones may shed light on their already ascertained higher awareness of perception and production of prestige norms, thus supporting earlier research on the topic (Milroy/Gordon 2003; Trudgill 1983; Wolfram/Fasold 1974) and earlier claims according to which Northern IndE varieties seemingly serve as superordinate norms in the student community (cf. Sections 5.1.3.1 and 5.2.1.1.2).

		1 f West Bengal		4 m Maharashtra		6 m Punjab		7 f Uttar Pradesh		2 m Tamil Nadu		3 f Karnataka L1: Konkani		5 f Karnataka L1: Kannada		8 m Andhra Pradesh	
		North	South	North	South	North	South	North	South	North	South	North	South	North	South	North	South
Home State	N	6	4	7	10	2	2	1	3	2	6	6	12			2	5
	%	18	15	21	38	6	8	3	12	6	23	18	46			6	19
North India	N	8	3	6	2	6	9	10	3	8	2	4	4	11	6	3	5
	%	24	12	18	8	18	35	29	12	24	8	12	15	32	23	9	19
Other (Northern states)	N	14	7	11	4	16	5	12	9	8	9	13	5	9	6	14	7
	%	41	27	32	15	47	19	35	35	24	35	38	19	26	23	41	27
North West India	N			1	0			1	0			2	0	0	1		
	%			3	0			3	0			6	0	0	4		
North East India	N			0	1							1	0	3	1	0	1
	%			0	4							3	0	9	4	0	4
West India	N			2	0	1	1							1	0		
	%			6	0	3	4							3	0		
East India	N					1	0			1	0	1	0	4	0	2	1
	%					3	0			3	0	3	0	12	0	6	4
Central India	N			2	1	1	1			2	0	2	0	1	2	3	0
	%			6	4	3	4			6	0	6	0	3	8	9	0
Central West India	N											1	0				
	%											3	0				
Central East India	N			1	0												
	%			3	0												
South India	N	2	9	4	1	4	4	8	4	11	2	3	4	5	5	9	4
	%	6	35	12	4	12	15	24	15	32	8	9	15	15	19	26	15
Other (Southern states)	N	4	3	0	6	2	4	2	7	2	7	0	1	0	5	1	3
	%	12	12	0	23	6	15	6	27	6	27	0	4	0	19	3	12
South West India	N					1	0					1	0				
	%					3	0					3	0				
South East India	N			0	1												
	%			0	4												
Total	N	34	26	34	26	34	26	34	26	34	26	34	26	34	26	34	26
	%	101	101	101	100	101	100	100	101	101	101	101	99	100	100	100	100

Tab. 5.1.19 Perceived ethnicity of the guises according to ethnicity

Ethnicity sheds new light on the degree to which the Northern and Southern participants recognise their in-group peers (cf. Tab. 5.1.19). Overall, the results suggest that people coming from either the same state of the guises or their same ethnic location tend to be more accurate in accent discrimination. As a matter of fact, the Northern informants recognise the Northern guises better (Speaker One: North 83 %, South 54 %; Speaker Four: North 77 %, South 65 %; Speaker Six: North 71 %, South 62 %; Speaker Seven: North 67 %, South 59 %), the Southern participants do so with the Southern ones (Speaker Two: North 44 %, South 58 %; Speaker Three: North 27 %, South 65 %; Speaker Five: North 15 %, South 38 %; Speaker Eight: North 35 %, South 46 %).

Table 5.1.20 shows the accent recognition indices according to the extralinguistic variable *time spent in Heidelberg*. On the whole, the reported results reveal that (i) the newcomers are better at recognising the guises and that (ii) those who have been living in Heidelberg longer have a tendency to mark Northern vs. Southern differences more strongly.

		1 f West Bengal		4 m Maharashtra		6 m Punjab		7 f Uttar Pradesh		2 m Tamil Nadu		3 f Karnataka L1: Konkani		5 f Karnataka L1: Kannada		8 m Andhra Pradesh	
		0.1-1	1.1-5	0.1-1	1.1-5	0.1-1	1.1-5	0.1-1	1.1-5	0.1-1	1.1-5	0.1-1	1.1-5	0.1-1	1.1-5	0.1-1	1.1-5
Home State	N	5	5	10	7	3	1	3	1	5	3	15	3			5	2
	%	13	24	26	33	8	5	8	5	13	14	38	14			13	10
North India	N	9	2	5	3	12	3	9	4	5	5	4	4	11	7	7	1
	%	23	10	13	14	31	14	23	19	13	24	10	19	28	33	18	5
Other (Northern states)	N	15	6	10	5	13	8	13	8	10	7	9	9	9	6	12	8
	%	38	29	26	24	33	38	33	38	26	33	23	43	23	29	31	38
North West India	N			1	0			0	1			1	1	1	0		
	%			3	0			0	5			3	5	3	0		
North East India	N			0	1							1	0	1	3	1	0
	%			0	5							3	0	3	14	3	0
West India	N			2	0	1	1							1	0		
	%			5	0	3	5							3	0		
East India	N					0	1			0	1	0	1	2	1	1	2
	%					0	5			0	5	0	5	5	5	3	10
Central India	N			1	2	2	0			2	0	2	0	1	2	2	1
	%			3	10	5	0			5	0	5	0	3	10	5	5
Central West India	N											0	1				
	%											0	5				
Central East India	N			1	0												
	%			3	0												
South India	N	5	6	5	0	4	4	8	4	10	3	6	1	9	1	7	6
	%	13	29	13	0	10	19	21	19	26	14	15	5	23	5	18	29
Other (Southern states)	N	5	2	4	2	3	3	6	3	7	2	0	1	4	1	4	1
	%	13	10	10	10	8	14	15	14	18	10	0	5	10	5	10	5
South West India	N					1	0					1	0				
	%					3	0					3	0				
South East India	N			0	1												
	%			0	5												
total	N	39	21	39	21	39	21	39	21	39	21	39	21	39	21	39	21
	%	100	102	102	101	101	100	100	100	101	100	100	101	101	101	101	102

Tab. 5.1.20 Perceived ethnicity of the guises according to time spent in Heidelberg

While the latter finding will be examined in depth in Section 5.1.3.4, there seems to be a tendency that people who have been living in Heidelberg less than a year are more accurate in accent discrimination (cf. Section 5.1.3.3.3). The newcomers are better at recognising the following guises: Speaker One (0.1–1: 74 %, 1.1–5: 63 %), Speaker Two (0.1–1: 57 %, 1.1–5: 38 %), Speaker Three (0.1–1: 56 %, 1.1–5: 24 %), Speaker Five (0.1–1: 33 %, 1.1–5: 10 %), Speaker Six (0.1–1: 72 %, 1.1–5: 57 %) and Speaker Seven (0.1–1: 64 %, 1.1–5: 62 %). Speakers Four (0.1–1: 68 %, 1.1–5: 81 %) and Eight (0.1–1: 38 %, 1.1–5: 44 %) are the only exceptions.

5.1.3.3 Correlation

The sum total of the guises from the Accent Identification Task recognised by each participant and the values attributed to the subgroups of the main extralinguistic variables are tested for correlations between them. A full account of the sum total of the guises as identified correctly by each participant is shown in Tab. 5.1.21, along with the values attributed to the extralinguistic variables at issue.[81]

Informant	Gender	Ethnicity	Time in HD	Integration index	Guises identified correctly		Informant	Gender	Ethnicity	Time in HD	Integration index	Guises identified correctly
RFmMa	1	1	1	3	7		NPfMP	2	1	2	2	4
SDfKa	2	2	1	4	7		DVfAP	2	2	2	3	4
JGMfKe	2	2	1	4	6		MGofUt	2	1	1	4	4
MMfKa	2	2	1	4	6		ATmDe	1	1	1	3	4
PPmKa	1	2	1	4	6		JDfMa	2	1	1	3	4
RNmKa	1	2	2	2	6		SSmKe	1	2	2	4	4
ABmDe	1	1	1	4	6		SLfUP	2	1	1	1	4
URmRa	1	1	2	4	5		SMfMa	2	1	1	4	4
DTfUt	2	1	2	4	5		SPmKa	1	2	1	3	4
TKfMa	2	1	2	4	5		MGfUt	2	1	1	2	4
GSmDe	1	1	2	2	5		SSmKa	1	2	1	3	4
TDfMa	2	1	1	2	5		SSmMa	1	1	1	2	4
SSmUt	1	1	1	3	5		APmTN	1	2	1	2	4
STfBi	2	1	1	4	5		SSfWB	2	1	1	0	3
ARmKe	1	2	2	4	5		SSmHa	1	1	2	3	3
KDmWB	1	1	1	3	5		HTmUP	1	1	2	2	3
VSmTN	1	2	1	4	5		PNmKe	1	2	1	3	3
DSfWB	2	1	1	4	5		BSmGu	1	1	2	4	3
BJmGu	1	1	2	4	5		SDfMP	2	1	1	2	2
PVfKa	2	2	1	3	5		ASmMP	1	1	2	4	3
AVmDe	1	1	1	4	5		NKSfTN	2	2	2	3	3
AHfKa	2	2	1	4	5		SAmKa	1	2	1	3	3
DLfMan	2	1	1	2	5		ASfKe	2	2	2	3	3
OFmTN	1	2	1	3	5		VJRfKa	2	2	2	3	3
PGfMa	2	1	1	3	5		RDfKa	2	2	2	2	3
SVmKa	1	2	1	4	5		RMfMa	2	1	1	2	2
KMmKe	1	2	1	0	5		MNmKa	1	2	2	4	2
SPfBi	2	1	1	3	4		VRmTN	1	2	2	3	2
JGfMa	2	1	2	4	4		SHfUP	2	1	1	1	2
KGfPu	2	1	1	2	4		SLmKa	1	2	2	3	2

Tab. 5.1.21 Correlation values for *gender*, *ethnicity*, *time spent in Heidelberg* and *network* male (1), female (2); North (1), South (2); 0.1–1 (1), 1.1–5 (2) Integration Index: highly unintegrated (0), unintegrated (1), somewhat integrated (2), integrated (3), highly integrated (4)

For this purpose, Spearman-Rho rank and Pearson's product-moment coefficient's correlation are performed on each of the main extralinguistic independent variable (i.e., *gender*, *ethnicity* and *time spent in Heidelberg*), on the dependent variable of *network* (analysed in Section 5.1.1.4) and on the results from the Accent Identification Task.[82] The aim of this correlation analysis is to

81 The same set of data will recur in Section 5.1.3.5, which deals with the implicational arrangement of the guises and the participants. However, they will be ordered differently for a different purpose. While the present section reveals the *strength* of the relationship between the variables, Section 5.1.3.5 will support the findings from the present section and will shed light on the *direction* of change in progress.

82 The Spearman's rank-order correlation is the non-parametric version of the Pearson product-moment correlation. Spearman's correlation coefficient, (ρ, also signified by r_s)

establish if there are possible connections between how the participants react towards accent variation and whether this is due to their gender, ethnicity, length of stay in Heidelberg or their network in-group affiliations.

Sections 5.1.3.3.1–5.1.3.3.5 will deal with the correlation analysis of each variable and will give some new insight into the ways in which the community's subgroups react towards accent variation.

5.1.3.3.1 Gender

The sum scores resulting from the addition of the values attributed to the gender of the informants on the y axis as well as the sum total of the guises as identified correctly by each participant on the x axis are shown in Fig. 5.1.37. The density plot shows the frequency of the values: the darker its shade, the higher its intensity and vice versa. The areas above and to the right of the plot represent histograms showing the distribution of the values on the x axis and the y one, respectively.

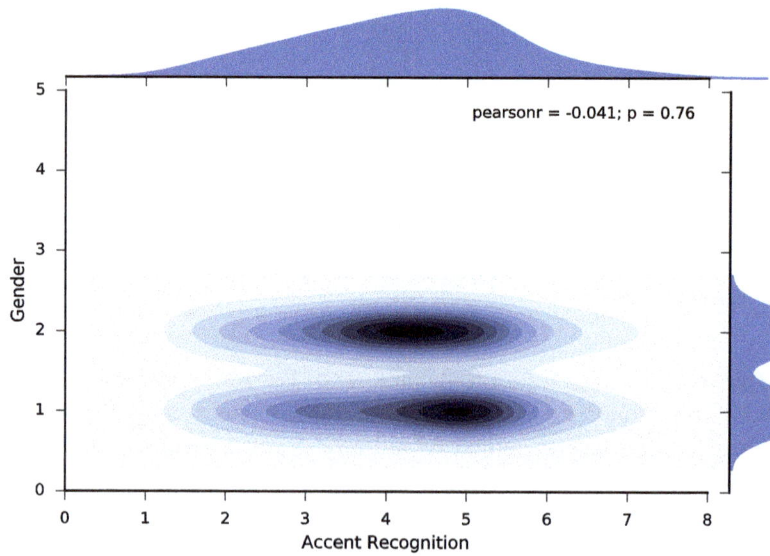

Fig. 5.1.37 Correlation between gender and accent identification ($r = -0.04$; $r_s = -0.05$; $r^2 = 0.0017$; $p = 0.76$)

measures the strength and the direction of association between two ranked variables. For a more detailed account of correlation analysis cf. Section 4.4.1.3.

By normal standards, the association between the two variables would not be considered statistically significant (p = 0.76). The plots are spread almost equally above y = 1 (male) and y = 2 (female). This means that *gender* and accent recognition show a linear relationship, i.e., one variable increases by approximately the same rate as the other. Moreover, they have a weak negative association ($r = -0.01$; $r_s = -0.05$), which indicates that above-average values of one tend to accompany below-average values of the other, i.e., one variable decreases when the other increases. This can be seen by the positioning of the darker shades of the plot: while y = 1 approximates x = 5, y = 2 does so with x = 4. In other words, male speakers are better at recognising the guises. This finding supports the results discussed in Section 5.1.3.2.

5.1.3.3.2 Ethnicity

Figure 5.1.38 shows that there is no significant correlation between *ethnicity* and accent identification (p = 0.94). The lack of correlation between the two may be due to the fact that the Northern participants recognise the Northern guises better, the Southern participants do so with the Southern ones. This fair balance between ethnicity-clustered participants and ethnicity-clustered stimuli may be the reason why the two variables do not correlate (cf. Section 5.1.3.2).

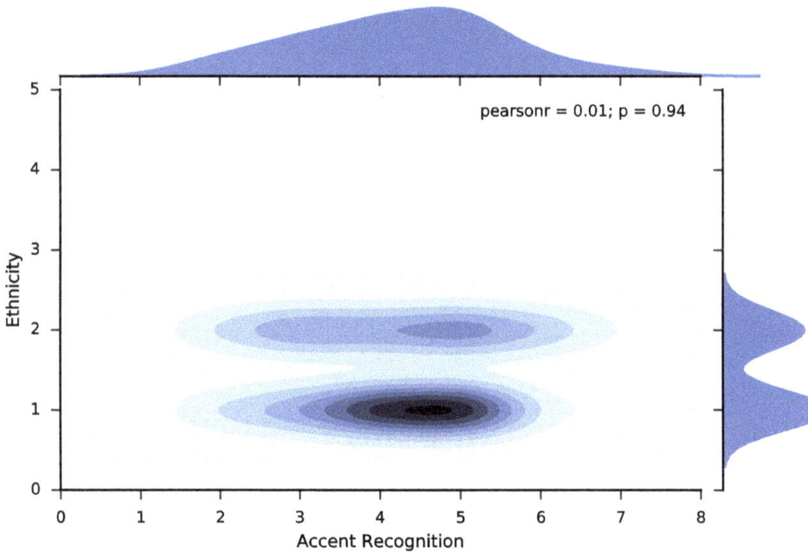

Fig. 5.1.38 Correlation between ethnicity and accent identification ($r = 0.01$; $r_s = 0.01$; $r^2 = 0.0001$; $p = 0.94$)

5.1.3.3.3 Time Spent in Heidelberg

The results from the Spearman-Rho rank and the Pearson's product-moment coefficient's correlation tests reveal that the correlation between *time spent in Heidelberg* and accent recognition is statistically significant (cf. Fig. 5.1.39; $r = -0.3$; $r_s = -0.3$; $r^2 = 0.09$; $p = 0.018$*). The association between the two variables is weak negative and, as is the case with *gender*, the high numerical values of one variable relate to the low numerical ones of the other. The density plot shows that at point (5,1) the shades are darker. Most of the informants who have guessed five guises correctly ($x = 5$) belong to the 0.1–1 subgroup. On a similar note, the peak of the histogram is at $x = 5$, which means that the highest accent recognition among all the samples is at $x = 5$. Likewise, the histogram to the right shows the same thing for the values on the y axis and, as expected, the peak is at $y = 1$. In other words, the lesser the time the participants have been spending in Heidelberg, the better they are at recognising the guises. This result is corroborated by the negative r and r_s values.

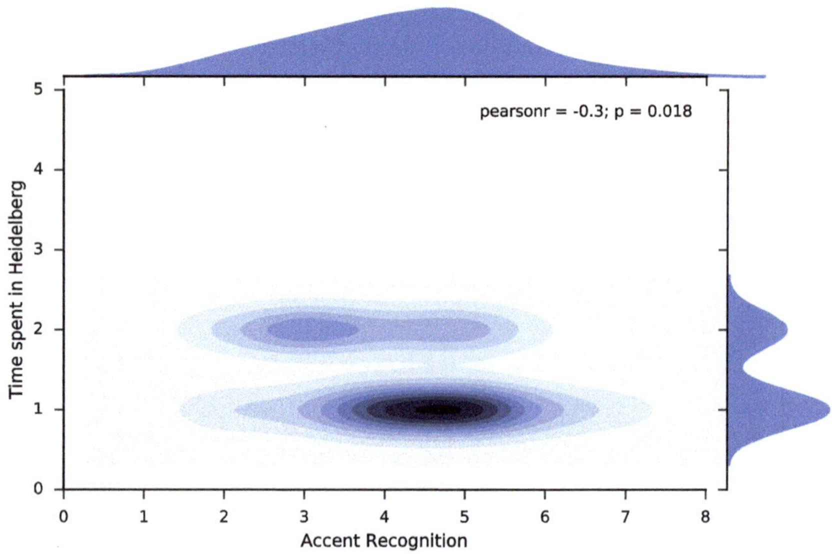

Fig. 5.1.39 Correlation between time spent in Heidelberg and accent identification ($r = -0.3$; $r_s = -0.3$; $r^2 = 0.09$; $p = 0.018$*)

An intuitive way of accounting for this result is that newcomers generally have stronger transnational ties and, thus, are seemingly keener on connecting with their mother country. The majority of them also top the scale for integration in the network-strength scale, just as they do for status. Moreover, the students who have lived in Heidelberg for between 1.1 and 5 years have had time to build up a local network as well, which decreases the impact of the mother country (cf. Section 5.1.3.3.4).

5.1.3.3.4 Network

The network-integration indices show a significant weak positive correlation between accent recognition and the sociometric status of the participants (cf. Figure 5.1.40; $r = 0.35$; $r_s = 0.35$; $r^2 = 0.09$; $p = 0.017$*). The density plot shows that at point (5,4) the shades are darker, i.e., the density of the values is higher. The majority of the informants who identify five guises correctly ($x = 5$) are highly integrated members ($y = 4$). On a similar note, the peak of the histogram is at $x = 5$, which means that the highest accent recognition among all the samples is at $x = 5$. Likewise, the histogram to the right shows the same thing for the values on the y axis and, as expected, the peak is at $y = 4$. Since the plot is more spread on the south-west of the figure, there is a linear correlation of variables on both axes, which is corroborated by the positive r and r_s values. Both variables move in the same direction, i.e., as one increases, the other increases as well.

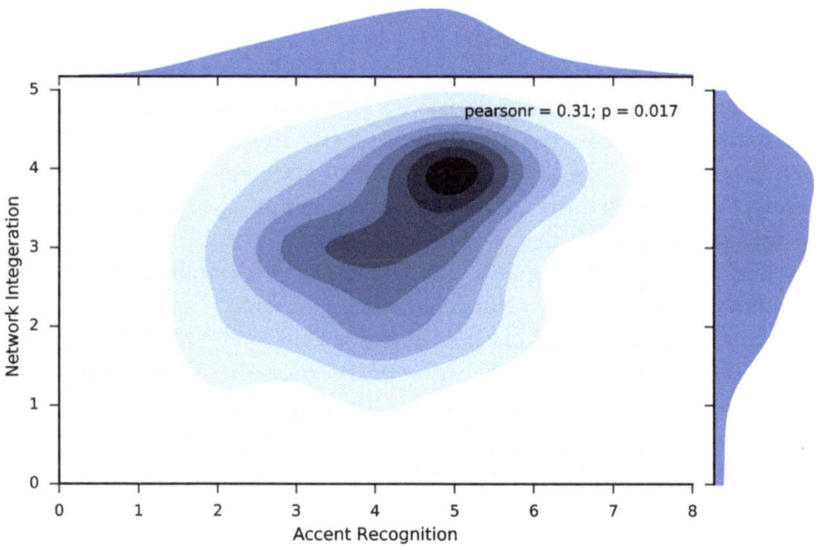

Fig. 5.1.40 Correlation between network and accent identification ($r = 0.31$; $r_s = 0.35$; $r^2 = 0.09$; $p = 0.017$*)

This result sheds light on the importance of network ties, accent perception and language variation within the Indian student community at issue since it shows that the more integrated the participants, the better they are at recognising the guises. Moreover, the present finding supports the correlation with *time spent in Heidelberg* investigated in Section 5.1.3.3.3. Highly integrated participants constitute the "ego" (Milroy 1980:46) or the core of the first-order network zone and are the ones usually responsible for language change. In this case, they index a higher level of awareness of accent variation.

5.1.3.4 Similarities and Differences

The Bonferroni-corrected results of the ethnicity-clustered guises presented in Section 5.1.3.1 show the following trends: (i) some informants have higher standards than others with respect to accent variation, and (ii) some find the differences between Northern and Southern stimuli more striking than others. The present section aims to analyse the similarities and differences of the ratings of the community members in order to have a broader perspective on what parameters they rely on in accent identification with regard to *gender*, *ethnicity*, *time spent in Heidelberg* and *network*. Most importantly, the section will provide some new insight in how the participants handle Likert scales overall and will shed light on their ratings of Northern and Southern IndE accents with regard to the correlations analysed in Section 5.1.3.3.

The data are interpreted on the averages of readiness-for-action, amiability and intellectuality traits. The analysis is performed as follows: Likert-scale mean values of Northern-clustered stimuli are deducted from the Southern-clustered ones. When positive, the result indicates that Northern guises are 'better'. There are few cases in which the result is negative, thus indicating that Southern stimuli are rated more positively than Northern ones. Differences between averages are presented as spaces between dots. The first level of the extralinguistic variables analysed, i.e., male (*gender*); North (*ethnicity*); 1 month -1 year (*time spent in Heidelberg*), is indicated by black dots, the second level, i.e., female (*gender*); South (*ethnicity*); 1.1–5 years (*time spent in Heidelberg*), by white ones.

Figures 5.1.41–5.1.45 show the similarities and differences of ethnicity-clustered stimuli according to *gender*. On the x axis, the values are ordered in ascending order. The primary and secondary axes indicate the speakers belonging to each subgroup. Overall, the data below show that the female students have higher standards than their male counterparts. Their ratings always top the scale for intellectuality, amiability and readiness for action and suggest that they exhibit stronger attitudes than men. This finding is in line with earlier sociolinguistic studies according to which women tend to show lower rates for stigmatised vernacular variants and higher ones for prestige forms (Trudgill 1983). In consequence, the female subgroup shows more awareness in their attitudes towards speech with regard to perceived accent variation (already in Wolfram/Fasold 1974).

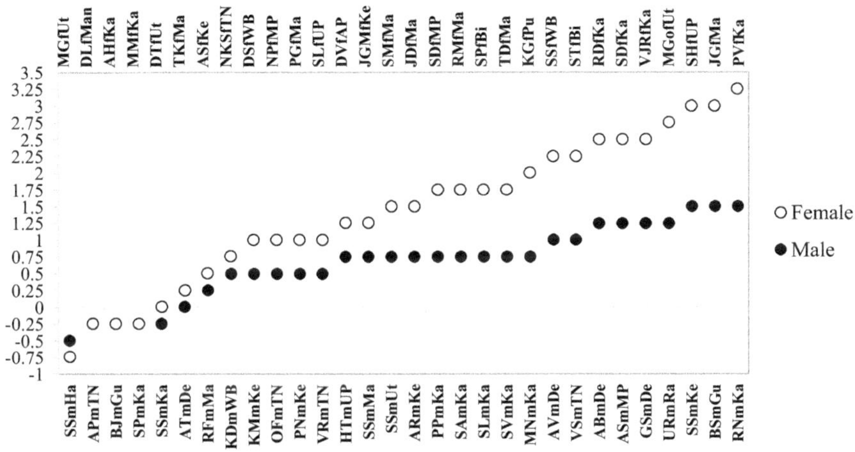

Fig. 5.1.41 Similarities and differences for ethnicity-clustered stimuli according to gender; Correctness (n = 60)

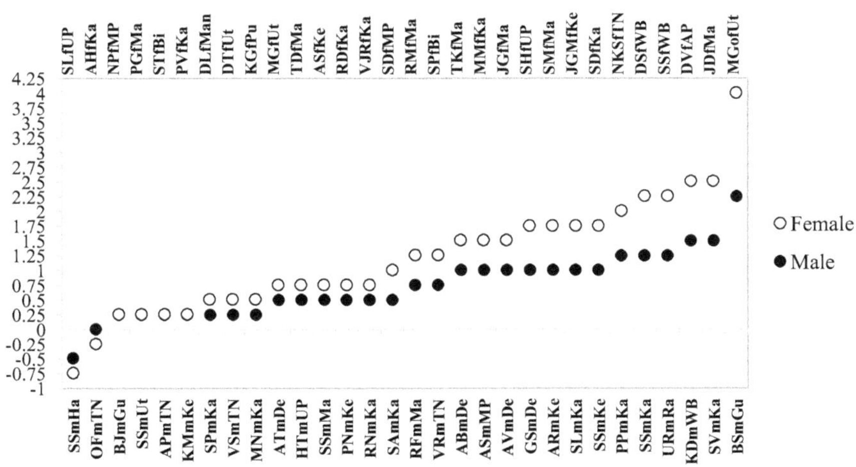

Fig. 5.1.42 Similarities and differences for ethnicity-clustered stimuli according to gender; Education (n = 60)

The male sample appears more unified in its ratings. The figures below show a rather flat representation of their attitudes towards ethnicity-clustered stimuli with few exceptions at either ends. This means that they handle Likert scales rather similarly. Again, this result concurs with earlier findings on the topic, characterising men as stylistically less flexible than women and with a tendency to develop narrower linguistic repertoires (Holmes 1997).

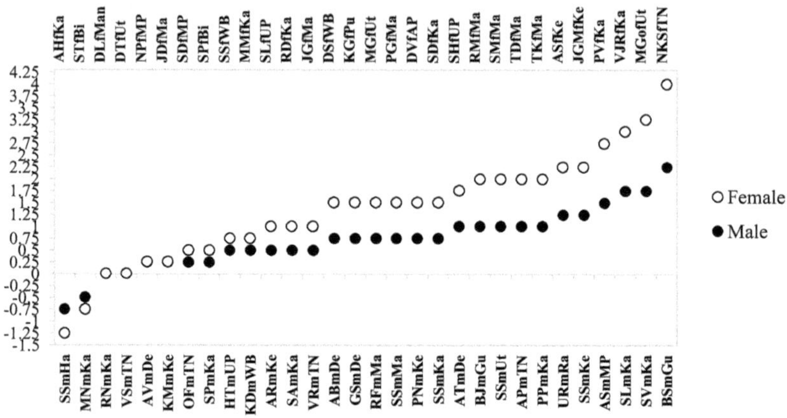

Fig. 5.1.43 Similarities and differences for ethnicity-clustered stimuli according to gender; Ambition (n = 60)

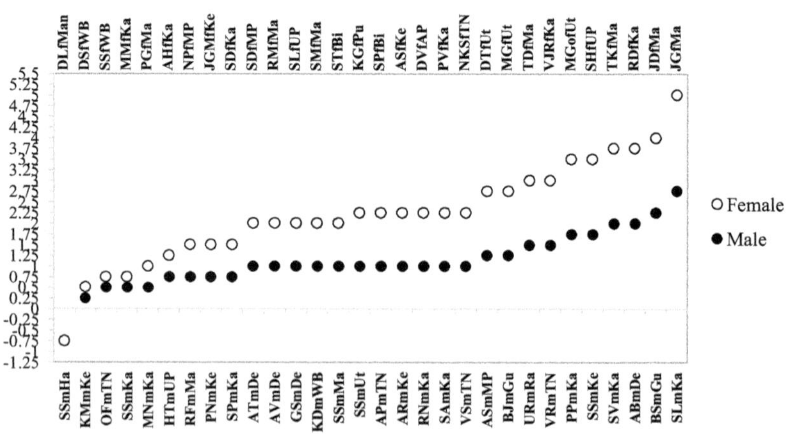

Fig. 5.1.44 Similarities and differences for ethnicity-clustered stimuli according to gender; Confidence (n = 60)

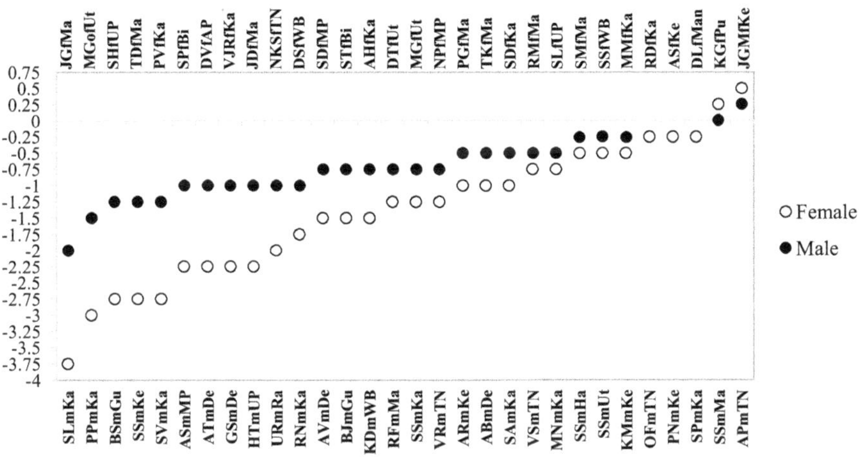

Fig. 5.1.45 Similarities and differences for ethnicity-clustered stimuli according to gender; Accent Improvement (n = 60)

Speakers' reactions towards Northern and Southern stimuli reveal interesting results with respect to *ethnicity* as well. As is the case with *gender*, the primary and secondary axes indicate the speakers belonging to each subgroup (North vs. South). Figures 5.1.46–5.1.51 suggest that the Northern participants tend to have more unified views about IndE accents.

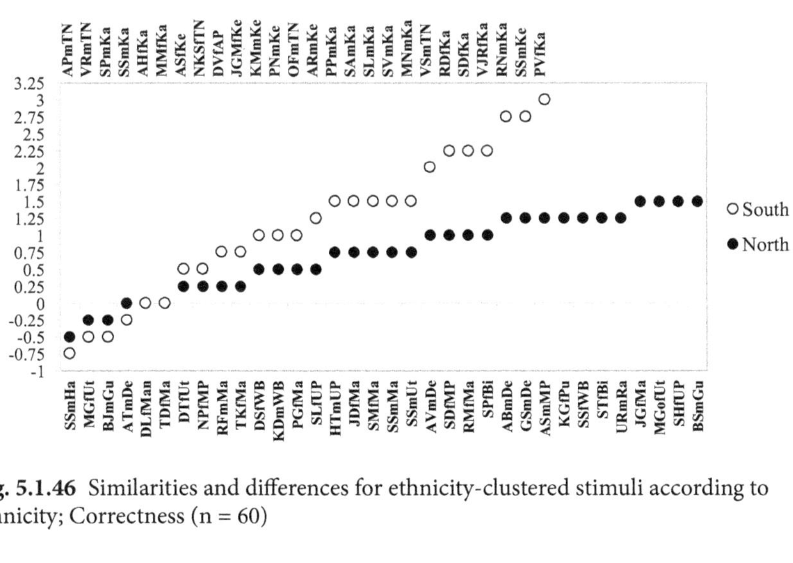

Fig. 5.1.46 Similarities and differences for ethnicity-clustered stimuli according to ethnicity; Correctness (n = 60)

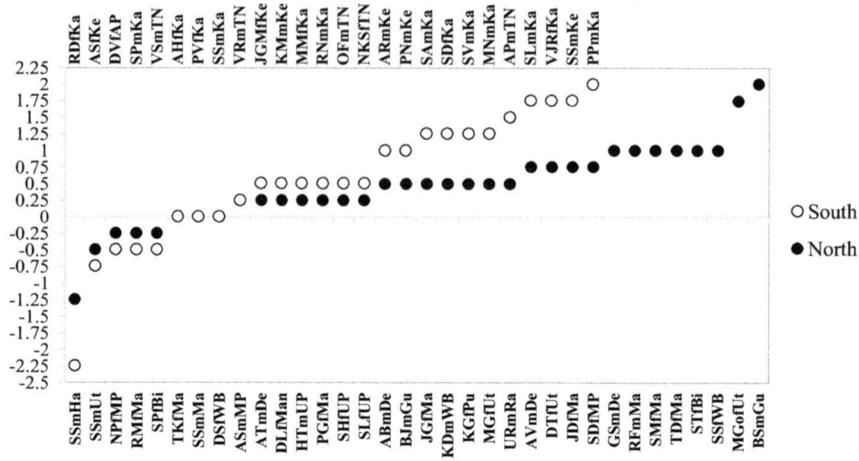

Fig. 5.1.47 Similarities and differences for ethnicity-clustered stimuli according to ethnicity; Intelligence (n = 60)

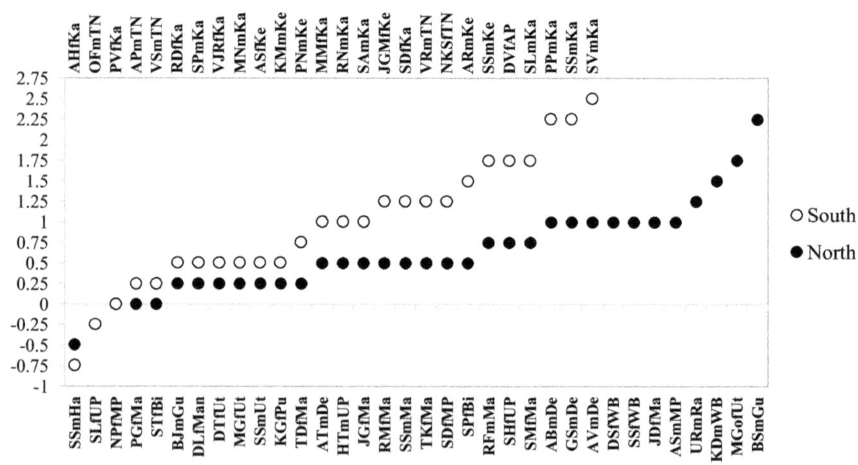

Fig. 5.1.48 Similarities and differences for ethnicity-clustered stimuli according to ethnicity; Education (n = 60)

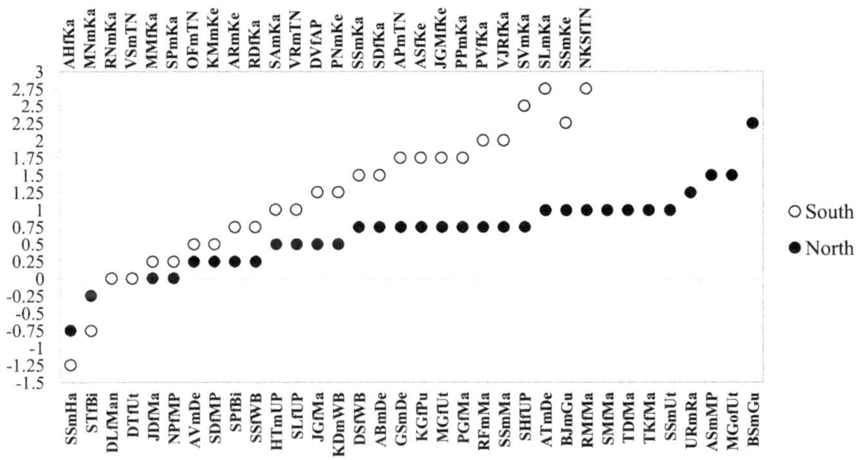

Fig. 5.1.49 Similarities and differences for ethnicity-clustered stimuli according to ethnicity; Ambition (n = 60)

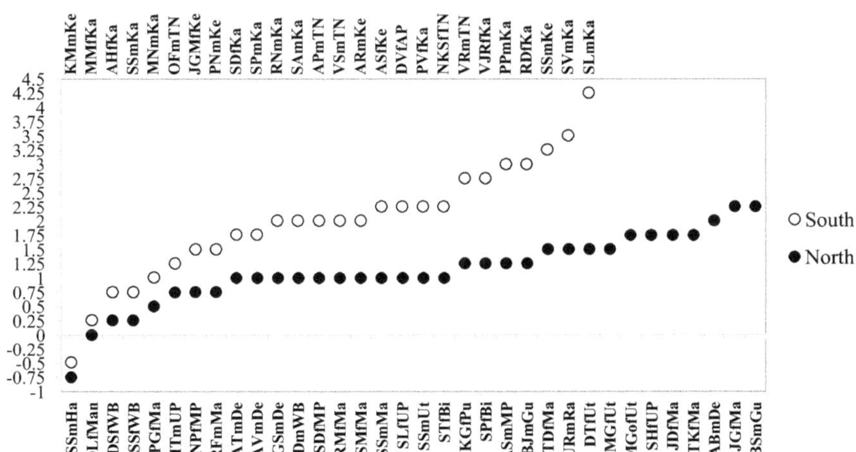

Fig. 5.1.50 Similarities and differences for ethnicity-clustered stimuli according to ethnicity; Confidence (n = 60)

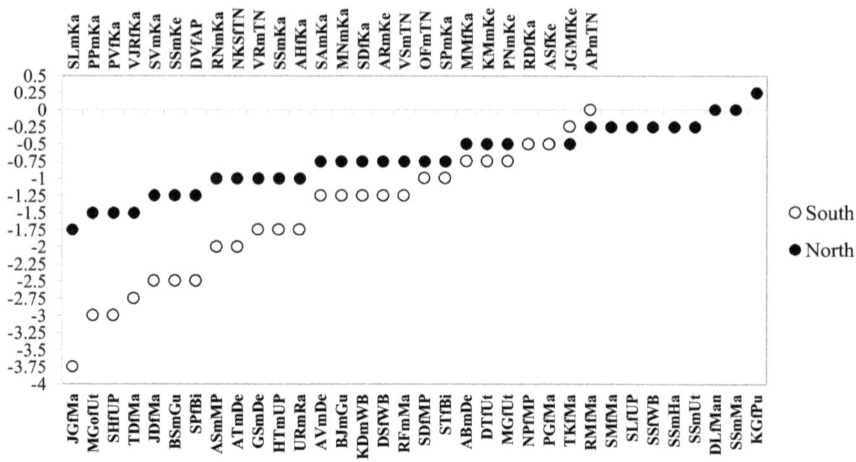

Fig. 5.1.51 Similarities and differences for ethnicity-clustered stimuli according to ethnicity; Accent Improvement (n = 60)

Overall, their language behaviour is in line with the male subgroup of the sample since both groups seem to respond to Likert scales similarly. This finding supports the statistical analysis discussed in Section 5.1.3.1 which shows that Southern speakers have taken over the stereotypes of the Northerners about themselves. This is particularly evident with respect to <accent improvement> (cf. Fig. 5.1.51): the massive differences between the Northern sample and the Southern one suggest that the latter holds strongly negative attitudes towards Southern IndE varieties. The ratings of the Southern subgroup shed light on the degree to which they perceive the Northern/Southern accent differences, which appear as massively demarcated and leaning towards the preference for Northern IndE accents. Subsequently, the Southern participants exhibit stronger language attitudes towards accent variation.

Figures 5.1.52–5.1.54 show the similarities and differences of ethnicity-clustered stimuli according to *time spent in Heidelberg*. At a first glance, the first level of the variable – corresponding to speakers who have been living in Heidelberg up to one year – constitute the more homogeneous sample. Their ratings are rather flat and, with some interesting exceptions which will be discussed below, suggest that the newcomers exhibit less strong attitudes towards accent variation.

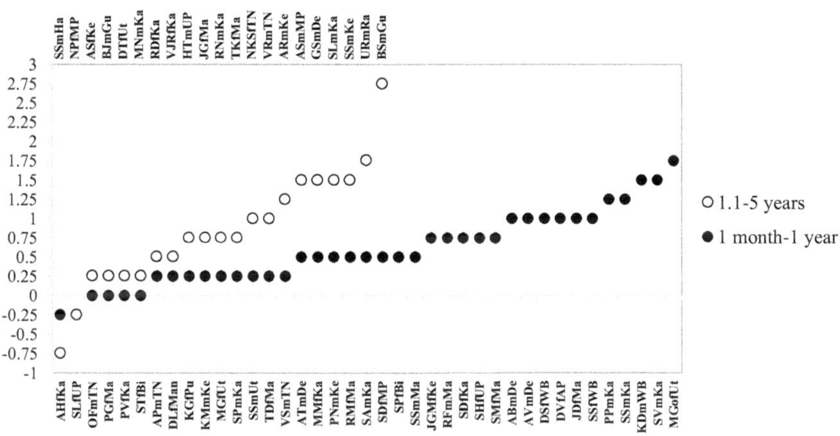

Fig. 5.1.52 Similarities and differences for ethnicity-clustered stimuli according to time spent in Heidelberg; Education (n = 60)

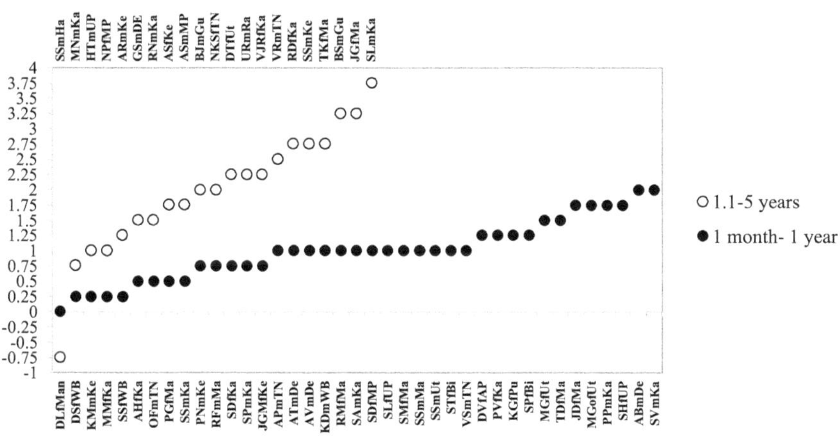

Fig. 5.1.53 Similarities and differences for ethnicity-clustered stimuli according to time spent in Heidelberg; Confidence (n = 60)

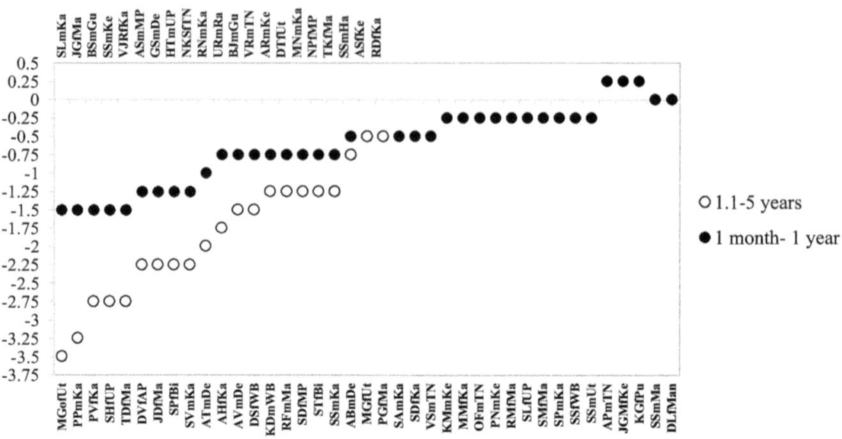

Fig. 5.1.54 Similarities and differences for ethnicity-clustered stimuli according to time spent in Heidelberg; Accent Improvement (n = 60)

However, a close look at the figures reveals that by correlating the ratings of *time spent in Heidelberg* with those of other extralinguistic variables, an interesting difference surfaces. The longer the Northern informants have been living in Heidelberg (and, hypothetically, have met other Indian ethnicities), the more the differences increase. This is most probably due to their assimilation into the German/international environment that Heidelberg offers. This finding is in line with earlier claims that Northern participants have stereotypical views about themselves and the South and seems to confirm and strengthen their stereotypes. On the other hand, the longer the Southerners have been living in Heidelberg and have had contacts with Northern speakers, the lesser their stereotypes and the more liberated from their former prejudices they get. In other words, while Northern stereotypes increase with time spent in Heidelberg, Southern ones decrease.

An additional correlation between *time spent in Heidelberg*, *ethnicity* and *network* sheds light on further underpinnings of the community structure. Among the 2–5 years group, there are ten Southern informants (ARmKe, ASfKe, MNmKa, NKSfTN, RDfKa, RNmKa, SLmKa, SSmKe, VJRfKa, VRmTN). According to the network strength scale discussed in Section 5.1.1.4, three of them are highly integrated (ARmKe, MNmKa, SSmKe) four are integrated (ASfKe, NKSfTN, VJRfKa, VRmTN), three somewhat integrated (RDfKa, RNmKa, SLmKa). The figures above suggest that the more integrated these students are, the less they perceive North/South differences, hence the lesser the stereotypes about Northern speakers and themselves. This result substantiates the hypothesis that *time spent in Heidelberg* increases the stereotypes of the Northerners about Southerners and decreases those of the Southerners about themselves.

Arranging the Likert scale values of the Accent Identification Task according to their similarities and differences allows for a deeper understanding of the structure of the Heidelberg Indian student community. This disposition aims to 'compensate' the statistical ordering presented in Section 5.1.3.1 which, although significant, lacks many possibilities to interpret the data. Furthermore, it allows to order equal values according to 'linguistic sense' and sheds new light on how the main extralinguistic variables influence network structure.

On closer analysis, the present data arrangement highlights some 'anomalous' individuals within the Northern sample. Their linguistic behaviour appears to be rooted in certain social attributes that distinguish them from every other member of the student community. Following Chambers' (2009:93) descriptions of such cases, it is possible to group these individuals in two broad categories:

> 'Oddballs', the subgroup whose attitudes mark them in some way as non-conformists both linguistically and socially, and 'Insiders', the subgroup that appears, paradoxically, to be marked by extreme conformity, or by total integration in the group.

While the former group seems to be constituted by a "fairly desperate lot" (2009:93) and is further divided into 'outsiders', 'aspirers' and 'interlopers', the latter is seldom recognised in social studies despite its members being the most linguistically significant individuals in their communities.

The figures above show two individuals who tend to disrupt the otherwise cohesive patterns of the value arrangement: SSmMa and BSmGu. SSmMa is a male speaker from Haryana who appears to be an integrated member of the student community according to the network-strength scale discussed above. BSmGu is a male speaker from Gujarat whose social status within the community network is that of a highly integrated member. At a first glance, the ratings that SSmHa attributes to the ethnicity-clustered stimuli indicate that he favours Northern Indian accents massively. Conversely, those of BSmGU are 'typical' values which, without this new data arrangement, would have gone unnoticed. According to the distribution of the values, SSmHa is an 'oddball', BSmGU an 'insider'. Closer inspection of these two students reveals that they are not simply anomalies although they stand apart from the majority of their group. SSmHa falls into a precise social sub-category of 'oddballs'. According to Chambers' criteria (2009:106), he is an 'interloper'. In purely sociophonetic terms, an 'interloper' is someone who has moved from one dialect area to another and whose abilities to master the new dialect depend partly upon his age. In language attitude studies, an 'interloper' might be someone who, from an early age, by moving from one dialect area to another, has gradually developed strong attitudes towards different accents on the basis of his experience. The content analysis of his sociolinguistic interview highlights some social factors which are at odds with his peers. Originally from Haryana, he was born in Delhi because his father was a defense officer. For this reason, he was requested to move around the subcontinent and, when SSmHa was in school-going age, his father got a new post in Mumbai (Maharashtra). However, when he was in 6th standard, his father retired and got a new post in Haryana, so the family had to move back. Since his son had always attended special schools for the children of defense officers, he had constantly been in touch with people coming from all over the subcontinent very early. For this reason, he confesses that he has become "negatively biased" towards Southern IndE varieties because he could not tolerate their so-called 'sing-song' accents (cf. Section 5.2.1.1). His sociolinguistic position within the student community justifies his categotisation as an 'interloper' since he is an integrated member (hence, he cannot be an 'outsider') and, although he favours Southern IndE accents in all attitude traits during the Accent identification Task (cf. figures above), he defines himself "negatively biased" towards them (this is the reason why he cannot be an 'aspirer' either).

'Insiders' tend to be hardly recognised within their communities. There appears to be a tendency for individuals who are at the centre of their network to run ahead of the group in their use of salient markers or, as in the present case, in their language attitudes. Generally speaking, 'insiders' are not necessarily core members or leaders of a network, but they are frequently central ones. What they usually have in common with the core members is a high degree of involvement in the affairs of the group. BSmGu is one such example. His ratings for all language attitude traits are fairly typical, yet significantly in favour of Northern IndE guises. Furthermore, although he is highly integrated in the student network, he is not among the most acknowledged members. His reactions towards ethnicity-clustered stimuli justify his categorisation as an 'insider' in that his elusiveness appears to arise from his very normalcy. Milroy and Milroy (1985:367) define such individuals as "early adopters", i.e.,

> [...] central members of the group, having strong ties within it, and [...] highly conforming to group norms; they frequently provide a model for other non-innovative members of the group.

In other words, 'insiders' are joiners and perhaps usually followers, yet they appear to be the ones who not only adopt linguistic changes but accelerate them.

Although there is no evidence that BSmGu has acquired his attitudes before his fellows, his ratings seem to be providing a linguistic model for the values associated with Northern (= 'somewhat positive') and Southern (= 'neutral') IndE accents in his community.

5.1.3.5 Numerical and Implicational Scales

The results indicate that the participants have a tendency to discriminate IndE accents on a North-to-South basis rather than on a state-to-state one (cf. Section 5.1.3.2). In order to detect patterns for accent recognition and to support this result, the findings from the Accent Identification Task have been ordered implicationally. Glauser (1991:15) interprets implicational scales as "[...] synchronic representations of change in progress, the direction of the change being derived from extralinguistic factors".[83] Hence, the aim of the section is to emphasise the sociolinguistic patterns that have guided community members in accent identification.

The section will draw attention to both recognition levels, i.e., state-to-state and North-to-South, although a major focus will be on the latter.

5.1.3.5.1 State-to-state Distinction

The guises are arranged along the horizontal axis and the informants along the vertical one. Guises with high total scores (right location, right ethnicity, wrong location, as computed from the original score, which is 1 for right location, 0.5 for right ethnicity and 0 for wrong location) are placed further to the left-hand side of the table, and participants with high totals are placed further to the top. Extralinguistic factors (*gender*, *ethnicity*, *time spent in Heidelberg*, *network*) and their mean values are in the rightmost columns (cf. Tab. 5.1.22).

83 For a more detailed account of implicational scales cf. Rickford (2002), Pavone (1980) and DeCamp (1968).

Tab. 5.1.22 Numerical arrangement of IndE accents: state-to-state distinction + right location; x right ethnicity; – wrong location a gender; b ethnicity; c time spent in Heidelberg; d network strength f female; m male; n north; s south;

sp.	4	1	3	6	7	2	8	5	a	b	c	d	Total
accent	N	N	S	N	N	S	S	S					
SDfKa	+	+	+	-	+	+	x	x	f	s	0.1–1	4	6
MMfKa	+	+	+	x	-	-	x	x	f	s	0.1–1	4	4.5
KDmWB	+	+	-	+	-	x	x	-	m	n	0.1–1	3	4
RFmMa	x	x	+	x	x	x	+	-	m	n	0.1–1	3	4
AHfKa	+	-	+	-	+	-	x	x	f	s	0.1–1	4	4
RNmKa	x	-	+	x	x	-	+	x	m	s	1.1–5	2	4
PNmKe	x	+	+	x	-	+	-	-	m	s	0.1–1	3	4
SSmUt	x	x	+	x	+	-	-	-	m	n	0.1–1	3	3.5
SPmKa	+	-	+	-	x	+	-	-	m	s	0.1–1	3	3.5
TKfMa	+	+	-	x	x	-	x	-	f	n	1.1–5	4	3.5
URmRa	x	+	-	x	x	+	-	-	m	n	1.1–5	4	3.5
ABmDe	x	-	+	x	x	-	x	x	m	n	0.1–1	4	3.5
SVmKa	-	x	+	x	-	+	-	x	m	s	0.1–1	4	3.5
TDfMa	+	x	+	x	x	-	-	-	f	n	0.1–1	2	3.5
OFmTN	-	x	-	+	x	x	+	-	m	s	0.1–1	3	3.5
ARmKe	x	x	-	+	-	+	x	-	m	s	1.1–5	4	3.5
PVfKa	+	x	+	-	x	x	-	-	f	s	0.1–1	3	3.5
PPmKa	x	-	+	x	x	x	x	-	m	s	0.1–1	4	3.5
JGMfKe	x	x	+	x	x	x	-	-	f	s	0.1–1	4	3.5
VSmTN	+	x	x	x	-	x	x	-	m	s	0.1–1	4	3.5
KMmKe	-	x	x	-	x	x	+	x	m	s	0.1–1	0	3.5
AVmDe	x	-	-	x	x	x	+	-	m	n	0.1–1	4	3
SPfBi	x	+	-	+	x	-	-	-	f	n	0.1–1	3	3
GSmDe	x	x	+	x	-	x	-	-	m	n	1.1–5	2	3
SSmKe	+	x	x	-	x	-	-	x	m	s	1.1–5	4	3
PGfMa	-	x	x	x	x	-	x	x	f	n	0.1–1	3	3
ATmDe	x	x	x	-	x	x	-	x	m	n	0.1–1	3	3
BJmGu	+	x	-	-	-	x	x	-	m	n	1.1–5	4	2.5
APmTN	-	-	-	x	-	x	+	x	m	s	0.1–1	2	2.5
MGfUt	-	x	-	x	x	+	-	-	f	n	0.1–1	2	2.5
STfBi	x	x	-	x	x	-	-	x	f	n	0.1–1	4	2.5
DTfUt	x	x	-	x	x	-	x	-	f	n	1.1–5	4	2.5
VRmTN	-	+	x	-	-	+	-	-	m	s	1.1–5	3	2.5
SSmHa	+	+	-	-	x	-	-	-	m	n	1.1–5	3	2.5
SAmKa	+	-	x	x	-	-	-	x	m	s	0.1–1	3	2.5
SSmKa	-	x	+	x	-	-	-	x		s	0.1–1	3	2.5
SLfUP	x	x	+	-	-	x	-	-	f	n	0.1–1	1	2.5

Tab. 5.1.22 Continued

sp.	4	1	3	6	7	2	8	5	a	b	c	d	Total
DLfMan	-	x	-	x	x	x	x	-	f	n	0.1–1	2	2.5
JGfMa	x	x	-	x	x	-	-	-	f	n	1.1–5	4	2
BSmGu	x	+	-	-	-	-	x	-	m	n	1.1–5	4	2
NKSfTN	x	-	-	x	+	-	-	-	f	s	1.1–5	3	2
SMfMa	x	-	-	x	x	x	-	-	f	n	0.1–1	4	2
JDfMa	x	x	-	-	x	x	-	-	f	n	0.1–1	3	2
KGfPu	x	x	-	x	x	-	-	-	f	n	0.1–1	2	2
MNmKa	+	-	+	-	-	-	-	-	m	s	1.1–5	4	2
RDfKa	-	-	-	x	-	x	+	-	f	s	0.1–1	2	2
RMfMa	+	x	x	-	-	-	-	-	f	n	0.1–1	2	2
HTmUP	+	x	-	-	-	x	-	-	m	n	1.1–5	2	2
ASfKe	+	-	-	-	x	-	x	-	f	s	1.1–5	3	2
DVfAP	x	x	-	x	x	-	-	-	f	s	1.1–5	3	2
SSmMa	-	x	-	-	x	x	x	-	m	n	0.1–1	2	2
NPfMP	x	x	-	x	x	-	-	-	f	n	1.1–5	2	2
MGofUt	-	x	-	x	-	x	-	-	f	n	0.1–1	4	1.5
DSfWB	-	x	x	-	-	-	x	-	f	n	0.1–1	4	1.5
SSfWB	x	x	-	x	-	-	-	-	f	n	0.1–1	0	1.5
VJRfKa	-	-	-	x	x	x	-	-	f	s	1.1–5	3	1.5
ASmMP	x	-	-	x	x	-	-	-	m	n	1.1–5	4	1.5
SDfMP	-	-	-	x	x	-	-	-	f	n	0.1–1	2	1
SLmKa	-	-	-	-	x	-	x	-	m	s	1.1–5	1	1
SHfUP	-	-	-	x	-	-	-	x	f	n	0.1–1	1	1
Total	30	26	22.5	22	21	19	16	7.5					

A first glance at the table shows that it is not possible to arrange stimuli and respondents implicationally. Thus, the table reveals a numerical arrangement corresponding to accent recognition. However, a closer look at the guises suggests that the informants operationalise differences on a North-to-South basis. Northern stimuli, in fact, top the left-hand side of the table, hence showing that they are the group of guises recognised most frequently (Speakers Four, One, Six and Seven received the highest total scores).

With respect to the social data of the informants, the numerical arrangement is in line with the correlation analysis described in Section 5.1.3.3 although there are many fallacies within the disposition of values. Men are generally placed towards the top of the table, i.e., they have higher scores than women, who cluster towards the bottom. In other words, the male informants are better at recognising the guises. Northern as well as Southern informants are located both towards the top and the bottom of the scale since their identification is ethnicity-based. While the Northern participants are better at recognising Northern guises, the Southern subgroup is better at identifying its peers. Informants who have been living in Heidelberg longer are situated towards the bottom of the table, which indicates that the newcomers are generally better at identifying the guises. The most integrated respondents top the scale, i.e., they are more aware of accent recognition.

Overall, the arrangement of the guises and the respondents does not show much regularity state-wise. Moreover, the extralinguistic variables do not match the fairly regular patterns uncovered by the correlation analysis discussed in Section 5.1.3.3. However, the left-to-right disposition of the guises sheds light on a further and, most probably, more reliable path to follow, i.e., the grouping of the guises according to their ethnicity rather than their state of origin (cf. Section 5.1.3.5.2).

5.1.3.5.2 North/South Distinction

Table 5.1.23 shows the implicational arrangement of guises and participants. The arrangement follows the one of Tab. 5.1.22, i.e., the guises are along the horizontal axis, the informants along the vertical one. In this scale, 1 means right location, 0 wrong location. Although the fit of this implicational scale is only approaching significance since there are more than 10 % error cells (Guttman Reproducibility Coefficient = 0.88; Rasch Scalability Coefficient = 6.1), it nevertheless allows to discover an interesting pattern in the process of accent recognition. Overall, Northern guises received higher scores than Southern ones.

Tab. 5.1.23 Implicational arrangement of IndE accents: North-to-South distinction + right location; - wrong location a gender; b ethnicity; c time spent in Heidelberg; d network strength f female; m male; n north; s south; (Guttman Reproducibility Coefficient= 0.88; Rasch Scalability Coefficient= 6.1)

sp.	4	1	6	7	2	3	8	5	a	b	c	d	Total
accent	N	N	N	N	S	S	S	S					
SDfKa	+	+	-	+	+	+	+	+	f	s	0.1–1	4	7
MMfKa	+	+	+	-	-	+	+	+	f	s	0.1–1	4	6
RNmKa	+	-	+	+	-	+	+	+	m	s	1.1–5	2	6
ABmDe	+	-	+	+	-	+	+	+	m	n	0.1–1	4	6
ATmDe	+	+	-	+	+	+	-	+	m	n	0.1–1	3	6
AHfKa	+	-	-	+	-	+	+	+	f	s	0.1–1	4	5
SSmKe	+	+	-	+	-	+	-	+	m	s	1.1–5	4	5
STfBi	+	+	+	+	-	-	-	+	f	n	0.1–1	4	5
KMmKe	-	+	-	+	+	+	+	+	m	s	0.1–1	0	6
PGfMa	-	+	+	+	-	+	+	+	f	n	0.1–1	3	6
SVmKa	-	+	+	-	+	+	-	+	m	s	0.1–1	4	5
RFmMa	+	+	+	+	+	+	+	-	m	n	0.1–1	3	7
DTfUt	+	+	+	+	-	-	+	-	f	n	1.1–5	4	5
VSmTN	+	+	+	-	+	+	+	-	m	s	0.1–1	4	6
KDmWB	+	+	+	-	+	-	+	-	m	n	0.1–1	3	5
TKfMa	+	+	+	+	-	-	+	-	f	n	1.1–5	4	5
ARmKe	+	+	+	-	+	-	+	-	m	s	1.1–5	4	5
PPmKa	+	-	+	+	+	+	+	-	m	s	0.1–1	4	6
AVmDe	+	-	+	+	+	-	+	-	m	n	0.1–1	4	5
OFmTN	-	+	+	+	+	-	+	-	m	s	0.1–1	3	5
DLfMan	-	+	+	+	+	-	+	-	f	n	0.1–1	2	5
JGMfKe	+	+	+	+	+	+	-	-	f	s	0.1–1	4	6
SSmUt	+	+	+	+	-	+	-	-	m	n	0.1–1	3	5
TDfMa	+	+	+	+	-	+	-	-	f	n	0.1–1	2	5
PNmKe	+	+	+	-	+	+	-	-	m	s	0.1–1	3	5
GSmDe	+	+	+	-	+	+	-	-	m	n	1.1–5	2	5
PVfKa	+	+	-	+	+	+	-	-	f	s	0.1–1	3	5
SPmKa	+	-	-	+	+	+	-	-	m	s	0.1–1	3	4
SLfUP	+	+	-	-	+	+	-	-	f	n	0.1–1	1	4
URmRa	+	+	+	+	+	-	-	-	m	n	1.1–5	4	5
JDfMa	+	+	-	+	+	-	-	-	f	n	0.1–1	3	4
SMfMa	+	-	+	+	+	-	-	-	f	n	0.1–1	4	4
MGfUt	-	+	+	+	+	-	-	-	f	n	0.1–1	2	4
VJRfKa	-	-	+	+	+	-	-	-	f	s	1.1–5	3	3
JGfMa	+	+	+	+	-	-	-	-	f	n	1.1–5	4	4

(*continued on next page*)

Tab. 5.1.23 Continued

sp.	4	1	6	7	2	3	8	5	a	b	c	d	Total
KGfPu	+	+	+	+	-	-	-	-	f	n	0.1–1	2	4
DVfAP	+	+	+	+	-	-	-	-	f	s	1.1–5	3	4
SPfBi	+	+	+	+	-	-	-	-	f	n	0.1–1	3	4
NPfMP	+	+	+	+	-	-	-	-	f	n	1.1–5	2	4
SSmHa	+	+	-	+	-	-	-	-	m	n	1.1–5	3	3
NKSfTN	+	-	+	+	-	-	-	-	f	s	1.1–5	3	3
ASmMP	+	-	+	+	-	-	-	-	m	n	1.1–5	4	3
SDfMP	-	-	+	+	-	-	-	-	f	n	0.1–1	2	2
SSfWB	+	+	+	-	-	-	-	-	f	n	0.1–1	0	3
SAmKa	+	-	+	-	-	+	-	+	m	s	0.1–1	3	4
SSmKa	-	+	+	-	-	+	-	+		s	0.1–1	3	4
MGofUt	-	+	+	-	+	-	-	-	f	n	0.1–1	4	3
RDfKa	-	-	+	-	+	-	+	-	f	s	0.1–1	2	3
APmTN	-	-	+	-	+	-	+	+	m	s	0.1–1	2	4
BJmGu	+	+	-	-	+	-	+	-	m	n	1.1–5	4	4
HTmUP	+	+	-	-	+	-	-	-	m	n	1.1–5	2	3
RMfMa	+	+	-	-	-	+	-	-	f	n	0.1–1	2	3
BSmGu	+	+	-	-	-	-	+	-	m	n	1.1–5	4	4
DSfWB	-	+	-	-	-	+	+	-	f	n	0.1–1	4	3
SSmMa	-	+	-	+	+	-	+	-	m	n	0.1–1	2	4
VRmTN	-	+	-	-	+	+	-	-	m	s	1.1–5	3	3
ASfKe	+	-	-	+	-	-	+	-	f	s	1.1–5	3	3
MNmKa	+	-	-	-	-	+	-	-	m	s	1.1–5	4	2
SLmKa	-	-	-	+	-	-	+	-	m	s	1.1–5	1	2
SHfUP	-	-	+	-	-	-	-	+	f	n	0.1–1	1	2
Correct	43	42	40	38	30	27	25	15					
Incorrect	17	18	20	22	30	33	35	45					
Total	60	60	60	60	60	60	60	60					
N correct	26	28	23	23	15	10	12	5					
S correct	17	14	16	15	15	17	13	10					
N incorrect	8	5	10	11	11	24	22	29					
S incorrect	9	13	11	11	19	9	13	16					
Total	60	60	60	60	60	60	60	60					

A first look at the horizontal dimension, i.e., at the frequency with which the guises are identified, shows that there is a large difference between the most frequently recognised stimuli and the least frequently recognised ones. Speaker Four, a male student from Maharashtra is most easily recognised. With a total score of 43, he is fairly close to the highest possible score of 60, i.e., the sum total of the participants. Conversely, Speaker Five, a female student from Karnataka is the least identified guise. She has a score of 15/60. In between these two poles, there is a gradual yet steady progression from the right to the left indicating the degree of accent recognition within the community. Interestingly, a sudden break appears with Speaker Three, a female student from Karnataka.

Overall, the results indicate that, although the community appears to have rather strong ideologies towards Southern IndE accents, it fails at their recognition, perhaps since Southern IndE accents are somewhat less salient than Northern ones with respect to their specific phonological patterns. The informants might be aware of the general speech pattern of Southern IndE varieties; they might have heard different Southern Indians speak English; they might even have come across these accents in their everyday lives. In short, they might be familiar with these accents and still be unable to recognise them. An intuitive attempt to account for this might be that all the guises are highly educated speakers who attended private English-medium schools back in India before moving to Heidelberg. Thus, the folk belief of the community may be related to more 'stereotypical' idiolects rather than real ones. Nevertheless, the result is striking in that it sheds light on the ease with which Northern IndE accents are recognised and on their more positive evaluation.

Table 5.1.23 also shows considerable numbers of wrong attributions, more strongly so with the Southern guises than with the Northern ones. However, the expectation that Northern guises mistaken for Southern ones produce Southern stereotypes and vice versa is only confirmed to some extent. The overall picture is much more complex than Trudgill's (1974) unidimensional connection between wrong geographical attribution and liking of a place since the guises are not taken as complex people, not just as Northerners or Southerners. While the geographical dimension does not seem to play a major role in accent discrimination, the intellectuality, amiability, readiness-for-action and reliability ones do (cf. Sections 5.1.3.1 and 5.1.3.2). The speakers rate the guises according to their personal preferences and whether they sound pleasant, correct, not so pleasant, not so correct, etc., perhaps even as resembling people they know. In other words, although it is tempting to juxtapose correct and incorrect attributions, the first tabulations in this direction show a very complex pattern that deserves a socio-psychological treatment that would lead far beyond the aims of the present work.

5.1.3.6 Cluster Analysis and Bubble Matrices

Sections 5.1.3.1–5.1.3.5 emphasises the participants' very strong overt reactions towards regional accents of IndE, based on stereotypes of speakers from certain regions being more friendly, pleasant, educated, etc. The analysis of covert attitudes shows that languages are not uniformly distributed along the poles of amiability (or solidarity) and intellectuality (or status) but rather are competing for both. Although individuals find certain accents more attractive than others, this usually has little to do with the pleasantness of the sound. Individual features of accents can be judged as prestigious for speakers coming from a given region and stigmatised for others. Since these generally recognised stereotypical attitudes towards certain IndE accents are conceptual rather than empirically founded, the question of what underlying factors are involved in the speakers' perceptions is still to be addressed.

The multivariate tools used in the present study are hierarchical cluster analysis and bubble matrices. As mentioned in Sections 4.4.1.4 and 5.1.2.2, factor analysis is not taken into account because it requires interval data and large-scale samples.

The present section will be organised as follows: Section 5.1.3.6.1 will draw attention to the clustering of reliability traits, i.e., <degree of certainty>, <degree of perceived difference>. Section 5.1.3.6.2 will deal with the intellectuality categories investigated, i.e., <correctness>, <education>, <intelligence>, <ambition>. Amiability scales, i.e., <confidence>, <pleasantness>, <politeness>, <friendliness> will be discussed in Section 5.1.3.6.3, and, finally, Section 5.1.3.6.4 will shed light on the cluster analysis of the only readiness-for-action attitude trait, <accent improvement>. As is the case with the clustering of the dependent variable <identity development> in Section 5.1.2.2, the metric used to calculate the distance is Euclidean, and the method employed is the Farthest Point algorithm, also known as the Voorhees algorithm (Jones *et al.* 2001). Moreover, each step at which a pair is merged is represented as a node in the tree diagram.

5.1.3.6.1 Reliability

The investigation of covert attitudes towards accent variation through the analysis of reliability categories aims to elicit speakers' metalinguistic awareness of accent recognition. The trait <degree of certainty> attempts to shed light on the speakers' accent categorisations, while <degree of perceived difference> aims to determine the extent to which the participants identify with selected IndE accents. Both traits are crucial in establishing groups.

5.1.3.6.1.1 Cluster I: Degree of Certainty

The dendrogram output of the agglomerative cluster analysis and the bubble matrix chart for <degree of certainty> are given in Fig. 5.1.55. The tree diagram on the x axis shows the hierarchical ordering of the guises based on similarities between the clusters, starting at the bottom of the tree. The colour of the guises designates their ethnicity (red: South India; green: North India). The further down the clusters join, the more similar the guises are perceived. Similarly, the agglomerative clustering of the y axis shows the similarities between the answers given by the informants. The colour of the label corresponds to their ethnicity (red: South India; green: North India). Bubble radiuses are proportional to the answer given, i.e., biggest bubble: 'very' (1); smallest bubble: 'rather not' (5). The colour of the bubble designates the answer given by each participant related to the alleged ethnicity of the guise (red: South India; green: North India).

The cluster analysis yields four subclusters: Cluster I_a, in purple, ranges from ASfKe to PPmKa, Cluster I_b, in sky blue, from JGmKe to SDfKa, Cluster I_c, in orange, from RNmKa to SDfMP and, finally, Cluster II, in green, from PVfKa to SSmUt. Cluster I_a, I_b and I_c are linked more closely than Cluster II; at first sight, one might favour a two-cluster solution (I and II). Nevertheless, there are also arguments to retain four subclusters: I_a and I_c have the most positive scores in the bubble matrix chart, thus indicating a higher degree of certainty about the origin of the guises. Whereas Cluster II is a straightforward daughter node, Cluster I has a more complex ancestry. SSmKa is an isolated cousin, I_c is a second-cousin node, I_a and I_b are third cousin nodes. As has been pointed out in the discussion of the influence of extralinguistic variables on the origins and clues that guided the informants in the recognition of the guises (cf. Section 5.1.3.2), there is a general tendency for Northern stimuli to obtain better scores.

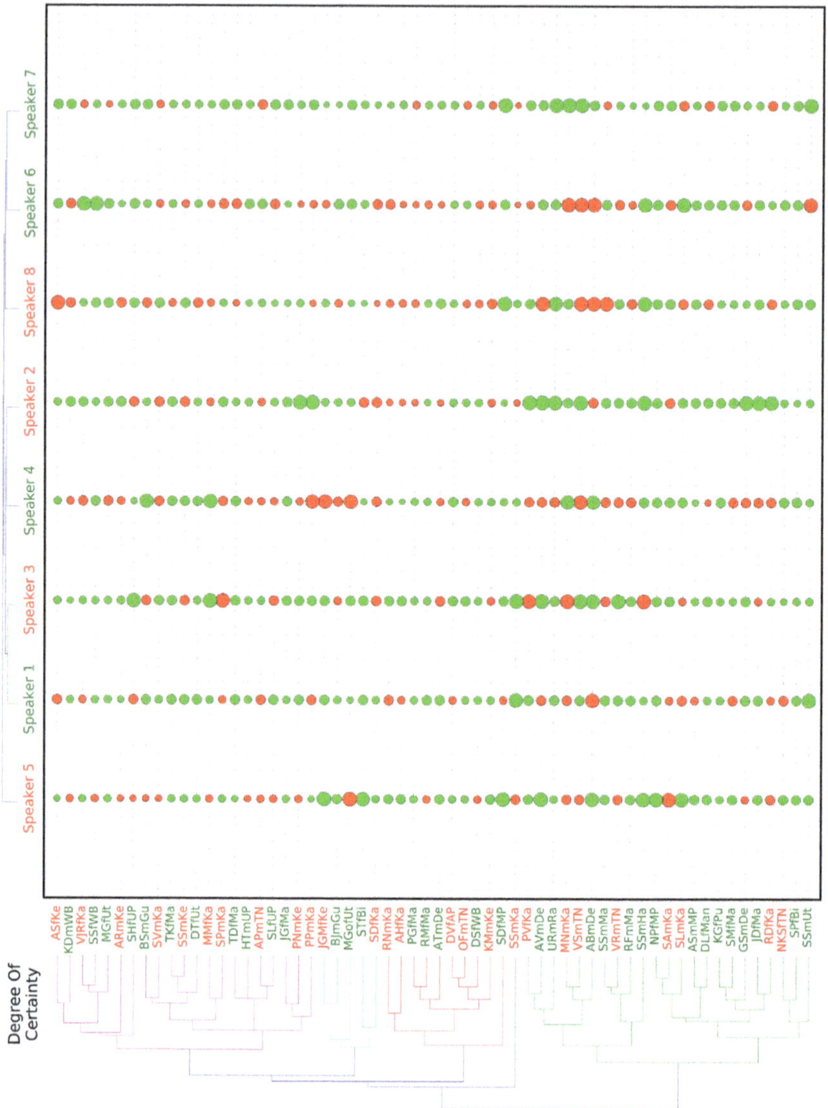

Fig. 5.1.55 Cluster analysis and bubble matrix for Degree of Certainty. Voorhees' algorithm, Euclidean distances. Colour of the labels and the bubbles: red= South India; green =North India. Radius of every bubble is proportional to the score (bigger bubble = closer to 1; smaller bubble = closer to 5)

As can be seen from the radiuses of the bubbles, the degree of certainty of the participants goes hand in hand with this result. The informants are surer about the origins of Speakers One, Four, Six and Seven. Interestingly, they are the ones who are recognised most often (cf. Tab. 5.1.23). A glance at the tree diagram on the x axis shows that the clusters are at more or less the same linking distance. However, despite the guises' different ethnicities, the community members react fairly similarly to Speakers One (West Bengal) and Three (Karnataka, L1: Konkani), Speakers Two (Tamil Nadu) and Four (Maharashtra) as well as Speakers Six (Punjab) and Seven (Uttar Pradesh). This is probably due to the informants' degree of exposure to these accents.

5.1.3.6.1.2 Cluster II: Degree of Perceived Difference

Figure 5.1.56 shows the tree diagram and bubble matrix chart for <degree of perceived difference>. A first glance suggests that the clustering of both axes is far more complex than that for <degree of certainty>. The cluster analysis of the vertical axis yields two dissimilar daughter nodes: Cluster I ranges from APmTN to MNmKa and II from SHfUP to MMfKa. Yet, the agglomerative clustering shows an intricate pattern of underlying similarities further down. While Cluster I retains two fairly similar subclusters (Cluster I_a from APmTN to SSmUt and Cluster I_b from ATmDe to MNmKa), Cluster II consists of two rather disproportional ones (Cluster II_a ranging from ShfUP to STfBi and Cluster II_b from PNmKe to MMfKa). Interestingly, I seems to be dominated by the Northern sample (in green), II by the Southern one (in red).

As has been pointed out in the discussion of the influence of some extralinguistic variables on the evaluative statements above (cf. Sections 5.1.3.1 and 5.1.3.4), *ethnicity* is among the main variables influencing the perception of accent variation. The bubble matrix chart shows that both Northern and Southern informants identify with the accents they rate most positively, i.e., those with bigger bubbles.

The dendrogram output of the hierarchical cluster analysis of the x axis shows two main Clusters: I combines Speakers One (West Bengal) with Seven (Uttar Pradesh) and Three (Karnataka, L1: Konkani), Cluster II does so with Speakers Four (Maharashtra), Two (Tamil Nadu), Six (Punjab), Five (Karnataka, L1: Kannada) and Eight (Andhra Pradesh).

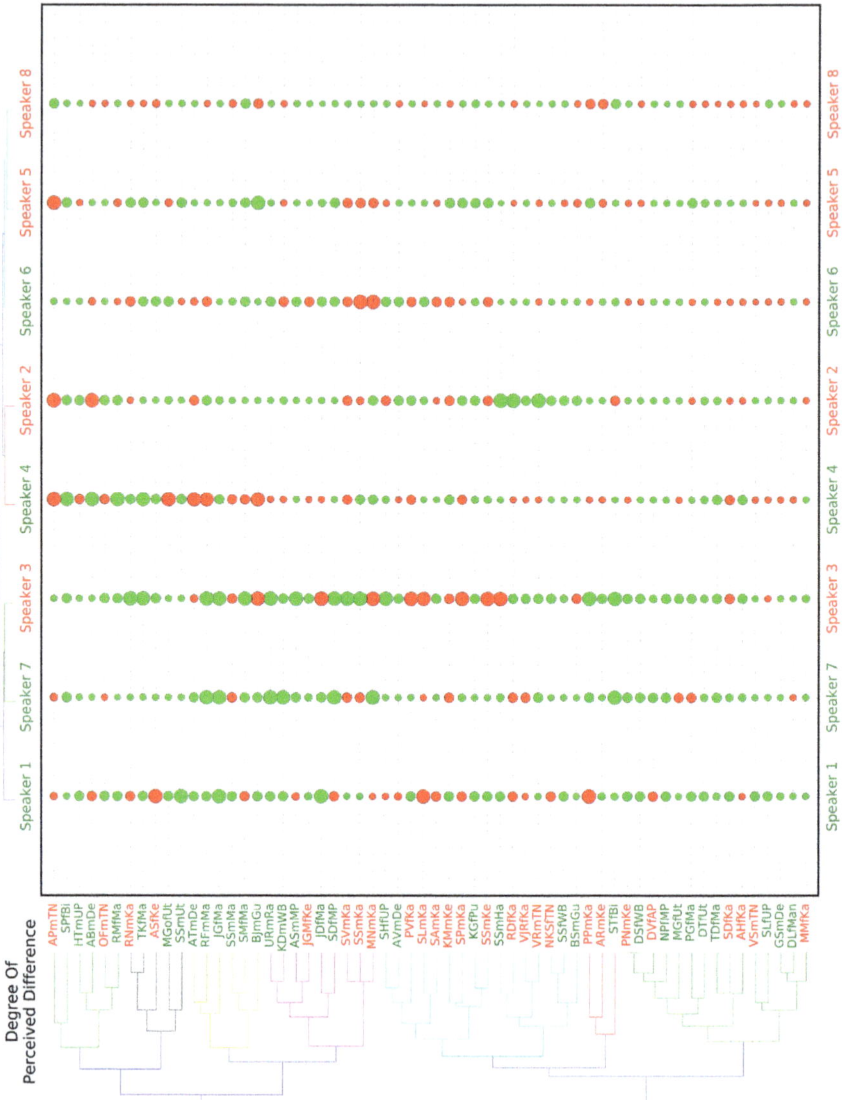

Fig. 5.1.56 Cluster analysis and bubble matrix for Degree of Perceived Difference. Voorhees' algorithm, Euclidean distances. Colour of the labels and the bubbles: red= South India; green =North India. Radius of every bubble is proportional to the score (bigger bubble = closer to 1; smaller bubble = closer to 5)

The high linkage distance between I and II confirms this trend. The components of Cluster II join at a lower linkage distance than those of Cluster I. This suggests that Speakers Four, Two, Six, Five and Eight are rated much more similarly than One, Seven and Three. Overall, the results substantiate earlier findings on the topic, i.e., Northern accents are rated more positively than Southern ones, and shed new light on the extent to which the participants identify with selected IndE accents. Moreover, the least relatable accents (Five and Eight) are the least recognised ones (cf. Section 5.1.3.5.2). On the contrary, Speakers One, Seven and Three are perceived as the standard everyone in the community can relate to. This indicates that the community members implicitly attribute global social authority to their own way of speaking English in relation to the perceived prestige that these accents carry.

5.1.3.6.2 Intellectuality

Traits used for attitudinal ratings are generally subdivided into two dimensions: one is intellectuality (or status); it contains traits such as 'correctness', 'ambition' and 'intelligence'. The other one is amiability (or solidarity); it includes traits like 'pleasantness', 'confidence' and 'attractiveness'. Both dimensions are fundamental in establishing groups. According to Hiraga (2005:289), the intellectuality dimension is the one responsible for determining the "perceived prestige of the accent".

The present section will be structured as follows: the cluster analysis of each status trait, i.e., <correctness>, <education>, <intelligence> and <ambition> is discussed separately. The results will be compared to the findings discussed in the sections above.

5.1.3.6.2.1 Cluster III: Correctness

The dendrogram output of the hierarchical cluster analysis for <correctness> is given in Fig. 5.1.57. At first sight, the cluster analysis of the y axis yields two fairly disproportional daughter nodes: I reaching from SLmKa to RMfMa, II from MNmKa to ARmKe. Daughter I has two similarly disproportionate daughters, cousin I_a from SLmKa to PPmKa and I_b from MMfKa further down to RMfMa. Clusters I and II join at a very high linking distance. The participants in Cluster II dissociate themselves from those in Cluster I for their generally high ratings of Speaker Six and Four, indicated by the large radiuses of the bubbles on the matrix chart.

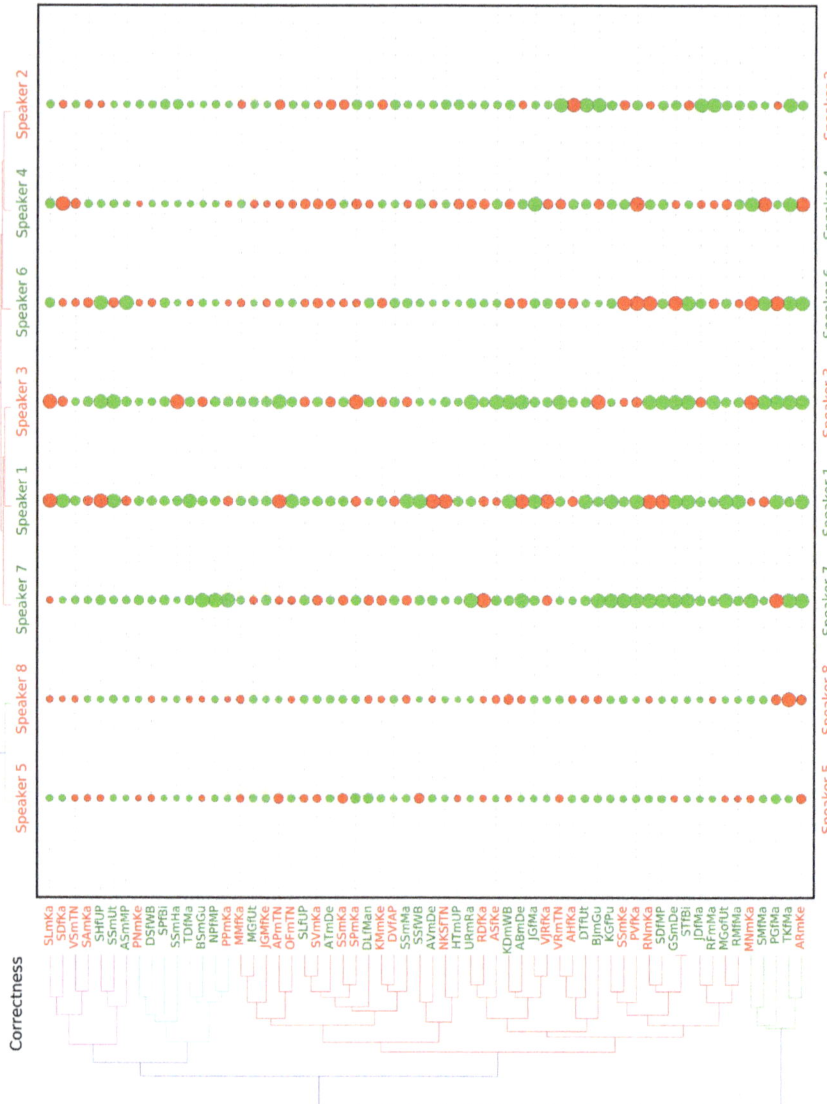

Fig. 5.1.57 Cluster analysis and bubble matrix for Correctness. Voorhees' algorithm, Euclidean distances. Colour of the labels and the bubbles: red= South India; green =North India. Radius of every bubble is proportional to the score (bigger bubble = closer to 1; smaller bubble = closer to 5)

The tree diagram on the x axis shows the hierarchical ordering based on similarities between the guises and suggests a linkage pattern similar to the one found in Fig. 5.1.56. Overall, there are two quite dissimilar clusters, which join at a relatively high linking distance. Cluster I consists of Speakers Five and Eight. Similarly to their clustering in Fig. 5.1.56, the two guises obtain the lowest ratings with respect to <correctness>. Interestingly, the tree diagram shows another cluster already described in Fig. 5.1.56: that of Speakers One and Three. Considering that the radius of every bubble is proportional to the Likert-scale scores, even with regard to <correctness>, the accents of the two guises are perceived as standards to follow.

5.1.3.6.2.2 Cluster IV: Education

The hierarchical cluster analysis for <education> shows interesting patterns of similarities on the x and y axes. The vertical one yields three major clusters (albeit that III is a daughter node and the other two are second cousins of two different cousin nodes). Cluster I_a ranges from ASmMP to ARmKe, Cluster I_b, from TDfMa to SPfBi, and, finally, Cluster II from SDfMP to AHfKa (cf. Fig. 5.1.58). The linkage distances between the clusters are too small to retain the clusters. Clusters I_a and I_b are linked more closely than I_a and II or I_b and II. Overall, the participants rate the guises fairly similarly. This supports earlier findings (cf. Section 5.1.3.1). The only exception is Cluster II. As can be seen from the bubble chart, the informants generally rate Southern Indian accents – and, particularly, Speakers Five and Eight – more positively than the group in Cluster I. However, this is not a statistically significant difference (cf. Section 5.1.3.1).

The cluster analysis of the guises on the x axis goes hand in hand with that of the y axis. There are two disproportional clusters, one consisting of Speakers Five and Eight, the other of Speakers Four, Two, Six, One, Seven and Three. Overall, the clustering of the guises shows the same trend for all the intellectuality traits, highlighting the massive discrepancy between Kannada English (Speaker Five) and Telugu English (Speaker Eight) as against the other IndE accents. With respect to <education>, the informants' ratings of these two stimuli seem to be inversely proportional to their ratings of Speakers One, Seven and Three, who still have the higher ratings.

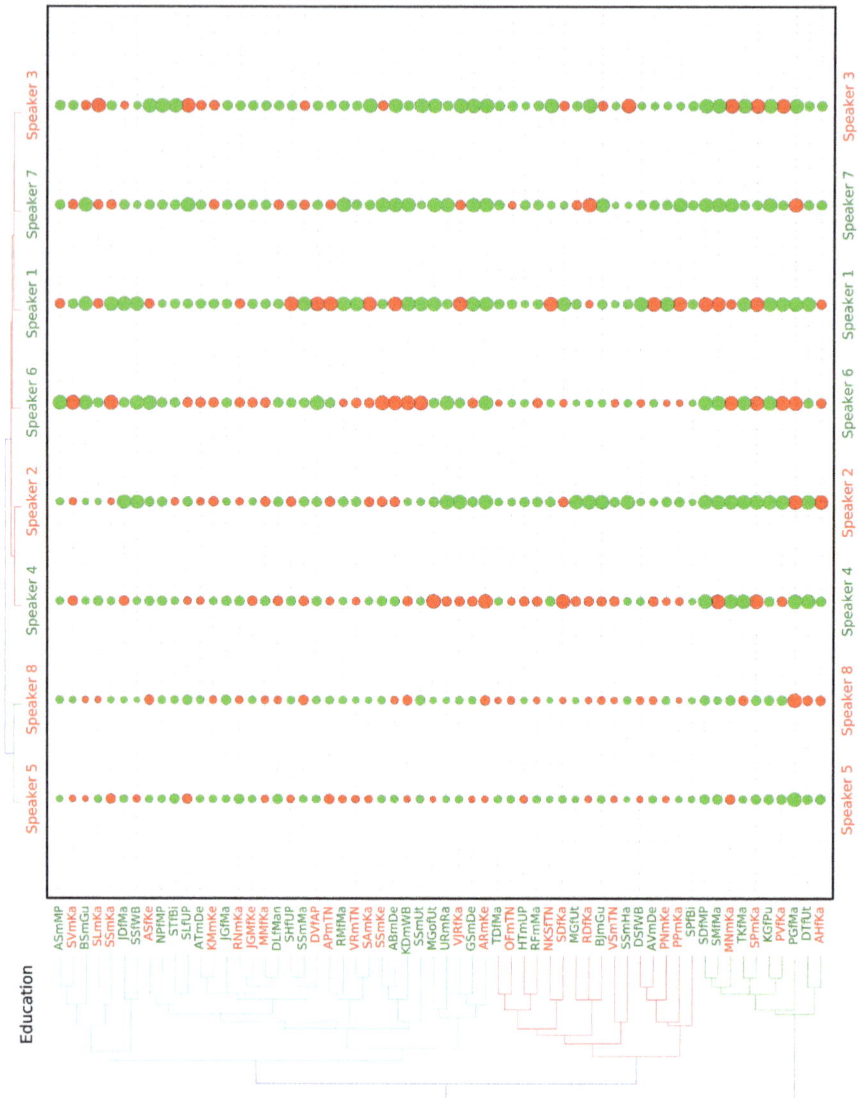

Fig. 5.1.58 Cluster analysis and bubble matrix for Education. Voorhees' algorithm, Euclidean distances. Colour of the labels and the bubbles: red= South India; green =North India. Radius of every bubble is proportional to the score (bigger bubble = closer to 1; smaller bubble = closer to 5)

5.1.3.6.2.3 Cluster V: Intelligence

Figure 5.1.59 shows the tree diagram and bubble matrix chart for the intellectuality trait <intelligence>. A first glance reveals that there are two main clusters on the vertical axis and two on the x axis. With respect to the y axis, Cluster I_a from SLmKa to PPmKa, I_b from MGfUt further down to SSfWB and Cluster II, ranging from PGfMa to ARmKe – the latter being a cousin, the former two second cousins – show interesting linkage patterns. Cluster I_a and I_b join at a high linking distance, thus suggesting a significant difference in the speakers' ratings of the guises. According to the bubble matrix chart, the participants clustered in I_a attribute higher ratings to Speakers One and Three, indicating their perceived high level of <intelligence>. While Cluster I_b mainly consists of Southern informants (in red), Cluster II predominantly includes Northern speakers. Interestingly, their reactions towards the guises differ the further down the tree diagram. Cluster II confirms the trend described in the clusters discussed above, i.e., the Northern guises generally receive high – and higher, in comparison to Southern stimuli – ratings. However, the participants in Clusters I_a and I_b have a tendency to rate all guises the same way despite their ethnicity, mostly attributing them lower scores.

Overall, the cluster analysis of the horizontal axis confirms the patterns of other reliability and intellectuality traits analysed, substantiating the massive difference in perception of Speakers Five and Eight who are rated fairly negatively by an overwhelming majority of the community.

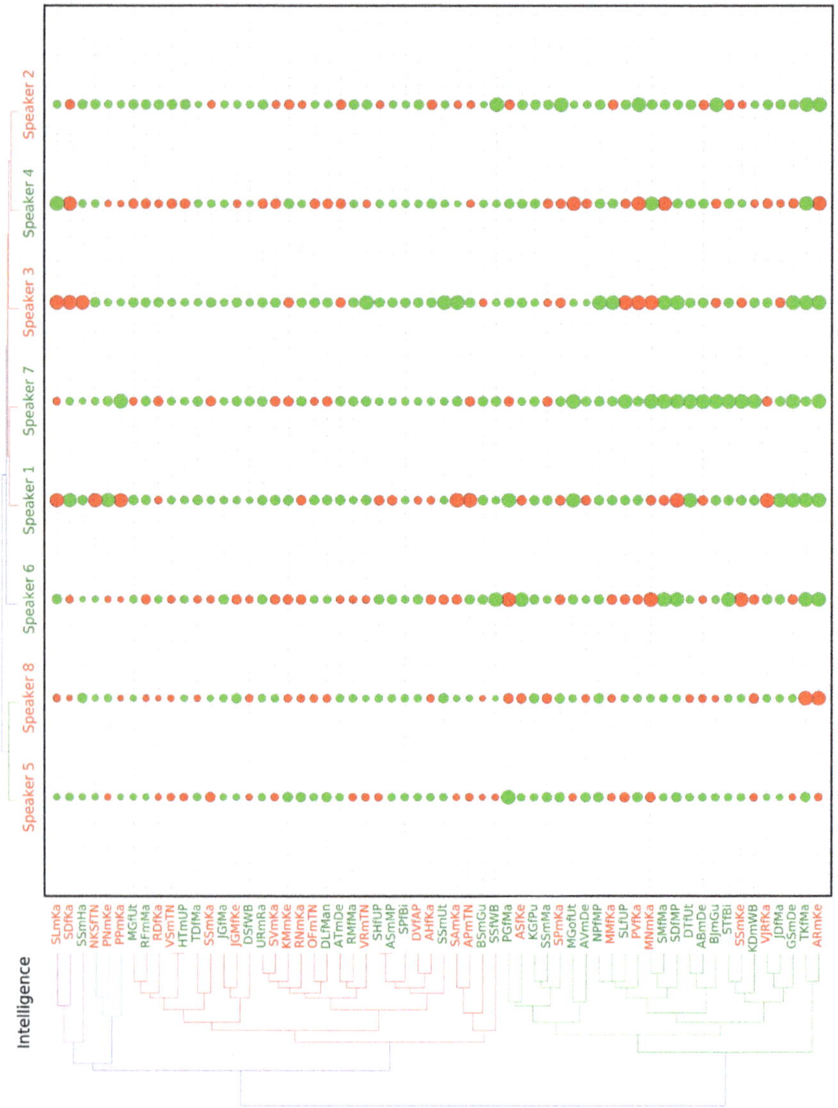

Fig. 5.1.59 Cluster analysis and bubble matrix for Intelligence. Voorhees' algorithm, Euclidean distances. Colour of the labels and the bubbles: red= South India; green =North India. Radius of every bubble is proportional to the score (bigger bubble = closer to 1; smaller bubble = closer to 5)

5.1.3.6.2.4 Cluster VI: Ambition

The dendrogram output of the hierarchical cluster analysis for <ambition> is given in Fig. 5.1.60. At first sight, the analysis of the vertical axis yields two fairly disproportional daughters and four cousins: Cluster I_a ranging from SSmMa to RDfKa and I_b from TDfMa to JGMfKe and Cluster II_a ranging from URmRa to SSfWB and II_b from KMmKe down to SSmUt. Both subclusters as well as Clusters I and II join at a high linking distance, thus indicating that the items are rather dissimilar. The bubble matrix chart substantiates the clusterings of the tree diagram since values tend to be proportional to the ethnicity of the speaker, i.e., Northern stimuli = higher ratings = bigger bubbles.

The cluster analysis for the horizontal axis confirms this trend. Since its hierarchical ordering is based on similarities between the guises, it comes as no surprise that Speakers Five and Eight form Cluster I and carry negative ratings. Cluster II shows higher scores and, subsequently, bigger bubbles, which indicate that the items are all rated fairly similarly. However, it is interesting to notice how some particular subclusters of Cluster II are in line with the results discussed in Section 5.1.3.1. <Ambition> marks a rather clear-cut distinction between Northern IndE accents (in green) and Southern ones (in red), which is not always present in the clusters analysed above. Speaker Three, for instance, is rated as somewhat confident overall, although she obtains several low scores.

The results account for the underlying similarities of the guises and the participants. They indicate fine-grained differences in the ratings of Northern and Southern IndE accents in a wide range of status traits. This shows that the respondents' norm-orientation is unidimensional since Northern Indian varieties seem to serve as a superordinate norm in the student community.

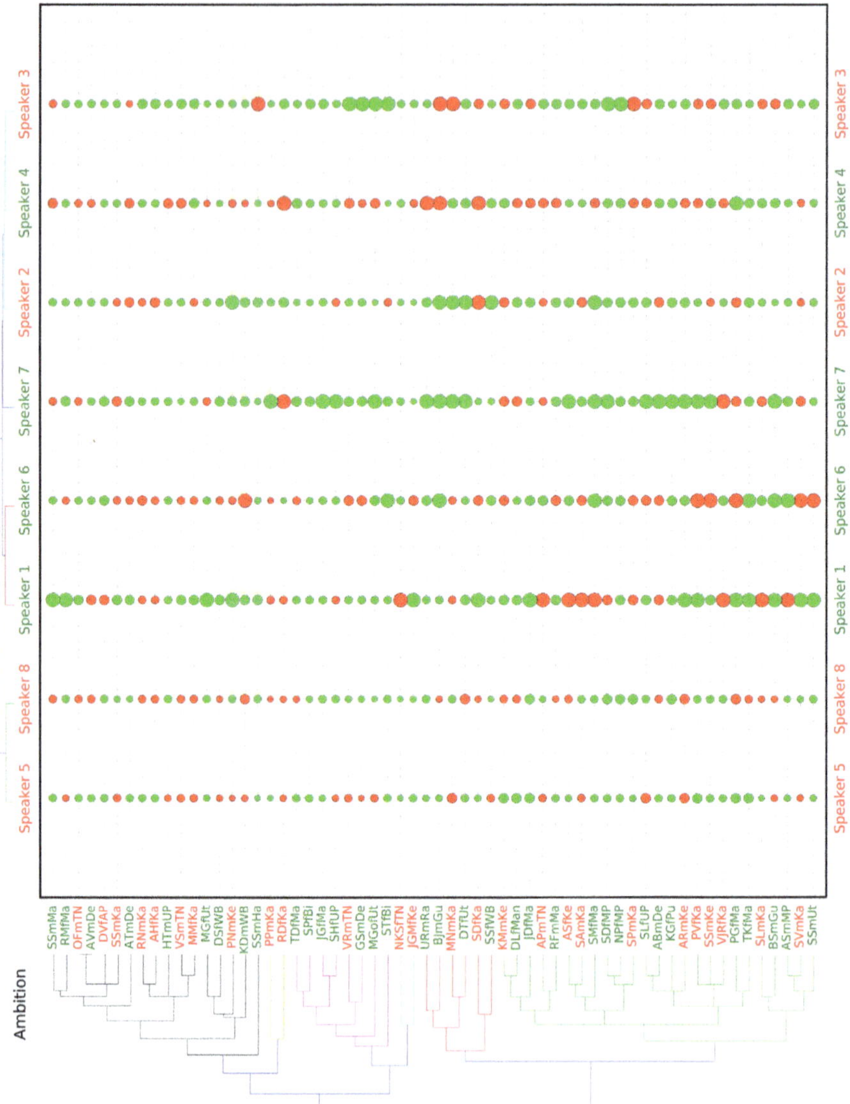

Fig. 5.1.60 Cluster analysis and bubble matrix for Ambition. Voorhees' algorithm, Euclidean distances. Colour of the labels and the bubbles: red= South India; green =North India. Radius of every bubble is proportional to the score (bigger bubble = closer to 1; smaller bubble = closer to 5)

5.1.3.6.3 Amiability

As mentioned in Section 5.1.3.6.2, intellectuality and amiability dimensions are fundamental in establishing groups. While the former usually reveals the perceived prestige of an accent, the latter determines "the extent to which an individual identifies with an accent" (Hiraga 2005:289). In doing so, the following amiability (or solidarity) traits have been selected in order to test the degree of metalinguistic awareness of the community members: <confidence>, <pleasantness>, <politeness>, <friendliness>, <attractiveness>. Results from the cluster analysis and the bubble matrices will be examined in relation to the findings discussed in Sections 5.1.3.1 and 5.1.3.4.

5.1.3.6.3.1 Cluster VII: Confidence

Figure 5.1.61 shows the tree diagram and bubble matrix chart for <confidence>. A first look at the tree diagram of the vertical axis shows a complex clustering. Overall, it yields three major clusters, I, ranging from SSmMa to MGofUt, II, from MGfUt further down to MMfKa and, finally, III from BSmGu to PPmKa. The Clusters I and II are cousin-nodes; III is a daughter node. Clusters I and II can be further divided to obtain four subclusters: Cluster I_a, from SSmMa to SSmKa, I_b, from PVfKa to MFGofUt, Cluster II_a, from MGfUt to SSmHa and II_b from SLfUP to MMfKa. Overall, the Clusters I and II are massively disproportional and only join at a high linking distance. The bubble matrix chart shows that the participants included in Cluster I and Cluster II_b react similarly to the guises, with the exception of Speaker Four, who is rated more positively by the first group.

The cluster analysis for the horizontal axis is more homogeneous in that it shows two fairly similar clusters: Cluster I, ranging from Speaker One (West Bengal) to Speaker Three (Karnataka, L1: Konkani) and Cluster II, from Speaker Five (Karnataka, L1: Kannada) to Speaker Two (Tamil Nadu). The linkage distance between the items in the two clusters shows that I is rated more uniformly than II since the items join at a lower level. The bubble matrix chart adds an attitude perspective since items from Cluster I are rated more positively than those in Cluster II. This indicates that, with the exceptions of Speakers Three (Cluster I) and Four (Cluster II), the tree diagram of the x axis operates ethnicity-wise (cf. Section 5.1.3.1). Northern IndE accents are rated more positively than Southern ones.

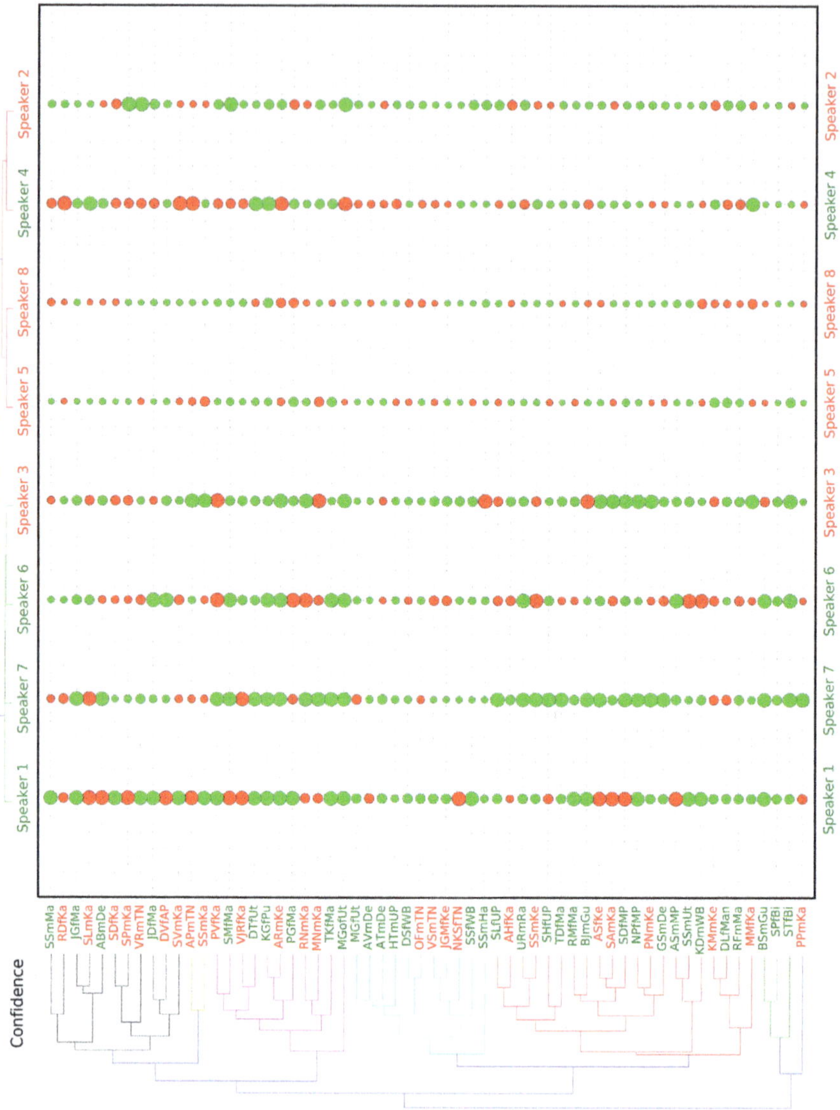

Fig. 5.1.61 Cluster analysis and bubble matrix for Confidence. Voorhees' algorithm, Euclidean distances. Colour of the labels and the bubbles: red= South India; green =North India. Radius of every bubble is proportional to the score (bigger bubble = closer to 1; smaller bubble = closer to 5)

5.1.3.6.3.2 Cluster VIII: Pleasantness

The dendrogram output of the hierarchical cluster analysis for <pleasantness> is given in Fig. 5.1.62. At first sight, the tree diagram of the vertical axis yields two disproportional clusters. Cluster I_a ranges from ASfKe down to SSmUt, Cluster I_b from PGfMa to DLfMan and Cluster II from MGofUt to AVmDe. However, Cluster II is a daughter, I_a and I_b are cousins. Overall, the participants have the same reactions towards the guises, marking the difference between Northern and Southern IndE accents with the two canonical exceptions of Speakers Four (rated farily negatively) and Three (rated fairly positively). The tree diagram of the x axis registers similarities between the guises according to their ethnicity. The clustering of the items shows the same pattern encountered in the tree diagram discussed in Fig. 5.1.61. This indicates that the participants perceive <confidence> and <pleasantness> similarly.

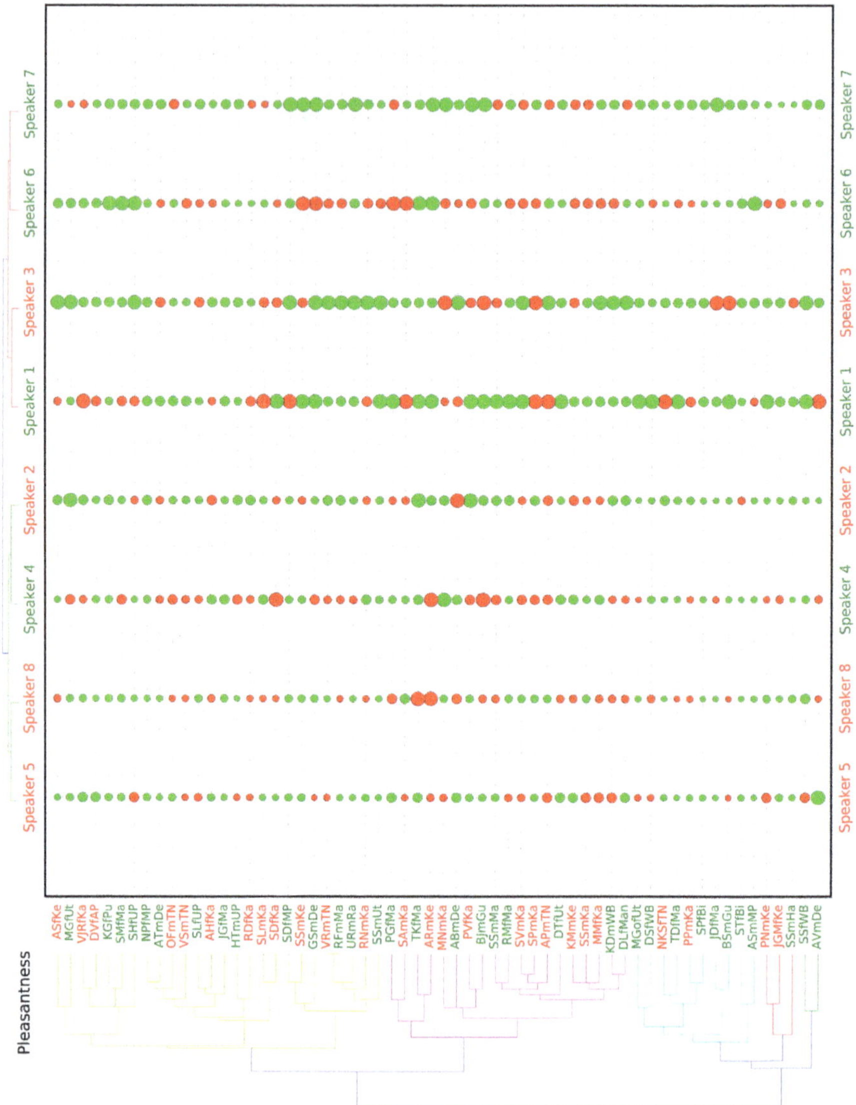

Fig. 5.1.62 Cluster analysis and bubble matrix for Pleasantness. Voorhees' algorithm, Euclidean distances. Colour of the labels and the bubbles: red= South India; green =North India. Radius of every bubble is proportional to the score (bigger bubble = closer to 1; smaller bubble = closer to 5)

5.1.3.6.3.3 Cluster IX: Politeness

The cluster analysis and bubble matrix for <politeness> are shown in Fig. 5.1.63. As discussed in Section 5.1.3.1, <politeness> is the only amiability trait that does not reach significance with respect to *ethnicity*. The respondents' ratings are rather uniform and do not mark any Northern vs. Southern distinction. The bubble matrix chart shows that, overall, each guise is rated somewhat positively, even the canonical 'negatively rated' Speakers Five and Eight. A first glance at the tree diagram of the vertical axis confirms this trend, showing that there are two major clusters, I ranging from OFmTN to PPmKa and II from SSmKe to ASfKe. While the items of Cluster II join at a low linkage distance, Cluster I can be divided further into three main subclusters: I_a reaching from OFmTN to BJmGu, I_b from VRmTN to RDfKa and I_c ranging from SSmHa to PPmKa. However, these differences are marginal.

The dendrogram output of the agglomerative cluster analysis of the x axis shows that the guises are rated fairly similarly. The two main Clusters I (including Speakers One and Three) and II (the other guises) show that the linkage distance between the items is rather low.

Overall, the underlying similarities and trends uncovered by the clustering of <politeness> seem to position the trait in-between the amiability and intellectuality dimensions discussed above. <Politeness> is the only category which is likely to reveal both the extent to which participants identify with an accent, i.e., both Northern and Southern guises, and the perceived prestige of the accents in question, i.e., Northern guises.

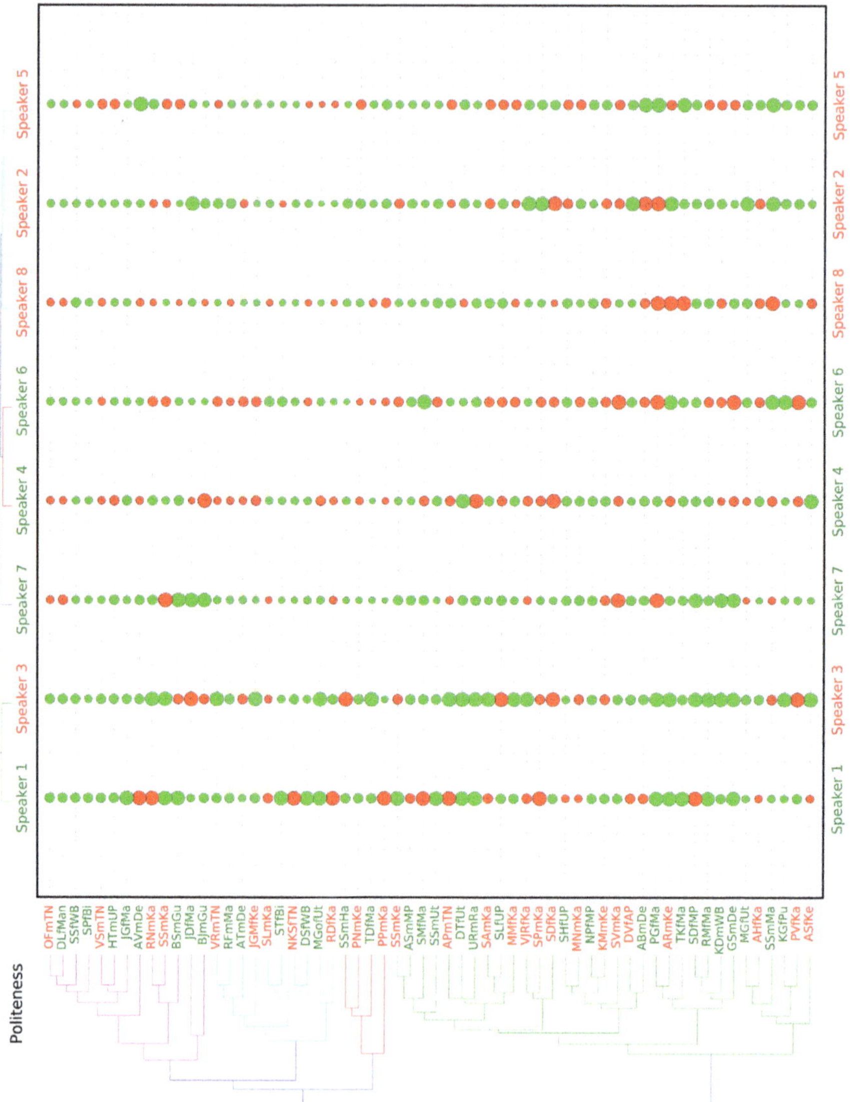

Fig. 5.1.63 Cluster analysis and bubble matrix for Politeness. Voorhees' algorithm, Euclidean distances. Colour of the labels and the bubbles: red= South India; green =North India. Radius of every bubble is proportional to the score (bigger bubble = closer to 1; smaller bubble = closer to 5)

5.1.3.6.3.4 Cluster X: Friendliness

A first look at the clustering of the y axis of Fig. 5.1.64 reveals a rather intricate pattern of similarities. Two dissimilar daughter nodes (Cluster I ranging from SSmKe down to PPmKa and Cluster II from MMfKa to BJmGu) join at a very high linking distance, suggesting that the participants' reactions towards the guises diverge considerably. Cluster I and Cluster II can be divided further into six clusters: Cluster I_a ranges from SSmKe to JGMfKe, I_b from KGfPu to PNmKe, I_c from ATmDe to AVmDe and I_d from NKSfTN to PPmKa. Cluster I shows considerable internal differences in its levels. Cluster II is structured much more straightforwardly; II_a from MMfKa to ARmKe and II_b from RNmKa down to BJmGu. Overall, the members of Cluster II have an expected and more uniform reaction towards the guises, i.e., Northern IndE accents being rated more positively than Southern ones. Conversely, the informants in Cluster I react differently towards the guises, rating all participants uniformly and generally attributing them low scores. Clusters I_b and I_d are the only exceptions and are in line with Cluster II. However, these differences are minimal and, although significant according to the Wilcoxon signed-rank test, they do not reach significance with the Bonferroni correction (cf. Section 5.1.3.1).

The cluster analysis of the x axis shows that the guises are rated similarly. Moreover, it shows the same clustering pattern as <politeness> (cf. Fig. 5.1.63). Two rather dissimilar clusters, Cluster I (including Speakers One and Three) and II (composed of Speakers Two, Five, Eight, Seven, Four and Six) join at a very low linking distance. The minimal differences in the clusterings of both axes indicate that <friendliness>, together with <politeness>, may not be a relevant attitude trait for the community.

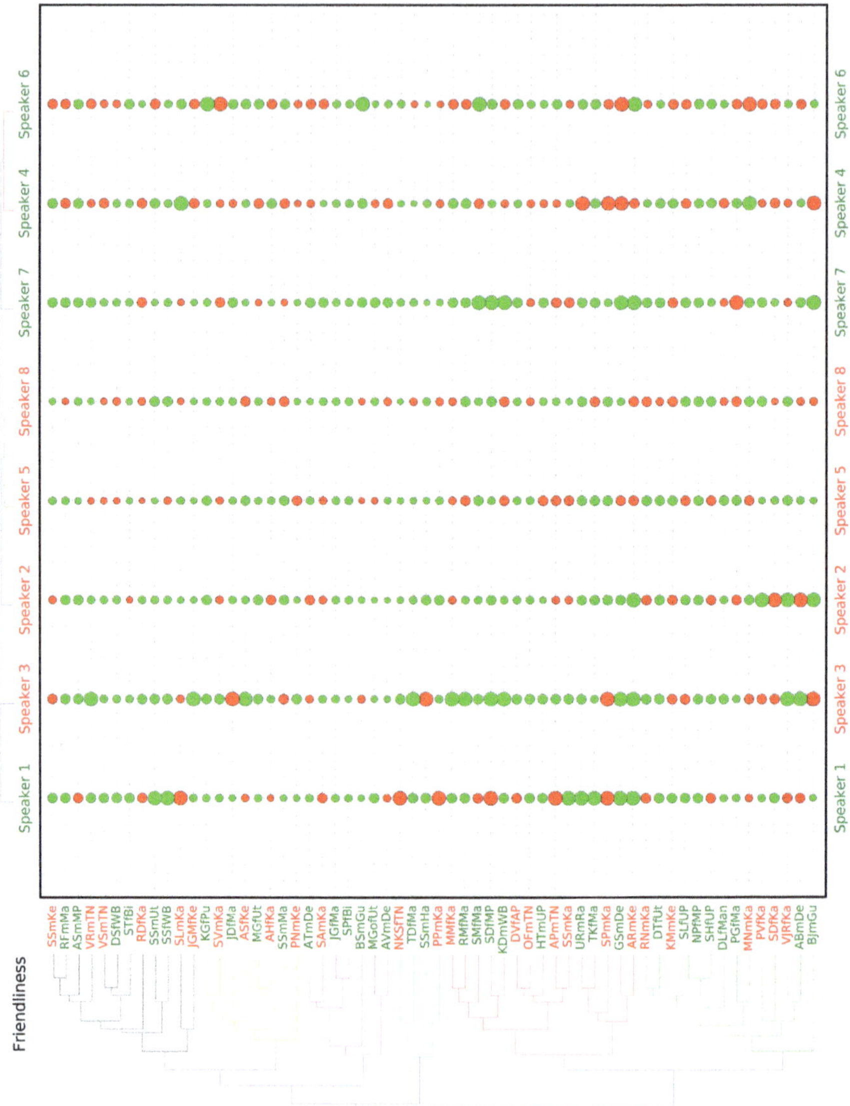

Fig. 5.1.64 Cluster analysis and bubble matrix for Friendliness. Voorhees' algorithm, Euclidean distances. Colour of the labels and the bubbles: red= South India; green =North India. Radius of every bubble is proportional to the score (bigger bubble = closer to 1; smaller bubble = closer to 5)

5.1.3.6.3.5 Cluster XI: Attractiveness

The agglomerative cluster analysis of <attractiveness> shows interesting patterns of similarities on the x and y axes (cf. Fig. 5.1.65). The vertical one yields three major clusters, although at different levels of relationship. Cluster I ranges from DVfAP to ARmKe, Cluster II from RNmKa to STfBi and Cluster III from BSmGu to TDfMa. Cluster I is the only node retaining two subclusters: I_a from DVfAP to SSmUt and I_b from SSmMa ARMKe. Interestingly, Clusters I, II and III seem to be mainly dominated by the Northern (designated in green), the Southern (in red), and, again, the Northern sample respectively. As has been pointed out in the discussion of the influence of some extralinguistic variables on the evaluative statements above (cf. Sections 5.1.3.1 and 5.1.3.4), *ethnicity* is among the main variables influencing the perception of accent variation. The bubble matrix chart shows that both Northern and Southern informants identify with the accents they rate most positively, i.e., those with bigger bubbles.

The dendrogram output of the x axis designates two main Clusters: Cluster I combining Speakers Four (Maharashtra), Two (Tamil Nadu), Five (Karnataka, L1: Kannada) and Eight (Andhra Pradesh) and Cluster II combining Speakers Six (Punjab), Seven (Uttar Pradesh), One (West Bengal) and Three (Karnataka, L1: Konkani). The components of both clusters join at a very low linkage distance. This suggests that, with the exceptions of Speakers Four and Three, the clustering of the guises follows an ethnicity-oriented distinction. Subsequently, Northern IndE accents are rated as more attractive than Southern ones.

Overall, the results substantiate earlier findings and add new light on the extent to which participants identify with selected IndE accents.

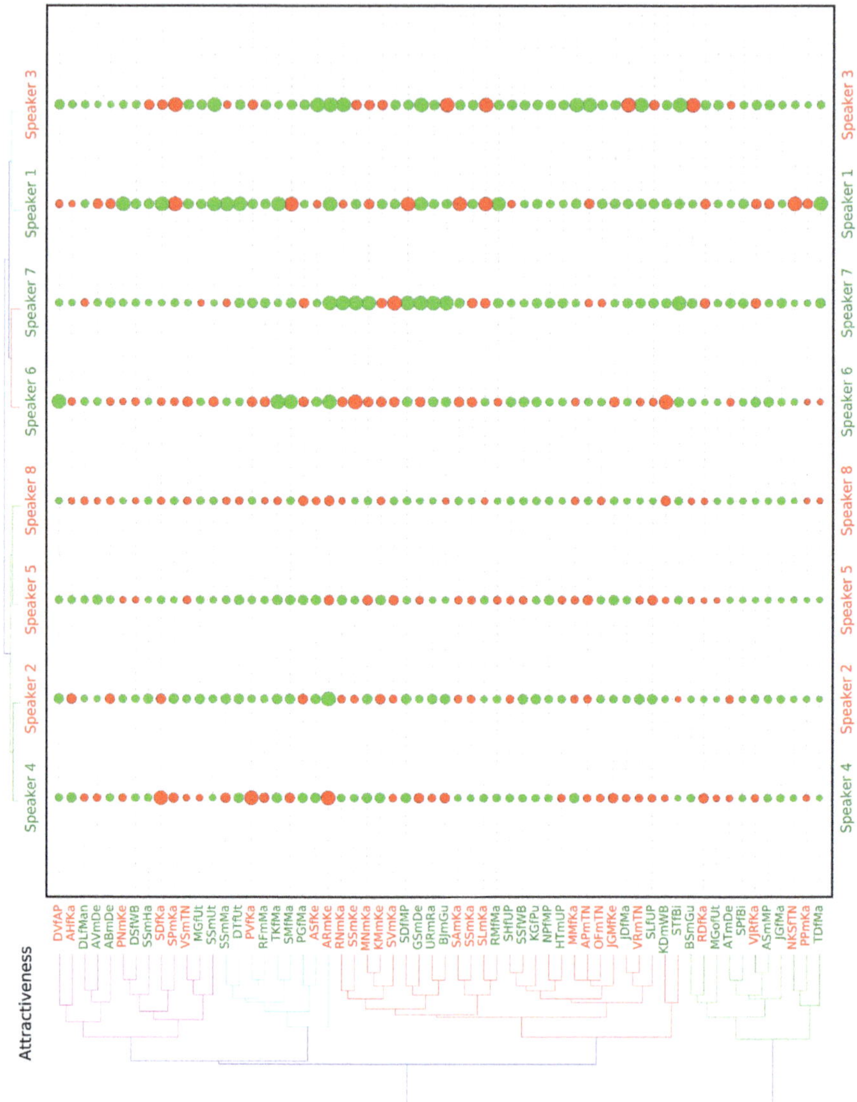

Fig. 5.1.65 Cluster analysis and bubble matrix for Attractiveness. Voorhees' algorithm, Euclidean distances. Colour of the labels and the bubbles: red= South India; green =North India. Radius of every bubble is proportional to the score (bigger bubble = closer to 1; smaller bubble = closer to 5)

5.1.3.6.4 Readiness for Action: Cluster XII: Accent Improvement

The investigation of covert attitudes towards accent variation through the analysis of the readiness-for-action trait <accent improvement> aims to determine the extent to which the participants identify with selected IndE accents and to reveal which ones have covert prestige. Figure 5.1.66 shows the hierarchical cluster analysis and bubble matrix of the trait.

At a first glance, the tree diagram on the y axis yields two quite dissimilar cousin clusters: I ranging from JGfMa to KGfPu and II from NKSfTN down to GSmDe. While the members in Cluster II join at a low linkage distance, Cluster I can be further divided into two more clusters: I_a ranging from JGfMa to RDfKa and I_b from SDfKa to KGfPu. The Clusters I_a and II are linked more closely than I_b and II because of the participants' similar reactions towards the guises of Cluster I displayed on the x axis (Speakers Four, Two, Five and Eight).

Although not statistically significant, I and II seem to be dominated by the Southern and the Northern sample, respectively. The bubble matrix chart confirms this trend on both axes: with the exception of Speakers Four and Three, the ratings of the guises follow their ethnicity. Northern guises, constituting Cluster II of the tree diagram on the x axis, are attributed significantly better scores, indicating, this time, that they do not need to improve their accents. On the contrary, Southern guises, constituting Cluster I of the clustering, obtain worse scores.

The results are in line with earlier findings according to which Northern IndE accents are generally attributed global social authority and are perceived as a superordinate norm in the student community. The lack of significance among the participants on the x axis indicates that the Northern Indian participants appear to have stereotypical views about themselves and the South and that the Southerners have by and large taken over the stereotypes of the Northerners about themselves. This is a clear example of how the linguistic power of the majority, i.e., the Northern Indians, is gradually accepted by the minorities, i.e., the Southern part of the community (cf. Section 5.1.3.4).

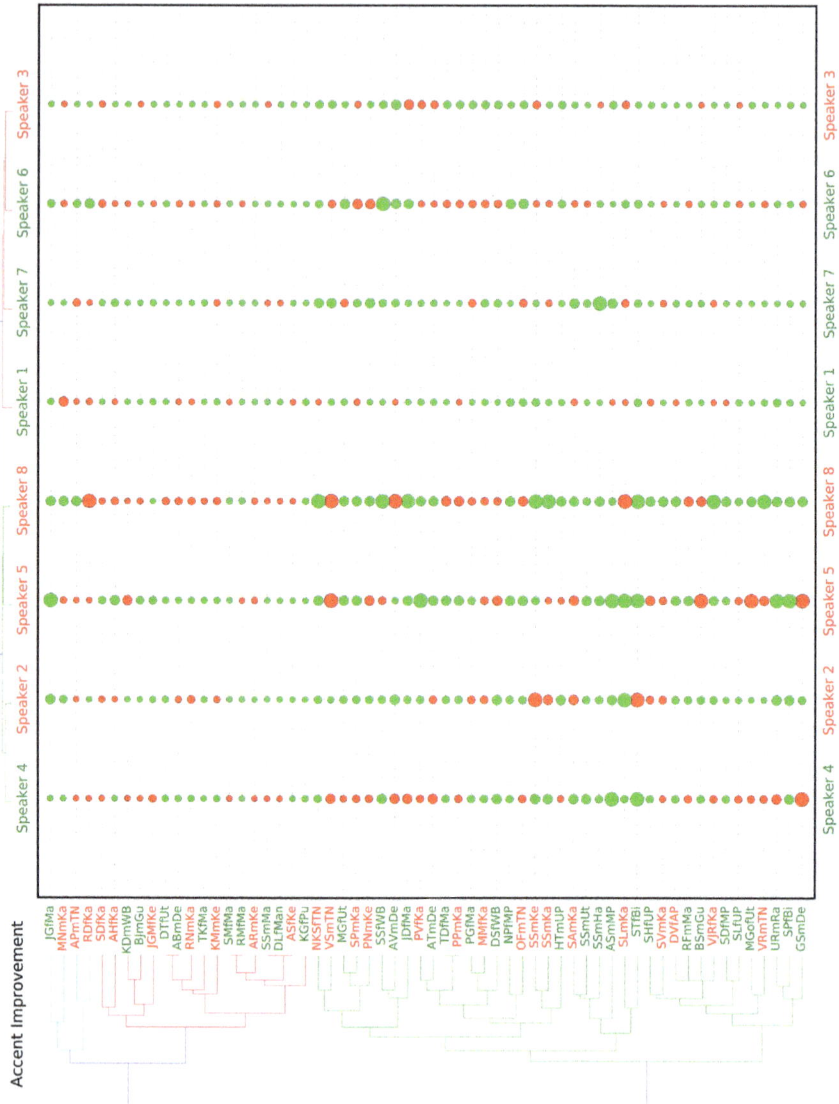

Fig. 5.1.66 Cluster analysis and bubble matrix for Accent Improvement. Voorhees' algorithm, Euclidean distances. Colour of the labels and the bubbles: red= South India; green =North India. Radius of every bubble is proportional to the score (bigger bubble = closer to 1; smaller bubble = closer to 5)

5.1.3.7 *Cognitive Maps*

In so far as dialect geography seeks to provide an empirical basis for conclusions about linguistic varieties occurring in certain areas, the most straightforward way of discovering what laypeople believe about language variation is to have them draw maps (cf. Section 4.2.3).

The present section presents findings based on the language regard methodology, i.e., speakers' awakening of a response, as devised and applied by Preston (1999; 1982), Preston and Howe (1987) and Niedzielski and Preston (2003). Before starting the Accent Identification Task, the participants were asked to "draw boundaries on the blank map below around areas where you believe English accents are different" and then to label the areas they outlined with an adjective (II.II.1). As mentioned in Section 4.2.3, since physical and political boundaries do not always coincide with dialect ones, it was necessary to provide the informants with a map showing state lines. This allows for a more detailed geolinguistic orientation. The aim of the task is to account for the overt attitudinal cognitorium of the participants with regard to popular beliefs about IndE regional varieties (cf. Section 5.1.3.7.1). Secondly, the participants listen to eight voices presented in a scrambled order on a "dialect continuum" (Preston 1999:xxxiv) and are instructed to assign each voice to the site they think it belonged (cf. Section 5.1.3.7.2). This step allows for eliciting covert attitudes towards IndE accent variation.

The results will be presented and discussed in two subsections (5.1.3.7.1 and 5.1.3.7.2). The first one corresponds to the *perception* of accent variation, i.e., the elicitation of the speakers' overt stigmatisation and stereotypes of IndE accents. Section 5.1.3.7.2 considers its *production*, i.e., the correlation between covert attitudes and accent variation, and corresponds to the Accent Identification Task of Survey II, part II (cf. Section 4.2.4), whose numerical data have been discussed in Sections 5.1.3.1–5.1.3.6. The first part of the map task, i.e., map labelling and characterisation, will be referred to as the 'label task', and the second section as the 'scales task'.

5.1.3.7.1 *Adjective Map*

In order to elicit dialect consciousness and to ascertain whether accent variation has salience for the community, the 'draw-a-map' task has proved to be an effective method. According to Tôjô (1954:11), "[t]he only way to establish dialect regions is to begin with the dialect consciousness of ordinary people and make additions and corrections on the basis of surveys of those special linguistic characteristics which are the basis for these perceptions". These perceptions may be referred to as dialect consciousness, i.e., "[t]he feeling that a dialect is different is something which everyone can relate to. Even if this is not a clear perception based on specific criteria, one may still have a vague feeling" (Tôjô 1938:29). In this sense, metalinguistic awareness should form the basis for the establishment of dialect areas.

As mentioned in Section 5.1.3.7, the participants were instructed to draw in what they felt to be the main English dialect regions of India (no maximum boundaries) and to supply labels they might typically use for these, which would characterise each of the dialects in terms of what they found to be most peculiar about them. In the questionnaire, IndE varieties were referred to as 'accents/ dialects' because it would have been unhelpful and confusing for the participants to become involved in such specialists' distinctions. Though major distinctions are drawn by linguists, i.e., with dialect inevitably subsuming accent, laypeople do not generally differentiate between the two terms, and the informants of the present study are no exception (cf. Section 5.2).

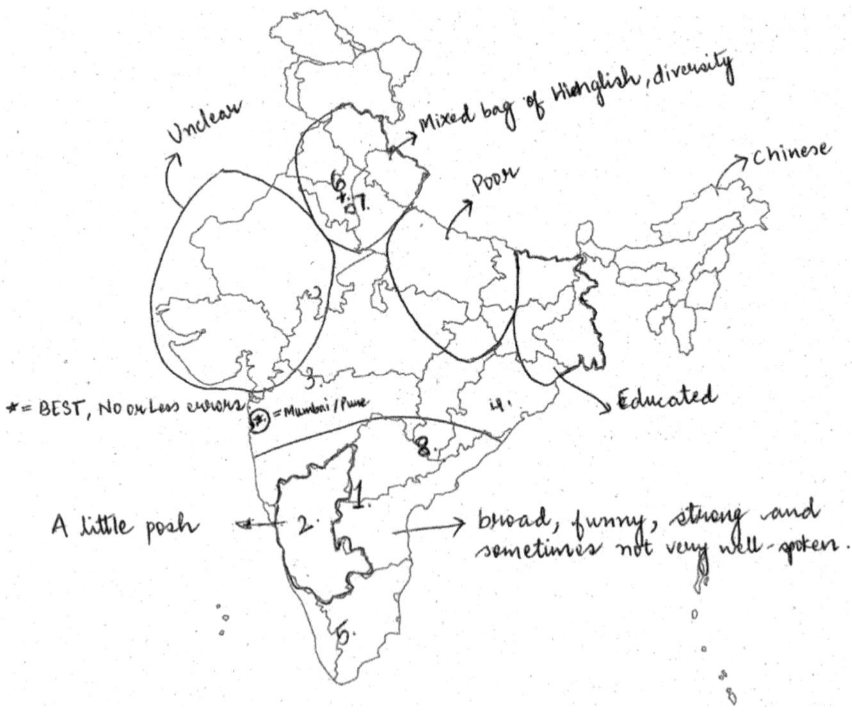

Fig. 5.1.67 A Delhi male respondent's hand-drawn map of IndE speech areas

Figure 5.1.67 is an example of a cognitive map drawn by a male student from Delhi who has been living in Heidelberg for less than one year; Fig. 5.1.68 is that of a male newcomer, native of the Southern state of Tamil Nadu. The details of the first map have somehow to be combined with the relatively limited information of the second one. As expected, many adjectives suggest that perceptions of accents and dialects in India are closely linked to social stereotypes about the people who speak them, e.g., 'educated', 'multicultural', 'posh', and many adjectives appear to be descriptions of ethnicities, e.g., 'Chinese', rather than accents or dialects.

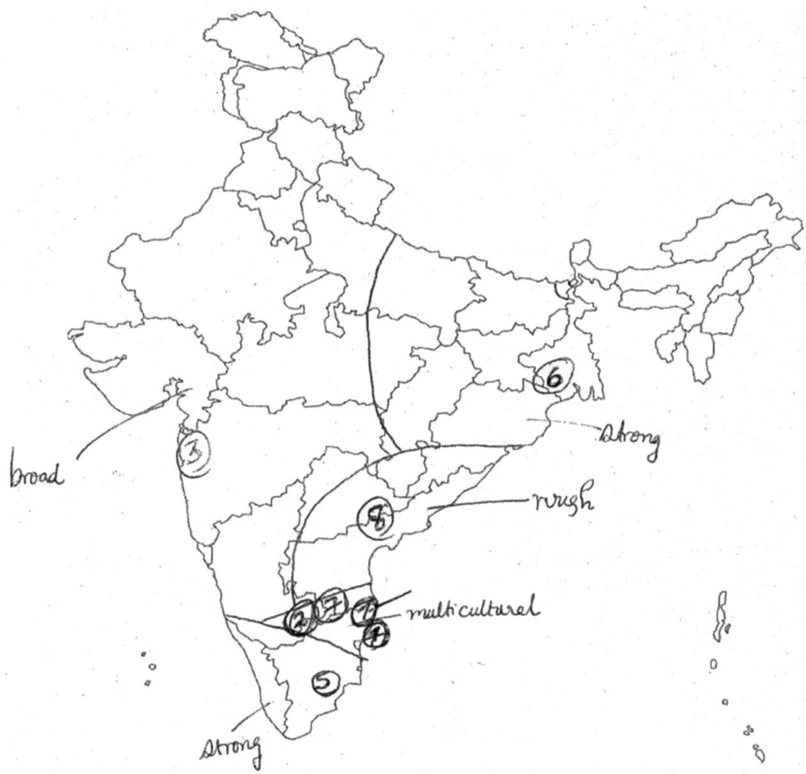

Fig. 5.1.68 A Tamil Nadu male respondent's hand-drawn map of IndE speech areas

The resulting 60 maps were analysed in order to create a composite map showing where the major dialect areas are perceived to be. Each respondent's boundary for each area have been treated as an isogloss.[84] Once it was seen that respondents from different geographical areas used more or less the same general cognitive template for area identifications, a way of determining isoglosses was devised. When the isoglosses from all informants for one area had been combined with hand drawing, bundles of isoglosses were identified and taken to be "that group's mental map outline of the dialect area" (Niedzielski/Preston 2003:47). The outlines of each respondent's areas were traced onto a standard map. Data were aggregated and processed using the GNU image manipulation programme GIMP (version 2.10.10).

The presentation and discussion of the findings below derive from the very basic notion that defining one precise linguistic border, i.e., where one dialect ends and the next one begins, is rather impossible since "there are generally no clear-cut boundaries between dialects" (Kristensson 1983:30). Yet, this does not prevent nonlinguists from agreeing among themselves that some boundaries define specific speech areas. As Glauser (1991:4) points out "[i]f speakers may harbour such fairly precise ideas about boundaries, the least linguists can do is to relate them to their networks in order to find out what criteria are made use of". To do so, it is fundamental to establish the main focal areas for dialects and the transition areas between them (Kristensson 1983).

Figure 5.1.69 shows the computer-determined mental map of IndE speech areas derived from the hand-drawn maps of the 60 Indian students. It shows different colours for each detected area, the darker sections indicating the 'cores'. The adjectives most commonly used to describe each area were added to the map, the size of the word being proportional to the frequency with which it is used, i.e., the bigger the size, the higher the frequency (font 12: > 50/60 speakers [> 83 %]; font 10: > 30/60 speakers [> 50 %]; font 8: > 20/60 speakers [> 33 %]). As briefly mentioned above, the participants used more or less the same general cognitive template for area identifications despite their different gender, ethnicity or time spent in Heidelberg. Though this finding allows for an easier determination of boundary lines and significantly reduces over-categorisations of data onto GIMP, it informs on the relation between overt and covert language

84 An isogloss is a boundary drawn on a dialect map, i.e., an (imaginary) line illustrating the geographical distribution of one or more linguistic features. Although major dialects are typically demarcated by bundles of isoglosses, such as the La Spezia–Rimini Line that divides the Northern Italian dialects from the Central Italian ones, an individual isogloss may or may not have any coincidence with a given language border. Cf. Chambers/Trudgill (2004) for further details.

attitudes of the community towards IndE accents. Figure 5.1.69 shows clear-cut aggregated dialect areas. Overall, speakers detect seven macro-areas in which English is spoken differently and provide specific adjectives describing each of them.

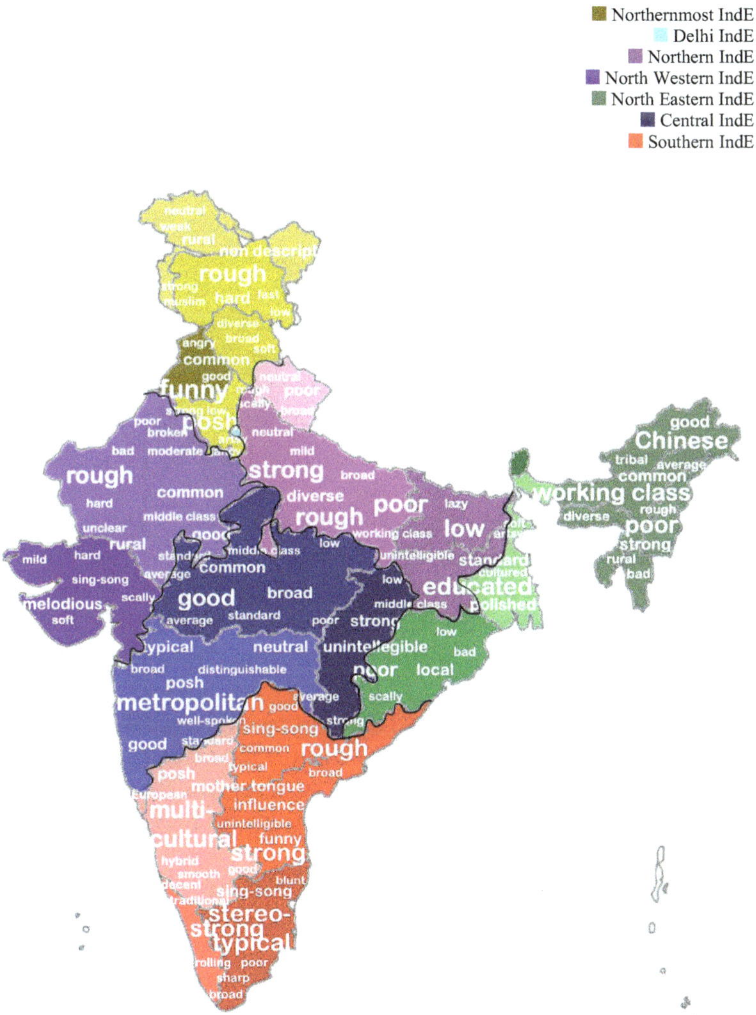

Fig. 5.1.69 Composite perceptual map of India, showing aggregated English dialect areas

The first one, which has been labelled 'Northernmost IndE', comprises the states of Jammu and Kashmir, Himachal Pradesh, Haryana and Punjab.[85] The darker section, represented by Punjab, indicates the 'core dialect area' of the region, i.e., the most stereotypical dialect/accent of the speech area. The territories around the 'grey area' of Jammu and Kashmir have not been identified frequently (hence, the lighter shade of yellow) and, when they have, they are described either as 'non-descript' and 'neutral' or as 'rural' and 'Muslim'. Himachal Pradesh English and Haryanvi English are rated 'broad' and 'diverse'. What emerges from the map is that, with the exception of Punjabi English, all 'Northernmost IndE' accents are closely linked to social stereotypes about the alleged educational level of their speakers, e.g., 'low' and 'weak' being some of the most common descriptors. Moreover, some adjectives appear to be descriptions of social status, e.g., 'rural', and religious affiliations, e.g., 'Muslim', rather than accents/dialects. Conversely, as its darker shade indicates, Punjabi IndE is identified by the majority of the sample as a 'funny', 'good' and 'common' accent of the 'Northernmost' speech area.

Delhi is another speech area detected by the informants. Marked in blue, it sheds light on one of the most common distinctions around social and regional accent variation: rural vs. urban. Delhi English is labelled 'posh', 'fancy' and 'artsy'. Yet, speakers perceive it as a near-standard and high-prestige variety of IndE (cf. Section 5.2).

The 'Northern IndE' speech area includes the states of Uttarakhand, Uttar Pradesh, Bihar and Jharkhand. 'Rough', 'strong', 'poor' and 'low' are features characterising these accents identified most commonly. Here, again, 'Northern IndE' accents are linked with social stereotypes about the alleged educational level of its speakers, their social status, e.g., 'working class', and their alleged personal qualities, e.g., 'lazy'.

'North Western IndE' is composed of Rajasthan and Gujarat. Gujarati English constitutes the 'core' of the speech area, being the most frequently perceived stereotypical accent of the two. More than 50 % of the sample considers it 'melodious' and, although some participants cluster it with Rajasthani English, they

85 Please note that the present map indicates political borders from the perspective of the Republic of India. The state of Jammu and Kashmir has been the subject of dispute between India, Pakistan, and China since 1947 (with Pakistan) and 1962 (with China). An agreement to resolve the Sino-Indian border dispute was attempted in 1996, including 'confidence-building measures' and a mutually agreed Line of Actual Control. At present, the dispute has not been resolved yet. However, the present map does not show the international boundaries, the internal administrative ones or the line of control between India and Pakistan and India and China. For a more detailed account of the border dispute cf. Orton (2010).

still differentiate them. However, these differences are not as perceptually salient as the ones demarcating the focal area of 'North Western IndE'.[86]

'North Eastern IndE' accents are represented by the so-called Seven Sisters' states, i.e., Arunachal Pradesh, Assam, Manipur, Meghalaya, Mizoram, Nagaland and Tripura, West Bengal and Orissa. The darker section, indicated by the Seven Sisters, displays the 'core dialect area' of the region. As with the 'Northernmost IndE' area, some of the adjectives appear to be linked to social stereotypes about the ethnicity of the speakers, e.g., 'Chinese', and their alleged educational level, e.g., 'poor'. However, unlike the 'Northernmost' area, the core of the Seven Sisters is labelled 'Chinese', 'working class' and 'poor' by more that 83 % of the respondents, suggesting not only that this region is highly stereotyped, but it is also among the more negatively connotated ones. The qualitative analysis of sociolinguistic interviews and the open-ended questions of Survey II, part I will provide a more detailed account of the topic, ultimately substantiating the findings of both the cognitive map task and the Accent Identification one (cf. Section 5.2). With respect to the other two accents of the 'Northern Eastern IndE' speech area, Orissa English is perceived fairly similarly to the English of the Seven Sisters. Bengali English is the only exception. Its lighter shade of green indicates that, despite being identified as 'Northern Eastern IndE', it is the least stereotypical one of the kind since it is associated with standardness, politeness, softness and higher literacy rates by more that 50 % and 83 % of the sample. An intuitive way of accounting for this result is that West Bengal has always boasted a rich literary heritage and a long tradition of folk literature and music. Hence, the speakers' perceptions of Bengali English are closely linked to the (positive) social stereotypes about the state (cf. Section 5.2).

The 'Central IndE' speech area includes Madhya Pradesh, Chhattisgarh and Maharashtra. Though some informants discriminate between the three states – clustering together Madhya Pradesh and Chhattisgarh only – the perceived difference is not as perceptually salient as the overall similarities recognised among the three IndE accents. For this reason, no isogloss demarcates Maharashtra as a speech area *per se* though, as is the case with Delhi, Western Maharashtra (and, particularly, Mumbai) is isolated from the rest with respect to the rural/urban accent distinction mentioned above. Subsequently, while more than 50 % of the participants label Marathi English 'metropolitan', 'posh', 'typical' and

86 The term 'focal area' is to mean the relative absence of isoglosses. For a detailed account of focal areas and transition ones cf. Glauser (2000, 1991).

'well-spoken', they describe Madhya Pradesh English and Chhattisgarh English as 'broad' and 'average'. Moreover, some adjectives appear to be descriptions of the alleged socio-economic status of the speakers, e.g., 'middle class', rather than their accents or dialects.

Finally, 'Southern IndE' accents are represented by the states of Goa, Karnataka, Telangana, Andhra Pradesh, Kerala and Tamil Nadu. 'Southern IndE' is the most heterogeneous area as compared to the other ones since it provides four different shades of red, indicating four different 'cores' or degrees of perceived stereotypical differences. The fairly detailed descriptions of Southern IndE accents come as no surprise, considering the commonly held folk belief in the community according to which Southern Indians have a distinctive accent when speaking English. Thus, a punctual observation of Southern IndE accents goes hand in hand with speakers' dialect consciousness. Tamil English constitutes the core dialect of the speech area; it is the 'Southern IndE' accent to be perceived as most stereotypical. More than 83 % of the sample agree on Tamil English being 'stereotypical', and more than 50 % consider it to be 'sing-song'. Interestingly, the second most stereotypical Southern IndE accent is Telugu English, spoken in both Telangana and Andhra Pradesh. This speech area is considered to be 'rough', 'strong', 'sing-song' and heavily influenced by the mother tongue. From a sociolinguistic and folk linguistic perspective, the adjective 'sing-song' carries interesting perceptual connotations, which will be looked into in more detail in Section 5.2. Interestingly, the adjective is used by more than 83 % of the informants to describe Tamil English and Telugu English, and by more that 33 % to connotate Gujarati English. Though the accents belong to two separate perceptual speech areas, i.e., 'Southern IndE' and 'North Western IndE', they pinpoint seemingly similar suprasegmental cues, which are most probably to be attributed to either speech rhythm (Regnoli forthcoming) or pitch correlates. However, further investigations are needed. Segmental cues seem to differentiate Malayalam English from the other 'Southern IndE' accents. 'Rolling' is the word most commonly used (> 33 % of the sample), indexing its excessive rhoticity due to L1 influence. In conclusion and in line with Delhi English and Marathi English, Karnataka English and Goa English are characterised by some 'multicultural' features which mark them as 'posh', yet 'smooth', 'hybrid', yet 'standard'. While the former is described as 'European' by more than 33 % of the participants – and is thus linked to social stereotypes about the original ethnicity of the speakers – the latter is perceived as a 'traditional' accent.

The present task accounts for the social stereotypes and overt attitudes of the participants towards accent variation in India. The above composite map shows seven transitional speech areas approximating the dialect or informal end of the continuum as low-prestige IndE and those closer to the national 'standard' or formal end as high-prestige IndE. Overall, the speech areas corresponding to 'Northernmost IndE', 'Northern IndE', 'Northern East IndE' (with the exception of Bengali English) and some areas of 'Southern IndE' are connotated negatively. On the contrary, the dialect areas of 'North Western IndE', 'Delhi IndE', 'Central IndE and some parts of 'Southern IndE' are seen positively. This happens because these varieties are associated with different levels of prestige depending on their status in society, and this degree of prestige has invariably been passed onto and associated with the speaker. As Trudgill (2000:8) argues:

> [b]ecause language as a social phenomenon is closely tied up with the social structure and value systems of society, different dialects and accents are evaluated in different ways. Standard English, for example, has much more status and prestige than any other English dialect. It is a dialect that is highly valued by many people, and certain economic, social and political benefits tend to accrue to those who speak and write it.

The seemingly contradictory perceptions of Southern IndE accents (carrying both positive and negative connotations) are due to a clear-cut difference that the respondents make between (heavily) accented speech and syntactic (in)accuracy. While this has been investigated elsewhere (Regnoli 2019a), it is important to mention that, although Southern IndE accents are often perceived as 'sharp' or 'rough', the general trend is to attribute Southern Indians a higher competence in, and command of, English than their Northern counterparts, either with reference to the higher literacy rate of major Southern states (cf. Karnataka in Figure 1.5.96) or to the status of the language as the *lingua franca* among the different Dravidian languages of the speech area.

Moreover, the perceptual urban/rural distinction emphasised by the participants appears to support actual dialect boundaries among states with better educational systems and higher literacy rates. This seems to go hand in hand with perceived standardness. Delhi, Maharashtra, West Bengal and some parts of Southern India are the speech areas connotated more positively. These accents are defined 'multicultural', 'hybrid' and, of course, 'standard', which means that they are overtly perceived as carrying much more status and prestige than other IndE varieties.

The fact that the informants use more or less the same general cognitive template for area identifications despite their gender, ethnicity or their time spent in Heidelberg substantiates the production counterpart of their perceptual cognitive map task (cf. Section 5.1.3.1). It shows how the linguistic power of the majority, i.e., the Northern informants, is gradually accepted by the minorities, i.e., the Southern part of the community. The stereotypical views of Northern

Indians about their own way of speaking (standard) English and that of Southern speakers are assimilated by their Southern counterparts, who have, by and large, taken over the stereotypes of the Northerners about themselves. Sections 5.1.3.7.2 and 5.2 will provide a more detailed account of the topic from a perception and a qualitative perspective, respectively.

5.1.3.7.2 Stimuli

The aim of the scales task is to obtain information on listeners' perceptions of production of different IndE accents. As discussed in Section 4.2.4, the participants are to listen to eight guises reading the same passage and, after each stimulus, are asked to "identify the ethnicity of the speakers and assign each voice to the site it belongs on the map provided" (II.II.1). Figures 5.1.22 and 5.1.23 show the numbering of guises according to their perceptually detected origin.

Data have been aggregated and processed following the method applied for the adjective map discussed in Section 5.1.3.7.1. The number of the guises that each respondent wrote down on the cognitive map was matched with the answer provided in II.II.1. The boundary for each state was treated as an isogloss, the one demarcating Northern and Southern India as a heterogloss.[87] For a better understanding of subjective dialect boundaries, the preliminary arrangement has been transferred into isopleth maps.[88] The data have again been aggregated and processed using the GNU image manipulation programme GIMP (version 2.10.10).

87 Although isoglosses are also called heteroglosses because they separate rather than connect points onto a map (Chambers/Trudgill 2004), the difference in the term is only kept in order to demarcate what was perceived as a wider boundary in accent variation.

88 An isopleth is a line drawn on a map connecting all points having the equal or corresponding value, amount or ratio of some geographical phenomena or linguistic variables. Cf. Chambers/Trudgill (2004) for further details.

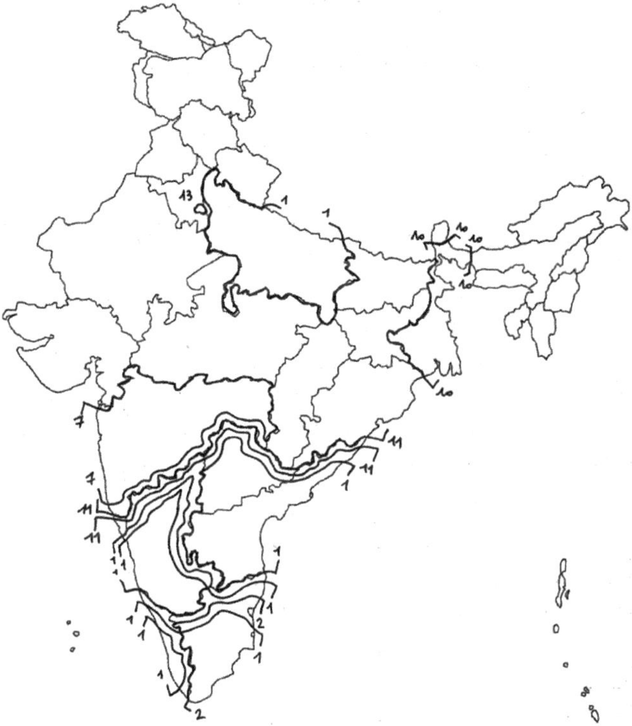

Fig. 5.1.70 Isoglosses, heteroglosses and isopleths indicating the alleged ethnicity of Speaker One: West Bengal

Figure 5.1.70 shows the distribution of heteroglosses and isopleths indicating the alleged ethnicity of Speaker One, a native of the North-Eastern state of West Bengal. The result is a cognitive map showing an interesting transition area between Maharashtra, Chhattisgarh and Orissa, and Goa, Karnataka and Telangana. West Bengal, Uttar Pradesh, Maharashtra, Tamil Nadu, Kerala, Andhra Pradesh, Telangana and Karnataka are bounded by seven isolated isoglosses. The Southern states of Karnataka, Kerala and Tamil Nadu form a focal area. Apart from the irregularities just mentioned, the lines form a very neat heterogloss between Northern India and Southern India. On the whole, Speaker One has been recognised as belonging to rather specific areas, yet 70 % of the sample correctly recognise her Northern ethnicity. 17 % identify the guise as native of West Bengal. The heterogloss demarcating Northern and Southern India clearly shows where the participants perceive the main dialect boundary. This supports earlier claims according to which "whatever reservations dialectologists may have about boundaries, they are certainly disconfirmed by dialect speakers who are quite willing to say where their speech form comes to an end" (Glauser 1991:4).

While the participants harbour rather precise ideas about dialect boundaries with regard to Bengali English, a first glance at Fig. 5.1.71 shows that this is certainly not the case with Tamil English.

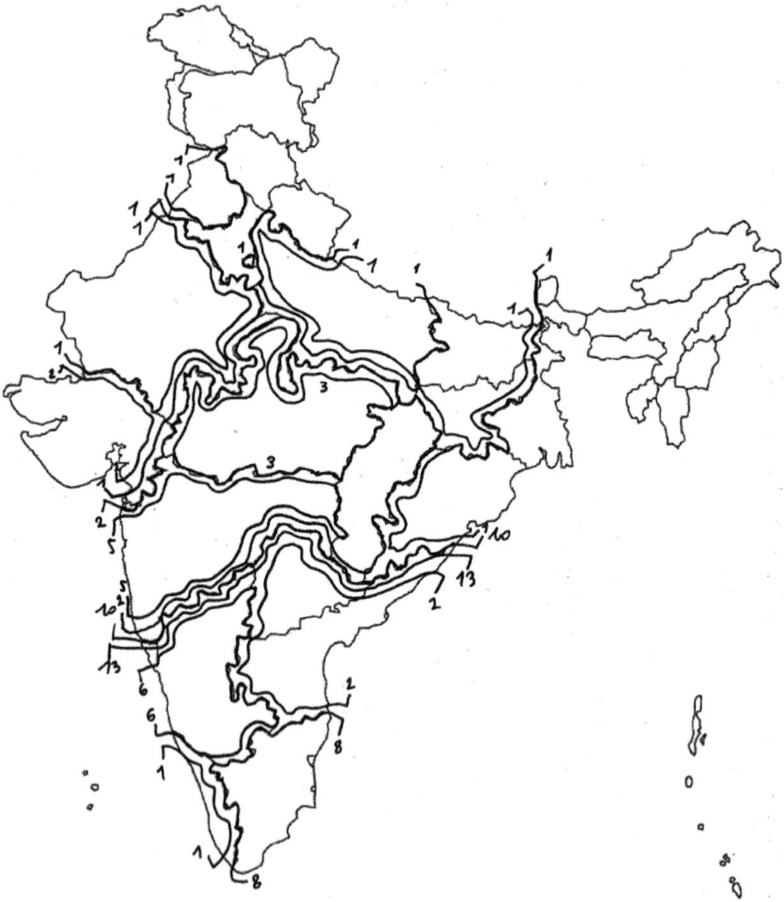

Fig. 5.1.71 Isoglosses, heteroglosses and isopleths indicating the alleged ethnicity of Speaker Two: Tamil Nadu

The distribution of isoglosses and heteroglosses separating single states and Northern India from Southern India resembles that of Fig. 5.1.70. On the whole, it is possible to detect five transition areas that separate North Western India, Northern India, North Eastern India, from Central India and Southern India. Although 13 % of the sample correctly identify the speaker as a native of the Southern state of Tamil Nadu, 50 % of the informants agree that Speaker Two is a native of Northern India, and, specifically, of the poorest states of the area. As discussed in Section 5.1.3.2, this claim substantiates earlier findings according to which the Southern guises are perceived as significantly less educated than the Northern ones (cf. Section 5.1.3.1).

From a perceptual dialectology perspective, the transition areas in Fig. 5.1.72 shed new light on the close connection between the (negative) social stereotypes about speakers of Southern IndE accents, i.e., less pleasant, educated, attractive, etc., and the inherently fuzzy dialect boundaries detected.

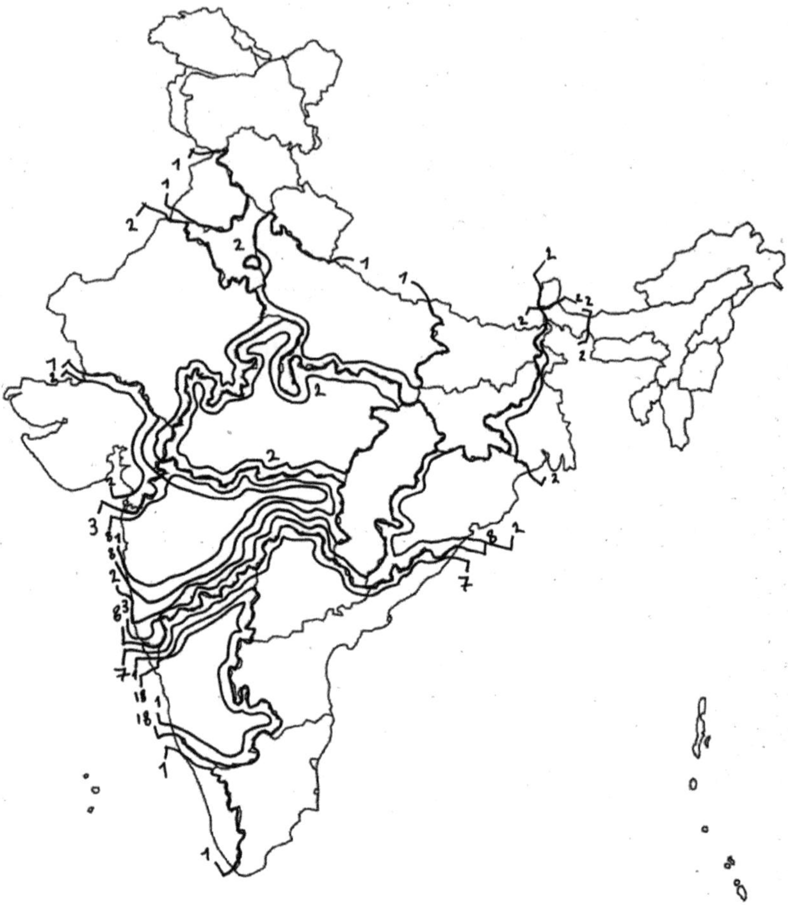

Fig. 5.1.72 Isoglosses, heteroglosses and isopleths indicating the alleged ethnicity of Speaker Three: Karnataka; L1: Konkani

The results from the Accent Identification Task show that Speaker Three has always been an exception with regard to the North vs. South distinction (cf. Sections 5.1.3.1 and 5.1.2). The composite perceptual map above seems to confirm this trend. The distribution of isoglosses, heteroglosses and isopleths shows the presence of two main transition areas. The first one separates Northern India from Southern India and the second one North Western India from the rest of the subcontinent. However, a close look at the map shows more transition areas than focal ones, thus underlying the participants' rather precise ideas about dialect boundaries. On the whole, although 30 % of the sample correctly locate the guise in her state of origin, i.e., Karnataka, the isopleths on the map show that an additional 10 % identify her as native of some North-Western, Central, Central-Western and South Western speech areas. Taking into account the state of origin of the guise, her L1, i.e., Konkani, and the main speech areas in which the latter is spoken, i.e., Maharashtra, Goa, Karnataka, the map below shows that the informants detect fairly accurate dialect boundaries.

Figure 5.1.73 shows the distribution of isoglosses, heteroglosses and isopleths indicating the alleged ethnicity of Speaker Four, a native of the Central state of Maharashtra, but with Gujarati origins.

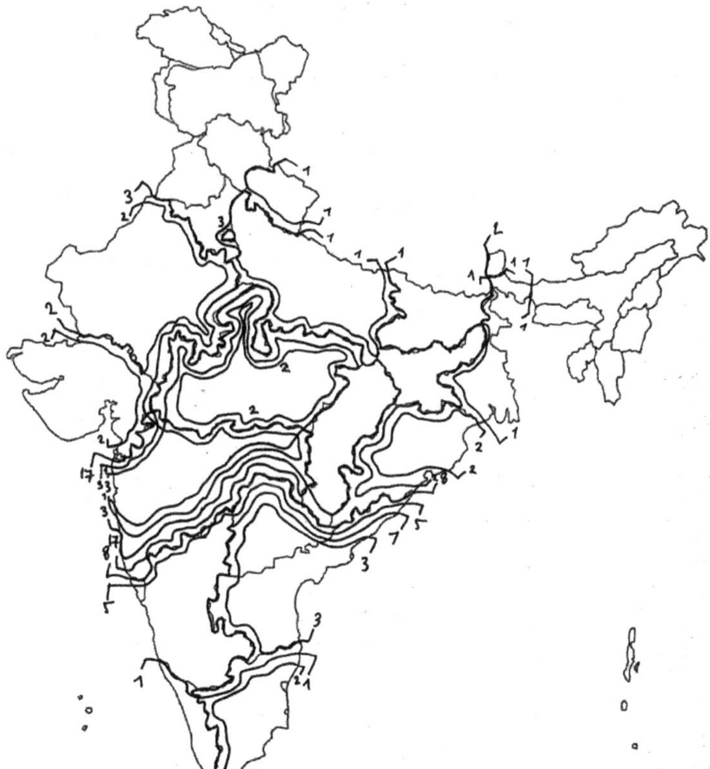

Fig. 5.1.73 Isoglosses, heteroglosses and isopleths indicating the alleged ethnicity of Speaker Four: Maharashtra

The result is a perceptual map showing a transition area similar to that of Speaker Three, but with a slightly more elaborate distribution of isoglosses. The complexity of these bundles of isoglosses is portrayed in the apparent 'confusion' of the participants with respect to the ethnicity of the guise. While 28 % of the sample correctly recognise him as native of Maharashtra, an additional 48 % identify his 'hybridity' (being a Maharashtrian with Gujarati origins) in terms of precise dialect boundaries. This result points to a conclusion common to all the guises and participants selected for the present study: while the former appear to be fairly representative of the standard IndE variety they are speaking, the latter show a high degree of language awareness, especially with regard to perceived accent variation.

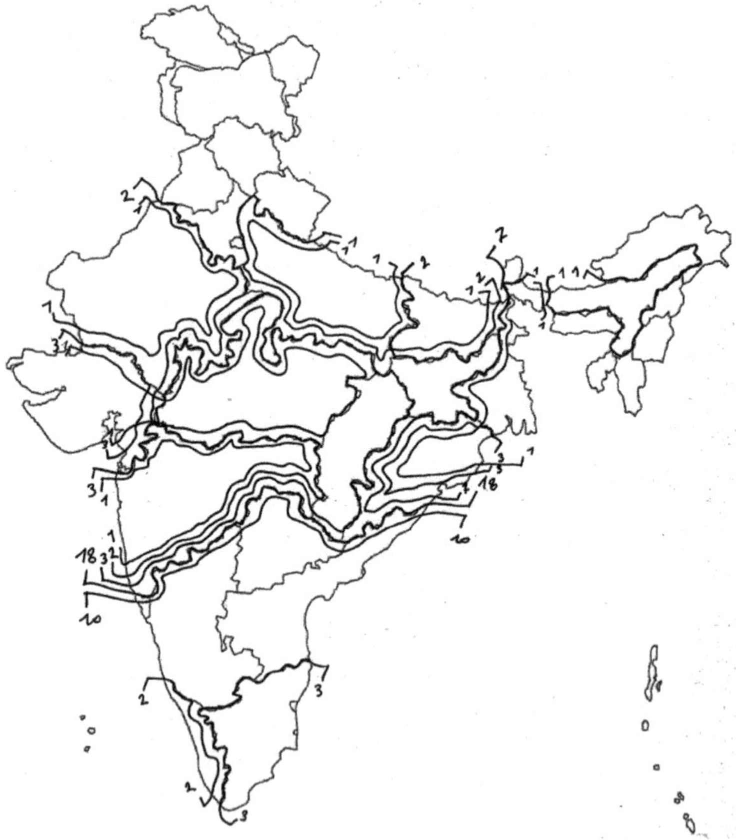

Fig. 5.1.74 Isoglosses, heteroglosses and isopleths indicating the alleged ethnicity of Speaker Five: Karnataka; L1: Kannada

Section 5.1.3.2 has shed light on Speaker Five, i.e., the guise recognised the least among the sample. Figure 5.1.74 shows the distribution of isoglosses, heteroglosses and isopleths indicating her alleged ethnicity. While no isogloss demarks the speech area she comes from, i.e., Karnataka, two isoglosses separating Northern India from Southern India and two isolated isoglosses each demarcating the Southern states of Kerala and Tamil Nadu inform on her correct ethnicity. Yet, the isopleths displayed on the map show that only 25 % of the sample agree on her Southern ethnicity. The remaining 76 % identify the guise as belonging to several speech areas located in Northern India, and particularly to some of the poorest states of the subcontinent, i.e., Assam, Bihar, Jharkhand. Though with fewer bundles of isoglosses, Fig. 5.1.74 shows a fairly similar transition area as Fig. 5.1.71. The isoglosses separating Northern India from Southern India show that 55 % of the sample recognise the guise as a Northern IndE speaker. Unlike other guises, and with the exception of Speaker Two, the North/South heterogloss indicates a massive discrepancy between the two speech areas, thus suggesting that Karnataka English is a rather difficult accent to pinpoint and locate.

Figure 5.1.75 shows how transitional the IndE dialect landscape can be with respect to the identification of Punjabi English. On the whole, the map shows a transition area between the North Western, the Central, the North Eastern and the Southern IndE speech areas. The Northern states of Punjab, Delhi, Uttar Pradesh, Bihar as well as Jharkhand (which form a focal area), the North-Eastern states of West Bengal and Orissa, the North Western states of Rajasthan and Gujarat as well as the Southern states of Karnataka, Kerala, Tamil Nadu and Andhra Pradesh and Telangana (which, again, form a focal area) constitute 12 speech areas marked by 12 isolated isoglosses. Despite the many bundles of isoglosses, the participants harbour fairly precise ideas about the ethnicity of the guise since 67 % of them recognised his Northern ethnicity (7 % of which identify the guise as native of Punjab). The isopleths displayed on the map suggest that a rather exiguous portion of the sample locate Speaker Six in Southern India (23 %). The remaining informants attribute the origin of the speaker to isolated states and speech areas in North-Eastern and North-Western India. The bundles of isoglosses mirror how transitional the IndE dialect landscape can be with respect to the identification of Punjabi English.

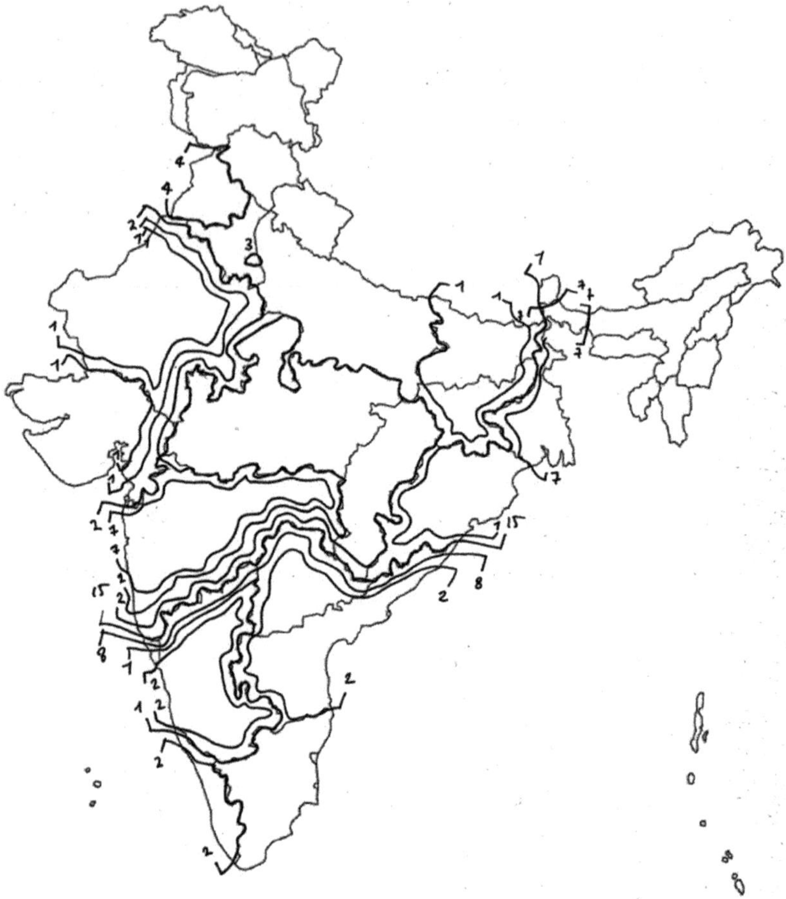

Fig. 5.1.75 Isoglosses, heteroglosses and isopleths indicating the alleged ethnicity of Speaker Six: Punjab

Figure 5.1.76 shows the same trend with respect to Uttar Pradesh English. The distribution of isoglosses, heteroglosses and isopleths indicates that, just like Speaker Six, only 7 % of the sample identify correctly the place of origin of Speaker Seven. The states of Uttar Pradesh, West Bengal, Punjab, Delhi, Madhya Pradesh, Maharashtra, Karnataka, Andhra Pradesh/Telangana (which form a focal area) as well as Kerala form nine isolated isoglosses. The resulting lines show a transition area between Madhya Pradesh, Maharashtra, Karnataka and

Telangana which forms a very neat boundary between Northern and Southern India. The isopleths displayed on the map indicate that 64 % of the participants have fairly accurate ideas about her ethnicity. On the whole, with the exception of an insignificant 2 % of the sample, the heterogloss differentiating Northern India from Southern India shows that the main accent boundary lies in between the transition area. This suggests that, with respect to accent recognition, the participants mainly rely on Northern vs. Southern IndE perceptual differences.

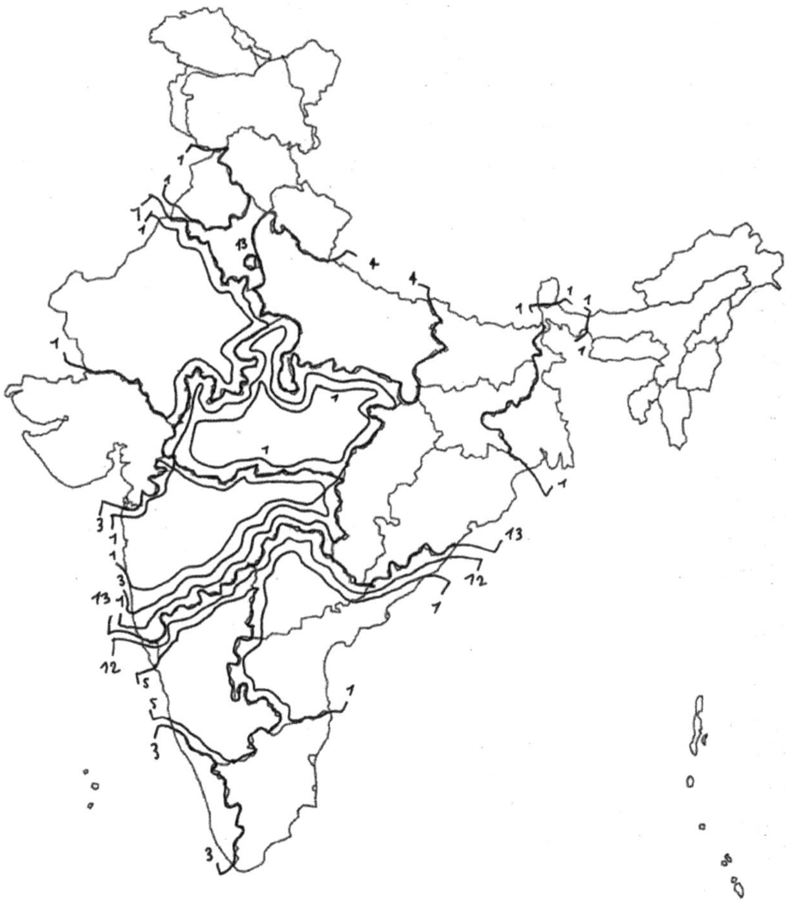

Fig. 5.1.76 Isoglosses, heteroglosses and isopleths indicating the alleged ethnicity of Speaker Seven: Uttar Pradesh

The perceptual map shown in Fig. 5.1.77 is no exception. The distribution of isoglosses, heteroglosses and isopleths on the map shows the ethnicity of Speaker Eight, a native of the Southern state of Andhra Pradesh, as perceived by the community members. The result is a transition area between Maharashtra, Chhattisgarh, Orissa, Karnataka and Telangana/Andhra Pradesh (which, as usual, form a focal area). The Southern states of Tamil Nadu, Karnataka and Telangana/Andhra Pradesh, the North Western states of Gujarat and Rajasthan, the Northern states of Bihar and Uttar Pradesh as well as the North Eastern states of West Bengal and Orissa form nine isolated isoglosses. With the exception of the focal area of Telangana and Andhra Pradesh (which was correctly identified by 12 % of the population) and apart from the irregularities indicated by the isolated isoglosses just mentioned, the lines form a very neat boundary between Northern and Southern India. As the isopleths show, 42 % of the sample recognise the (correct) Southern ethnicity of the guise while another 46 % indicate that he is from Northern India. The remaining 12 % locate him in the following speech areas: Central India, North-Eastern India and East India. As with Speakers Two and Five, Speaker Eight is often perceived as coming from the poorest states of India, i.e., Bihar, Jharkhand and, generally, Eastern India. This finding substantiates earlier claims according to which Southern IndE accents tend to be perceived as less prestigious on a massive number of attitude scales (cf. Sections 5.1.3.1 and 5.1.3.2).

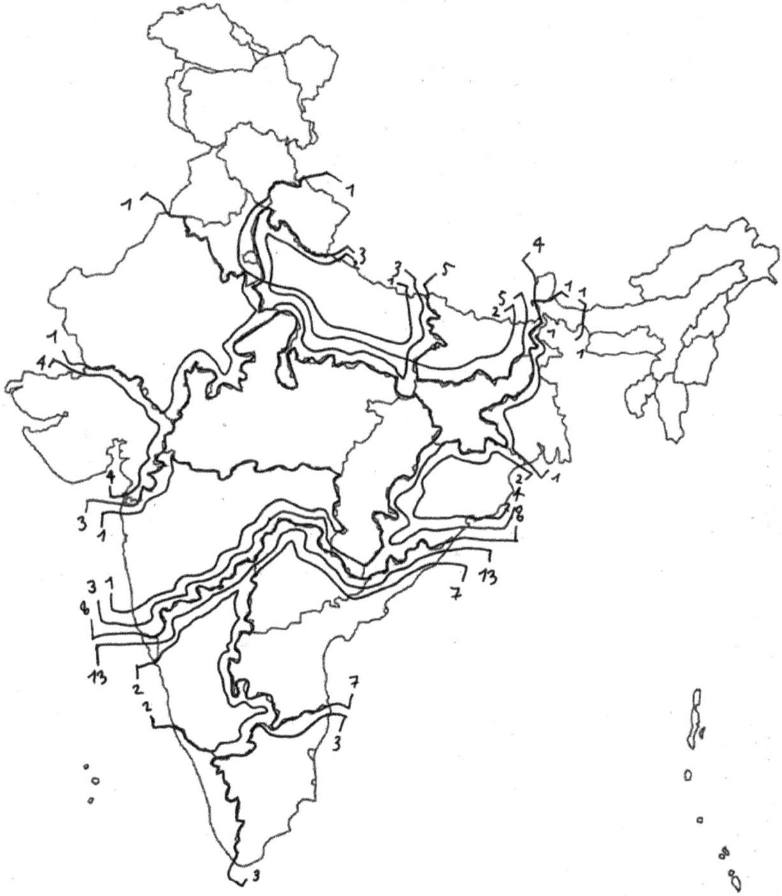

Fig. 5.1.77 Isoglosses, heteroglosses and isopleths indicating the alleged ethnicity of Speaker Eight (Andhra Pradesh)

On the whole, the discussion of the assignment of the guises to the site they are perceived to belong on the blank map points to a general conclusion – common to all the guises selected as well as the participants. However transitional the IndE dialect landscape appears to be, there are folk conceptions such as Northern IndE, Southern IndE, Central IndE, North-Eastern IndE, North-Western IndE and Delhi English which cannot remain unnoticed, whatever reservations dialectologists may have about boundaries. Although linguists try to fill them with certain characteristics which, at times, appear rather fuzzy (cf. Section 5.1.3.2), these cognitive boundaries exist and need to be addressed and related to their networks in order to understand what sociolinguistic stereotypes are at stake and what criteria are made use of in such discriminations.

Moreover, though this conclusion can potentially be extended to all the IndE accents selected for the present study, there are some that tend to be less identifiable than others. The analysis of the Likert scales presented in Section 5.1.3.1 and the implicational arrangement of the guises and participants with respect to the Accent Identification Task (cf. Section 5.1.3.5.2) suggest that Southern IndE accents are the least recognised ones. The cognitive map task substantiates these findings and adds a new perspective to the topic: the higher the recognition, the less fuzzy the boundaries. In other words, the informants harbour more precise ideas about dialect boundaries when the guise is from Northern India. This may justify the folk beliefs of the community according to which Southern Indians have a distinctive IndE accent to the extent that social stereotypes play a fundamental role in accent recognition. Section 5.2 will provide a detailed account of the speakers' classification of local speech and assessment of IndE varieties.

5.2 Qualitative Analysis

The essentially quantitative approaches used in the sections above are supplemented and expanded on here based on data gathered in Survey II, part I and the interviews. As discussed in Section 4.4.2, a bottom-up approach has been preferred in order to let the data 'speak for themselves'. The topics for the qualitative part have been prepared and analysed by applying a revised form of the qualitative content analysis developed by Mayring (2014). The data are first determined and described, and, in a second step, the relevant passages are located and grouped for each (sub)topic. These passages mainly correspond to either one or more questions in the survey or in the semi-structured interviews. However, quite often, the informants have also commented on a topic at an earlier or later stage of the survey or the interview. Thus, all passages in which the participants relate explicitly to a given topic have been analysed.

The qualitative data analysis software MAXQDA (version 2018.2) has been used in the organisation and the structuring of the data. Specifically, the data are first imported and transcribed when needed, and then coded. The assignment of a code to a particular part of a document follows a bottom-up approach. Finally, the data segments of the retrieved codes are collected and exported into a list of results. Table 5.2.1 shows the code system of both Survey II,I and the interviews.

Tab. 5.2.1 Code system of II,I and sociolinguistic interviews (MAXQDA 2018.2)

Code System	**2781**	
1. Indexicality	92	/575
- Accent and belonging	133	
1.1 State-to-state distinction	20	
1.2 North-South distinction	36	
1.2.1 Northern IndEs	111	
1.2.1.1 Northern commentary	70	
1.2.1.2 Southern commentary	41	
1.2.2 Southern IndEs	183	
1.2.2.1 Northern commentary	61	
1.2.2.2 Southern commentary	67	
1.2.2.3 Compliment	55	
2. Metalinguistic awareness	250	/1306
2.1 Degrees of consciousness	306	
2.1.1 Markers	16	
2.1.1.1 Phonetics	15	
2.1.1.2 Lexicon and syntax	1	
2.1.2 Stereotypes	137	
2.1.2.1 Phonetics	126	
2.1.2.2 Lexicon and syntax	11	
2.2 Diaspora consciousness in Heidelberg	124	
2.2.1 Change of accent	60	
2.2.1.1 Yes	26	
2.2.1.2 No	24	
2.2.1.3 Unsure	10	
2.2.2 HISA	65	
2.2.3 Indians in Heidelberg	63	
2.2.4 Networking	90	
2.2.5 Transnational ties	53	
2.3 Language embarrassment	62	
2.3.1 Grammar improvement	45	
2.3.2 Accent improvement	87	
2.3.3 Neutral accent	17	
2.4 Ideologies	56	
2.4.1 Ideologies of nativeness	55	
2.4.2 Best English/education	69	
2.4.3 Urban/rural distinction	57	

As can be seen, all the sub-codes detected are clustered into two main topics: indexicality and metalinguistic awareness. While most topics are implicit in the design of the questionnaire, it emerged during fieldwork that this is not true for all of them. One advantage of the qualitative design is that these recurrent issues (which are deemed important in the eyes of the informants) may be incorporated into the interpretation of the results. The main issues, covered in Sections 5.2.1 and 5.2.2, will be treated as dependent variables and interpreted in relation to the quantitative data analysed in Section 5.1. As described in Section 4.1, this explanatory sequential design allows for a quantitative strand to receive the greatest emphasis, i.e., sequential timing was preferred during individual tasks, beginning with a quantitative strand, and for its results to be followed up with a qualitative phase.

II,I and the interviews will be analysed dependently and concurrently. The main issues covered by II,I concern accent and identity and are devised to measure the extent to which informants identified with their home town/state/geographic location in terms of accent perceptions. The main aim of the questionnaire was to elicit respondents' awareness of their own accents in English according to Silvertein's (1981) five conditions enhancing and predicting folk scrutiny, i.e., unavoidable referentiality, continuous segmentability, relative presuppositionality, decontextualised deducibility and metapragmatic transparency (cf. Section 4.2.2). The main issues covered by the sociolinguistic interview task are structured in three modules and are coded accordingly: (i) demography; (ii) accent and identity, language attitudes and regard; (iii) Heidelberg and networking.

Figures 5.2.1 and 5.2.2 show the list of frequencies of the topics detected in II,I and the interviews, respectively, enabling a comparison of the flow of codes for each participant. Both document comparison charts show the participants on the y axis and the paragraph numbers according to which the answers are ordered on the x axis. The cells show the codes that exist in each paragraph for each participant with a bar assigned the same colour as the code it represents. Each code present in the paragraph is represented by a coloured section of the bar. Each colour is equivalent to all the topics and sub-topics already presented in Tab. 5.2.1. When a code is used more than once in a paragraph, it is still only visualised once. When multiple codes appear in the same paragraph, the colours of both codes are listed in the respective cell. By default, each paragraph is the same width, regardless of how many characters it includes. In the case of several codes, the available space is assigned proportionally to the coded segments in the paragraph, reporting how frequently a code had been assigned in the paragraph – not how extensive the segment was. If a code occurs three times in the paragraph and another one only once, the first code gets ¾ of the area, the second only ¼.

A first glance at Fig. 5.2.1 shows that metalinguistic awareness is the topic discussed more frequently in Survey II,I. This comes as no surprise considering that the main aim of the questionnaire was to elicit the respondents' awareness of their own accents in English. Interestingly, more than 50 % of the sample connect metalinguistic awareness with language embarrassment (in blue) and, inevitably, with overt commentaries regarding Northern and Southern IndE varieties. The high frequency of the sub-code diaspora consciousness (displayed in green) shows that the majority of the community members address the topic extensively, and always in relation to whether they have known some Indians who changed their accents after moving to Heidelberg (II.I.14; cf. Section 5.2.2). The other main topic of interest, indexicality, is addressed by almost all the informants and, if not commented upon alone, it was either connected with metalinguistic awareness or accent and belonging.

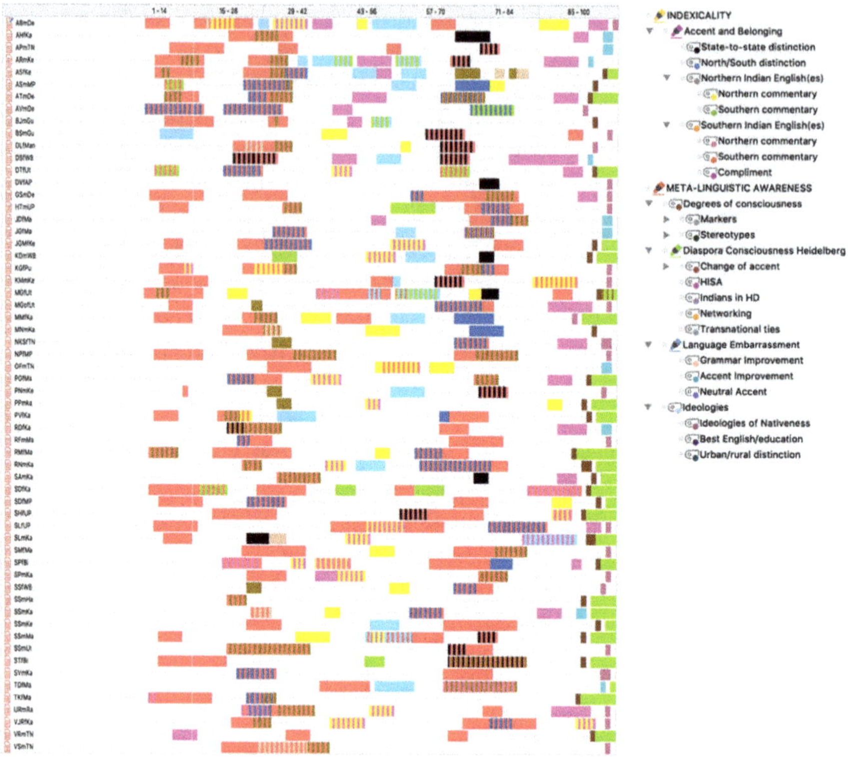

Fig. 5.2.1 Document comparison chart of II,I

In contrast to Fig. 5.2.1, Fig. 5.2.2 shows a higher number of topics and subtopics in progression as a result of the more complex nature of sociolinguistic interviews. Yet the document comparison chart shows a stable pattern of codes and sub-codes which yields four major topics: commentaries about Southern IndE varieties (displayed in dark pink for Northern informants and in red for Southern ones), accent improvement (in turquoise), networking in Heidelberg (in orange) and HISA (in purple). With some exceptions which will be addressed in the following sections, the topics are in linear progression since the interview task is semi-structured and follows the three modules described above.

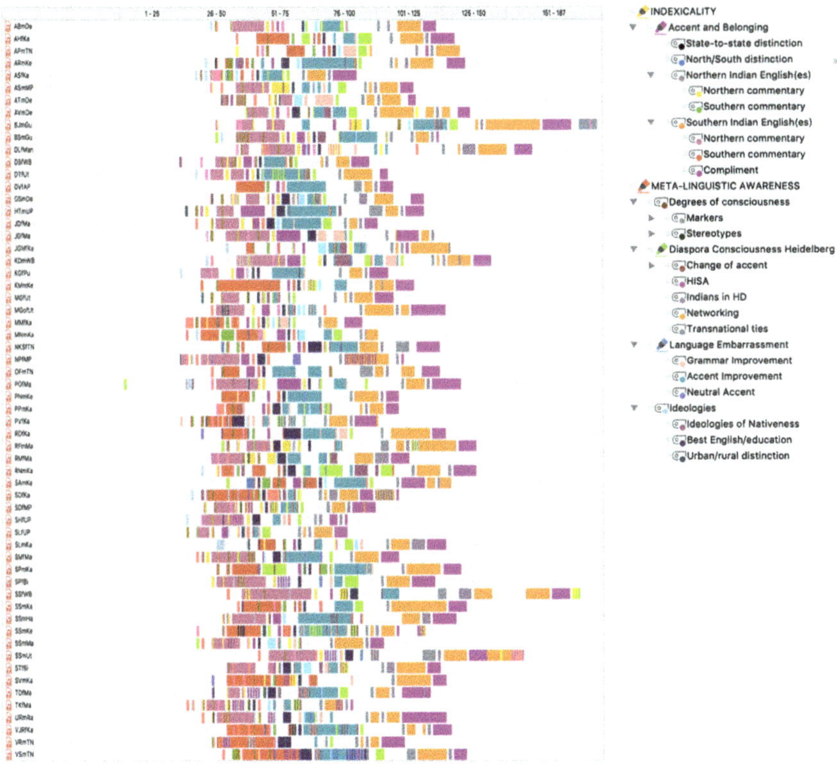

Fig. 5.2.2 Document comparison chart of sociolinguistic interviews

On the whole, the main issues detected in Figs. 5.2.1 and 5.2.2 will be discussed as follows: Section 5.2.1 will treat folk scrutiny and indexicality and will shed new light on the qualitative counterpart of the data concerning the classification of local IndE speech, the exploration of language attitudes towards IndE varieties and the role of identity within the community. Section 5.2.2 will raise the following issues: diaspora consciousness, accent awareness, the role of language ideologies on the attitudes analysed in the earlier section – especially in relation to nativeness and the 'neutral' accent – as well as network affiliations and transnational ties.

5.2.1 Folk Scrutiny and Indexicality

As suggested earlier, in the world outside linguistics, people who are not engaged in any study of language talk about it all the same. The present section will address such overt knowledge of and comments about language, i.e., folk metalanguage (cf. Section 2.4.2) on a consciousness continuum. As discussed in Section 2.3.2, folk awareness of language may, in addition to having a cline of availability, range along a continuum of detail, from the specific to the global. As Niedzielski and Preston (2003:305) argue:

> [...] these global sorts of folk linguistic comments may be internally motivated ones, for they seem to be based on the respondent's awareness of a difference between his or her language use and that of the others, however unspecified the details of the difference may be.

Although it has been argued that folk linguistics is only concerned with "'superficial' results of deeper [linguistic] operations" (Niedzielski/Preston 2003:304), it occasionally draws attention to other ways of expressing metalanguage belief. The present section will shed light on how laypeople's comments about accent variation suggest that a major sociopsychological factor which motivates the folk notice of language lies in institutionalised or conventionalised regulations, i.e., language ideologies. Positing that all performed speech requires a focus on and reference to language itself and that, when embedding an imitation of a group or an individual, one implicitly refers to an exophoric 'cultural script', Section 5.2.2 will address how identities and associated stereotypes are also awakened by such performances. Results from the analysis of these performances will be correlated with those retrieved from the Accent Recognition Task and discussed in Section 5.1, with the ultimate aim of comparing the extent to which the stimuli selected awaken any recognition of a caricaturist sort to the speakers' overt reactions to variation.

5.2.1.1 Classification of Local Speech

The informants' sociolinguistic awareness of local speech is the subject of the largest group of questions in Survey II,I and the sociolinguistic interviews. On the whole, these questions deal with (i) the informants' overt consciousness of the existence of particular forms of local IndE varieties; (ii) the labels attributed to these forms, their scope and delimitation; (iii) the participants' attitudes towards and assessment of their knowledge of local forms of speech and (iv) their perception of dialect/accent variation. In order to answer these questions, the present section has been divided into four subsections: the first one will deal with the recognition and classification of local IndE varieties; the second part will treat the assessment of IndE varieties within the Heidelberg Indian student community and the last two will be concerned with attitudes towards local speech including beliefs about language and speakers. Each sub-section, and especially the last two, will include different components of the threefold attitude model discussed in Section 2.4.

Since language, society and awareness are closely related to identity (cf. Section 5.1.2.1) and, of course, interrelated, the present section will finally provide a description of the extent to which the informants' sociolinguistic awareness can be made explicit by themselves and through the interpretation of their speech performances.

5.2.1.1.1 Distinctiveness of Speech

The present section has local speech as the attitude object. As discussed in Section 2.4, the exploration of language attitudes in the present study is based on a threefold attitude concept in which the cognitive, affective and conative components interact to form a super-attitude towards different attitude objects. Here, cognitive attitudes will be taken into account with respect to the classification of IndE varieties. Since the cognitive element corresponds to beliefs about language attitudes, it has been considered important to assess how the participants perceive Indian varieties of English before investigating their perceptions of their own speech (cf. Section 5.2.2.1). The terms used by the participants to refer to local IndE speech or forms of local IndE speech have been elicited through the following questions:

- *Are there different accents in India? (II.I.10)*
- *If there are, what are they? Do you like them? Can you tell them apart easily? (II.I.11)*

While II.I.10 is a multiple-choice question (yes, no, unsure), II.I.11 is an open one and thus produces a number of different answers, which are categorised with the help of the qualitative content analysis (cf. Section 4.4.2). Table 5.2.2 shows that, with the exception of one Southern female informant who has been living in Heidelberg for less than a year, all community members agree on the existence of different Indian accents of English. The mere acknowledgement and occurrence of some IndE varieties which have distinctive features is enough to count as a 'performance' of them and qualifies any use of them whatsoever as a likely trigger of metalanguage response.

Tab. 5.2.2 Awareness of IndE accents according to the community, gender, ethnicity and time spent in Heidelberg[a]

Are there different accents in India? (II.1.10)	**N**	**%**
Yes	59	98
No	0	0
Unsure	1	2
Total	60	100

(a) according to gender	Male		Female	
	N	%	N	%
Yes	30	100	29	97
No	0	0	0	0
Unsure	0	0	1	3
Total	30	100	30	100

(b) according to ethnicity	North		South	
	N	%	N	%
Yes	34	100	25	97
No	0	0	0	0
Unsure	0	0	1	3
Total	34	100	26	100

(c) according to length of stay in Heidelberg	0.1–1		1.1–5	
	N	%	N	%
Yes	38	97	21	100
No	0	0	0	0
Unsure	1	3	0	0
Total	39	100	21	100

a Percentages have been rounded.

This question enables the participants to dig deeper and to provide a classification of local speech through II.1.11. Although they did not have to choose from a given selection of terms, the variety of answers is surprisingly small and follows, on the whole, the same cognitive pattern of identification/ discrimination, i.e., geographical variation:

(1) Yes, with the vast diversity of local languages in India, these local languages have their influences on English, which often at times is the second language. Most often, I feel I can tell them apart. (ABmDe) surv.[89]
(2) Yes, there are. I like all the Indian accents. I think one can broadly distinguish between North and South Indian accents. For me, it's a little hard to further distinguish between within South Indian accents, but I understand that they exist. I find distinguishing between North Indian accents a little more hard than South. Because South India has more languages than North. Hindi is kind of the lingua franca of North, and for that reason most of us North Indians would have been raised learning the same accent. Whereas in South Indian, as you have more languages (which are very different from each other), I guess that's why there are more distinguishable accents. I could tell them apart, at times. (GSmDe) surv.
(3) There are definite differences in southern and northern accents. Especially the north-eastern and eastern. I think that I can tell the differences, at least some of them. I can do that because I know how they generally sound due to frequent interaction and exposure to many of them, especially during my stay in Delhi for two years and Mumbai for 3 years. (RMfMa) surv.
(4) I can tell the difference between a south Indian and north Indian accent but not the difference between different north Indian states as I do not come from that region. But I do think each one us has a different accent. (MMfKa) surv.

These examples seem to confirm the results from the Accent Recognition Task and the cognitive maps, analysed in Sections 5.1.3.1 and 5.1.3.7, respectively. Community members tend to differentiate on a North vs. South basis first, and then, depending on their "frequent interaction[s] and exposure to many of them [accents]", they operationalise differences on a more local/ethnic level. The following examples contribute to shedding light on the topic:

(5) In my personal opinion, these are the following accents prevalent in India: 1. Punjabi/Haryanvi 2. Malayali & Tamil 3. Telegu 4. Bengali and North-Eastern 5. Metropolitan. (DSfWB) surv.

---

89 The present quotations are all unchanged. When present, short hesitations are indicated as _, while long ones are mentioned in round brackets. Further comments are in round brackets as well. For a detailed account of the transcription conventions cf. p. xviii. The quotations are indicated as int. if they are taken from interviews or surv., if from the survey tasks.

(6) I think it is fascinating to hear different accents and each and every one of them is interesting by itself. I think I am able to roughly tell where a person is from by their accent. I would generally categorise them as: South Indian, generic north Indian, metropolitan, rural/northern hinterlands, Eastern, Bengali, Gujarati, Marathi. (MGfUt)
(7) Malayalam: They pronounce the 'o' differently. Can be noticed in office, orange. And they roll their tongue a lot. Tamil: Sharp cuts between words, again due to how Tamil is. Kannadiga: Closer to Tamil accent according to me. Sharp cuts, and usage of some Kannada connecting words. Telugu: The one that remains out of the other southern accents. Hindi: 'z sound.' Machine. Rural areas they add 'iss' before school, smile. Yes. (ASfKe) surv.
(8) Yeah, Kannada English, Tamil English, Hindi English...it depends on each state but usually I divide them into Northern or Southern accents. Basically the North accents have a lot of Hindi words used when they are speaking or there are grammatical mistakes in their English. In the South we are more correct and fluent and the accent is more multicultural. (PVfKa) surv.

What emerges from the examples above is that some local varieties of IndE are more easily recognised than others. This may be one of the factors among other social ones which marks certain community in-groups (and their ordinary language behaviour) as 'folk objects' in some cultural settings. As seen in Section 5.1.3.2, even on a more cognitive level, the participants are better at identifying certain IndE varieties. The reported results show that the speakers' covert perceptions and overt statements coincide since they agree on Bengali English and Kannada English being among the most recognisable and distinctive local varieties of IndE.

Moreover, this is very clearly a discourse which has indexicality and metalanguage as its main topic ("I think I am able to roughly tell where a person is from by their accent"). The examples above shed light on the participants' accurate discriminations between Northern and Southern accents. GSmDe, for instance, points to the importance of Hindi as a *lingua franca* in Northern India and to the subsequent possible reason why Northern IndE accents sound pretty much the same. Doubtless all of this is true, but from a folk linguistic perspective, an excursion into GSmDe's folk philosophy of language reveals interesting overt metalanguage comment. The presupposition behind this statement, i.e., that Northern IndE accents are more compact systems compared to Southern IndE ones, is shared by the majority of community members (DSfWB, ASfKe, PVfKa, MMfKa are among others). In addition, it generally forms the backbone of mutual understanding within the community. It goes without saying that the deeper the sense of the community, network density and shared culture among the participants, the more likely the numbers of presupposed beliefs play a crucial role.

The data from the Accent Identification Task and the 'scaling task' discussed in Sections 5.1.3.2–5.1.3.4 and 5.1.3.7.1 respectively suggest that GSmDe's overt and covert attitudes towards Northern and Southern IndE accents share a solid common ground. Both tasks, II,I and the sociolinguistic interview show that he perceives strong and clear-cut differences between Northern and Southern IndE accents. On a more cognitive level, the data show that he judges that Northern accents are 'better' than Southern ones on a number of attitude traits. Overall, the qualitative content analysis substantiates the findings of the quantitative one with respect to the North vs. South accent/dialect distinction. In addition, it provides further insight into the acknowledgement of a similar cultural model shared by the community members. As D'Andrade (1987:112–13) contends "[one] result of intersubjective sharing is that interpretations made about the world on the basis of the folk model are treated as if they were obvious facts of the world". For the community members, language itself seems to be the very real (though admittedly ideal) fact which dominates language use. Yet, the only possible usage which derives from this ideal is 'good' language. All other forms seem to be deviations from what *a* norm ought to be. The difference between Northern and Southern IndE varieties seems to follow the same pattern. Section 5.2.1.1.2 will delve into an enriched understanding of the underlying folk beliefs the informants have about the nature of IndE varieties.

5.2.1.1.2 Assessment of Indian Varieties of English within the Community

To gain insight into the assessed vitality of local speech, module II of the interview task (Accent and Identity; Language Attitudes and Regard) focused on the elicitation of information on how informants perceive Northern and Southern IndE varieties. Participants have first been asked to comment upon the Accent Identification Task just completed and to provide the clues/cues they used to discriminate the guises and then to elaborate on the commonly held folk belief about Southern IndE accents. Specifically, the following questions have been asked:

- *Many people from the Indian community here in Heidelberg say that Southern Indians have a peculiar speech. What do you think about that? Is it true in your opinion? Why? (int. II.4)*
- *Can you tell if someone's from the South of India by the way he talks? How can you tell? (int. II.5)*
- *How about, in comparison to say, Northern India? (int. II.7)*

Conversational data concerning the Accent Identification Task show a great number of metalanguage comments and attitudinal responses to language. The following examples show the speakers' awakening of response to IndE accent variation:

(9) RFmMa: For, at the beginning it was difficult because I was not able to understand what I have to do and secondly I've met many less people in (pauses) my life, not less people but I guess I met people only of my religion or from North India. I have met many less people from South India because I live in Pune, and Pune, in Pune mostly Maharashtrian live, and where I live, it is always dominated (laughs) by Maharastrian's people, so. And in my school and my college, it was nearby my, near in my, in, in, in, in, nearby area only, so I guess that time also, I, I met very less people but after coming to Germany I met people of various caste and religion, so I guess, I'm able to identify them a little bit now.
GR: Do you think you were able to discriminate speakers geographically just from the audio clips? RFmMa: I guess I can now (pauses) after this exercise I can now, because I've never thought of it but I, I can differentiate between North and South Indians but I cannot differentiate in states, like 'this might be from this state' because as I said, in my (pauses). int.

(10) Uhm, it was very difficult in terms of, 'cause I have these images and ideas in my head which might not always be true, then, what I actually think, what is actually there. So, listening to those things, when I was making the map, in my head 't was much different than when I was actually hearing someone, some people talk because, I mean (pauses). Everything, there's no boundary as such as 'okay this is South there', I mean, somewhere there is, but then there is no boundary 'okay this is where, this is where they're coming from, this is what' so at least, where boundary lies and they meet together, so (pauses). And but if, there's no set thing, you know, it's not like 'okay this is a box, this is a box'. So, I feel it was somewhat, it was quite easy actually to do, the thing I felt I was, I could strongly tell 'okay this is maybe from the South or not' broadly speaking and lot, lot of things I could catch on because with my, because in my university I have friends from all over the country right now as well as back in India, in school. So, I felt that I could do because of my interactions I could understand the differences in terms of how, what people said, what people spoke of and how this, how they talk. So, they was, it wasn't very difficult, but (nods). (ABmDe) int.

Although diaspora consciousness and accent awareness will be investigated in Section 5.2.2, it is important to note that these comments trigger an interest in metalanguage *per se* and naturally lead the interview to general topics such as language variation and change and to more specific ones, like IndE accent variation. On the whole, the examples above inform on the participants' cognitive boundaries. RFmMa overtly states that he differentiates IndE accents on a North vs. South basis and that he considers his home state, Maharashtra, Northern India. GSmDe questions the exact location of the North vs. South 'boundary of the mind' ("there's no boundary as such as 'okay this is South there', I mean, somewhere there is") coming to the conclusion that "there's no set thing" as such. Although they both address the issue from two different standpoints – the first claiming the clear existence of a North vs. South boundary, the second rejecting the idea – they share the same presupposition that, nevertheless, the North vs. South boundary exists.

The elicitation of metalanguage comments emphasises another social factor playing a central role in accent recognition: ethnicity. The qualitative content analysis shows that the latter is most often connected with education. The following extracts from the interviews are one such example:

(11) Ah, yeah I think it was pretty difficult for me [carrying out the task] (pauses) and, I feel that, okay for South Indians they do have some accent and I might can understand 'okay, he comes from South' but I don't know which part, and to locate exactly which place in South it's very difficult, and then also in the North I feel that the way people are educated, is it a convent school? Is it a government school or private school? This can have a lot of influence in the way they speak or, even their surroundings, so from place, within a same city there can be different accents, I feel that. (ASmMP) int.

(12) APmTN: (pauses) It wasn't very difficult, yeah. You can, you can get a rough idea of (pauses) the education background of the (pauses) pupil, or (pauses) yeah, the region from where they come from, yeah. It was, it wasn't difficult, and it wasn't easy as well.
GR: Do you think you were able to discriminate speakers geographically?
APmTN: (pauses) Geographically discriminating was a little difficult, but (pauses) I could, I could (pauses) try to guess the education background they come from and, yeah. int.

The unasserted belief behind much metalanguage overt comments in both examples above is that Southern IndE speakers are perceived as less educated compared to their Northern counterparts. Comparing the 'Best English/education' code (cf. Tab. 5.2.1) with the cluster analysis of the intellectuality trait <education> (cf. Fig. 5.1.58) and interrelating the results from the 'scaling task' of the map-making with the Likert-scale values shows an interesting mismatch between the speakers' production and perception. Section 5.1.3.2 shows that the speakers almost always attribute a Northern ethnicity to those Southern guises they perceive as less educated by locating them in some of the poorest states of Northern India. The qualitative content analysis reveals that the North vs. South distinction is far more complex in terms of educational practices since many Southern states have the highest literacy rates:

(13) PVfKa: I mean the peculiar speech [Southern IndEs] (pauses) yeah, I mean (pauses) because yeah, as I told most of the people in South they're well educated and they try to always send their children to English-medium schools and, or else they try to give them (pauses) knowledge in English. So, the mode of communication nowadays, when I was studying it was always the mother tongue, only in school we used to speak (English). Right now, even the small childrens they speak in English everywhere, and we, we get stung by listening to their pronunciation and the vocab they use, so maybe. In North it's not that much as because maybe in the North India counts many states (laughs) in general when we consider. South India I think it's just us right now, like, maybe, 6 states because of Telangana one more, so, like, but 6 states they have good (pauses) I mean, the education and also the parents try to make sure that their children learned the language, which is mostly required for them to (pauses) know and it will help in future. And (pauses) and also, it's because of the culture I can say. People in South they always try to get multicultural, try to im _ like, learn or adopt the culture of other people, but in North it always happens that they're very, like, close and only in few parts of North India there are people where, where they open up and they accept the multiculture or else, where in most of the places in North India it is a case where they're not so much open and they don't send their children to school and they don't make them educated, because of which they don't get a knowledge of English, and they just learn it from either, like, using the social networks or something, yeah, with grammatical mistakes and stuff always be there, with _ if they learn it through like that, yeah.
GR: So, broadly speaking, you're able to recognise Southern speakers _
PVfKa: Oh yeah, we can recognise, except, like, it's very easy to recognise the Kerala people. They have a strong mother tongue influence in their English whenever they speak it's very easy to identify 'okay this person is from Kerala'. Ah, and the North, yeah, they have this speak _ the different languages but they mostly speak Hindi and that influence is also there. int.

According to the majority of the informants, education does play a role in accent variation, but it is not its main trigger. PVfKa is trying to 'justify' the apparent distinctiveness of local Southern IndE speech by either pointing to its undoubted multiculturalism – which is due to the coexistence of many local languages and which subsequently results in people willing to send their children to English-medium schools – or by contrasting the latter to the relative scarcity of cultural openness in Northern India. The presuppositions which lie behind this metalanguage commentary may be translated into the following statements, one being the effect of the other: (i) cultural and linguistic openness must be related to English and (ii) English equals higher education. These unasserted beliefs are implicit in what Shuck (2004) postulates as the 'ideology of nativeness', which constructs the categories of 'native English speakers' as contiguous with British or Americans, and 'non-native English speakers' as contiguous with foreigners (Regnoli 2019b). What needs to be assessed, however, is the participants' perceptions of the degree of non-nativeness in India with respect to accent variation. Section 5.2.2.2 will attempt to shed light on this topic.

Apart from education, a further sociolinguistic factor that PVfKa is linking to ethnicity is indexicality. In the second part of the extract above, she anticipates the discussion about the features characterising Southern IndEs by commenting on the distinctiveness of Kerala English and its subsequent immediate recognition ("whenever they speak it's very easy to identify 'okay this person is from Kerala'"). Being a Southern IndE speaker herself, PVfKa is able to identify Southern IndE accents at the state level, but not Northern IndE ones, ultimately recognising Northern IndE as a monolithic variety with a superordinate L1 influence: Hindi ("Ah, and the North, yeah, they have this speak _ the different languages but they mostly speak Hindi and that influence is also there").

The perceived difference of Southern IndE speech is discussed soon after the conversation about the Accent Identification Task. Int. II.4 aims firstly at eliciting whether informants agreed on the existence of this folk belief – which is acknowledged during the pilot study (Regnoli 2016) – and then at gathering information about both terms and perceptions of local speech. The following examples correspond to the prototypical metalanguage comments of the community:

(14) It is unique, it is unique, and I would not say peculiar, but it is different from the North. It's definitely because of the mother tongue influence (pauses) it is also because (pauses) the very basics tip for the South Indian languages are one, I personally believe are one and not from Sanskrit, though they have got Sanskrit in _ by themselves, I believe it's not to a big extent. So, I believe these South Indian languages belong to a different family set of languages (pauses) So, they are different from the North. I wouldn't have said they are peculiar, but they are different. (VSmTN) int.

(15) After doing here (laughs) accent thingy [the Accent Identification task] I don't think (laughs) but, frankly speaking, I would also _ I would agree to what others said [that Southern Indians have a distinctive speech in English], I mean, I have met some of my South Indian friends and it is very easy for me to distinguish from where they are coming from, just because to _ how they speak, just from hearing that, and sometime even from looks, so I don't know. But yeah, in general, I would agree to what others said as well. (TKfMa) int.

(16) Like, I would say that is true because that, so the lan _ what I know, for what I know, they have certain alphabets in the, in their mother tongues which they use more often while speak in their mother tongue that other people generally do, so those accents or those dialects and those syllables are more pronounced in their speech and maybe that's why they have this _ a bit of distinctive accent than the other people in the country. (SHfUP) int.

(17) Okay, you are asking me that, okay (laughs) yeah, yeah, I don't think it's, like, very peculiar. Sometimes it's peculiar sometimes _ it depends on the person (pauses) mostly but, like, at least, again, half of the people will be having a kind of a peculiar kind of accent, which comes with every State, I would say (pauses) yeah, it is (pauses) the Southern accent is more, like, (pauses) hard and, I mean, like they try to pronounce each and every word in a (pauses) twisted way, I can say. Well, in the North, Northern side it's, like, stronger, like (pauses), yeah, strong kind of an accent, yes. Yeah, it's quite peculiar but, like, it depends on the person again. (OFmTN) int.

The qualitative content analysis shows that all community members agree on a distinctive speech characterising Southern IndE accents/varieties. A common denominator to all such metalanguage comment is indexicality ("it is very easy for me to distinguish from where they are coming from, just because to _ how they speak, just from hearing that"). This 'pragmatic force of words' allows for a deeper understanding of the community. According to Duranti (1997:211–2):

> [i]f talk helps establish what is going on, what one particular interaction is about, who the speakers are or who they would like to be, indexes are the basic tools that help participants negotiate such issues.

In this sense, Southern IndE varieties index a particular 'folk object', i.e., Southern IndE speakers and their ordinary language behaviour. The indexical relations between linguistic expressions and features are conveyed by specific terms used to characterise the Southern IndE speech. 'Hard', 'peculiar', 'distinctive', 'unique', 'twisted' and 'different' are the adjectives used most frequently during the interview task. Moreover, their classification confirms the adjective map discussed in Section 5.1.3.7.1.

Two further points emerge from the examples above: (i) there are as many Southern IndE accents/varieties as there are Southern languages and (ii) there is considerable variation even within one dialect/accent, and idiolects should be taken into account as well. The fact that the informants are able to provide such sophisticated metalanguage detail substantiates earlier claims which emphasise their high level of awareness towards Indian varieties of English despite their gender, ethnicity and time spent in Heidelberg. Yet, as briefly mentioned above, ethnicity plays a pivotal role in the description of the features of Southern IndE varieties. The qualitative content analysis shows that the coding of both interviews and survey II,I require a further sub-coding allowing for the description of metalanguage comments based on the ethnicity of the participants. Subsequently, both codes 'Northern Indian English(es)' and 'Southern Indian English(es) include the sub-codes 'Northern commentary' and 'Southern commentary'. The sub-codes are visible in Tab. 5.2.1. A first glance at the table shows that Southern IndE varieties/accents (n = 183 segments) are addressed more than Northern IndE ones (n = 111 segments). As expected, ethnicity plays a role even in the simple discussion of Indian varieties of English. While Southern speakers (n = 67 segments) are more prone to talk about their own varieties/accents than Northern ones (n = 61 segments), Northern participants prefer discussing Northern IndE varieties/accents (n = 70 segments) over Southern ones (n = 41 segments). On the whole, the segments selected suggest that the Northern speakers (n = 131 segments) are slightly more inclined to engage in metalanguage discussions on IndE dialect/accent variation than their Southern counterparts (n = 108 segments), but that Southern informants are the ones leading the conversation with respect to the folk metalanguage on their varieties/accents (cf. Section 5.2.2.1).

In order to elicit metalanguage comments on *what* trigger such perceived distinctiveness in Southern IndE speech, the following question has been asked: "Can you tell if someone's from the South of India by the way he talks? How can you tell?" (int. II.5). Not only does the question aim to obtain information on the interrelation between indexicality and metalinguistic awareness, but it has been designed to shed light on the potential linguistic features causing such a clear-cut distinction. Specifically, considering that research on indexicality and contextualisation has primarily focused on phonological variants and associated aspects of styles as well as on intonation and discourse markers, the present question has the further aim of assessing whether phonological aspects are the main perceived triggers of accent variation (cf. Regnoli 2019, forthcoming, 2016).

Data from the qualitative content analysis suggest that phonology is the main linguistic category to be addressed with regard to language variation. In a folk linguistic perspective, laypeople rarely discuss "phonology qua phonology" (Niedzielski/Preston 2003:261), but they reveal beliefs about some phonological concerns in their discussions of dialects and varieties as well as of second and first language acquisition. However, this is not surprising since language structure tends to be placed as a presupposed background to more 'fronted' folk linguistic concerns, e.g., correctness. The following examples show metalanguage response to Southern IndE accents/varieties from the Northern speakers, i.e., the sociolinguistic 'other' according to the results from Sections 5.1.3.1 and 5.1.3.4.[90] Their progressive ordering follows Silverstein's (1981) conditions enhancing folk scrutiny (cf. Section 4.2.2) and Labov's (1994:78) distinction between degrees of consciousness of variables, including markers, i.e., topics "not at the same high level of awareness", yet, with "consistent stylistic and social stratification" and stereotypes, i.e., "overt topics of social comment" showing "both correction and hyper-correction" (cf. Tab. 5.2.1, code: Degrees of Consciousness; subcodes: Markers and Stereotypes).

The three examples below suggest that the folk seem to reflect both the 'relative presuppositionality' and 'decontextualised deducibility' positions (Silverstein 1981):

(18) [...] (pauses) (laughs) I told you, the South Indian people have some different accent, like, they (pauses), I feel like they sing while they are speaking (laughs) in English because it's really different tone. (STfBi) int.

(19) So, like, (pauses) I mean (pauses) like I said for South Indians, they have a very sing-songy kind of accent, like, because that, that's how their own languages, when they speak their own language they they tend to be, like, more (pauses) sing-songy (laughs). (HTmUP). int.

(20) So their English is fluent, they have a very fluent English and a perfect grammar and (pauses) but there is, like, a certain tone, a certain tone, you know, which is kind of a giveaway that _ yeah, this, this particular person belongs to South India, so there is influence of the mother tongue, so. (NPfMP) int.

Here, the awareness of alleged first-language influence on different South IndE accents or dialects and the capacity of describing specific features of these

90 Metalanguage comments of Southern speakers and Northern speakers towards their own varieties will be discussed in Section 5.2.2.1, whose main topic will be accent awareness.

dialects/accents shed light on some of the phonological cues the community members use to differentiate IndE accents/varieties. 'Relative presuppositionality' is often equated, in folk terms, with 'mother tongue influence', and optimal 'decontextualised deducibility' would appear to be a presupposition about the existence of a singsong 'tone', indexing, nevertheless, the influence of the mother tongue. Both STfBi and HTmUP above are eager to note that "they" (presumably, the Southern IndE speakers) sing while they speak because "that's how their own languages" are. NPfMP adds to the discussion an indexical perspective, claiming that this is the "kind of a giveaway that [...] this particular person belongs to South India". These metalanguage comments evolve into what Silverstein (1981) defines as 'metapragmatic transparency', i.e., the immediate recognition and subsequent imitation of (specific features of) a specific dialect or accent:

(21) So, the _ the _ there is some kind of (pauses) stress that they put in- towards the end of each word, I mean, some words are more stretched, like, like, when, when they ask a question, like, "what is the?", like, there's some kind of stretch in their words or the sentence there. (TKfMa) int.
(22) That's what I said. They emphasise on particular word a lot, like, they speak 'keep this here from there to here' (stopping after every word, emphasising all the syllables). They are having that kind of accent, the way they speak Tamil. (JDfMa) int.
(23) [...] (pauses) Like, I said, like, it's more emphasis on several words, like, so it, like, and I have, like, I have had some teachers from Kerala who were just pronounce 'mziam' so those kind of extra things which comes into the normal speech which you don't really listen or get to hear from a person from North India. So those are, would be, like, my first cues to look at if I want to distinct _ if I want to identify where the person is from. Otherwise, it's more general the tone, because in some part of the country the tone is a bit more stronger than how the others [...]. (SHfUP) int.

The examples above suggest that the particular 'tone' and singsong accent may be due to non-functional suprasegmental features, including stress, intonation and word juncture. While TKfMa is typically referring to stress correlates, JDfMa and SHfUP are most probably hinting at speech rhythm and, more specifically, at the peculiarity of syllable-timed languages and varieties (such as standard IndE) to exhibit isochrony at the syllable level, i.e., syllables tend to have the same duration. In purely linguistic terms, rhythm being primarily a perceptual phenomenon, what JDfMa and SHfUP are referring to, apart from signalling alleged intonation and pitch influence, may address rhythmic contrast in Northern and

Southern IndE varieties (Regnoli forthcoming). The examples below are more explicit statements of such folk metalanguage perception:

(24) Rhythm in terms of the South there is like, is like quicker, it's like, you know, act like [ta| ta| ta| ta|] and here it's like [ta↑ ta↓ ta↑ ta↓ ta↑], you know, taking the time kinda, so. (ABmDe) int.
(25) You can say in South India, sometimes. And they have this very peculiar accent in South India. They have this melody as well somewhere, like [ah↑ ah↓ ah↑]. They somehow speak something like that, people from Chennai, so like that. (BSmGu) int.
(26) Ah (pauses) if there is a statement such as 'What are you doing?' in North India, someone would 'What are you doing?' [wɒt↑ ɑr↓ ju:↑ duɪŋ↓], so this is ac #_# accurate Delhi 'What are you doing?' [wɒt↑ ɑr↓ ju:↑ duɪŋ↓]. In South it, like 'What are you doing?' [ə:↑ vɒt:↑ ɑr↓ ju:↑ duɪŋ↑]. So, this is different, no? (ATmDe) int.
(27) ASmMP: I think it's true (pauses) yes. And (pauses) I cannot recall right now what was, those words be, but they do have, let's say, when they, when the sentence end, it's, it lingers a little and it doesn't stop, okay? Now, full stop. It still continues a bit, like, maybe they are extending the last letter a bit. And this, for me, is some South Indian accent.
GR: Can you give me an example? What do you mean by their lingering at the end?
ASmMP: (pauses) Let's say, if they want to say 'No', they would say 'No' [no:↑↓↑] Maybe like that. int.

Stereotypes are the highest degrees of consciousness according to Labov (1994, 1972a) and often manifest themselves in overt imitations (Sharma 2005). The instances above are one such example. The singsong accent and the 'tone' remarked on in the earlier examples are here addressed once again through their direct and explicit imitations. The alternation of higher and lower pitch – indicated in some of the sentences above as pronounced by the informants – provides valuable folk metalanguage comments about the intonation patterns of Southern IndEs. It is worth noting that what the folk define as 'tone' is used in their descriptions of intonation. The reported examples clearly refer to the pitch movement found on the nucleus or tonic syllable in an intonation unit within each utterance ("when they, when the sentence end, it's, it lingers a little and it doesn't stop"). On the whole, the continuous rising and falling intonations as detected by the community members serve a pragmatic 'indexical function' (Wells 2006) since they act as a marker of social identity. According to the Northern speakers, this "melody" is typical of Southern IndE varieties/accents and is adopted subsequently by that specific in-group. However, although intonation is primarily a matter of pitch variation, it is important to be aware that functions attributed to intonation such as the expression of social identities and attitudes almost always involve concomitant variation in other prosodic features such as rhythm, loudness and tempo. For this reason, folk comments on suprasegmental variation should be treated as a whole. Section 5.2.2.1 will elaborate on what Southern IndE speakers have to say about this matter and whether and, if so, the extent to which they agree with the claims discussed above.

As was the case with the suprasegmental level, at the segmental one, the folk seemingly reflect the 'relative presuppositionality' and 'decontextualised deducibility' positions expressed by Silverstein (1981). Yet, contrary to what happens at the suprasegmental level, here both positions seem to be encoded into the doctrine of 'correctness'. While variation in intonation and rhythmic correlates is tolerated and, at times, acclaimed for its indexical force of distinctiveness and uniqueness, variation in segmental phonology does not seem to be accepted. Two further professional positions, in addition to those proposed by Silverstein (1981), need to be addressed: 'ease of articulation' and 'perceptual separation' (Ladefoged 1975). 'Ease of articulation' is often equated with laziness, and 'perceptual separation' concerns the quality of the 'standard', hence the inability to pronounce certain phonemes. The examples below provide some insight into the topic:

(28) Yeah, I think they have a strong and a thick accent which comes naturally from their mother tongue, like, you can see, like, they, like for example in Hindi there is the sound /d/ but it's not that common in the South India and it's find it hard to say [d] and they end up saying [ɖ], like this, so this is how you can tell somebody from South India I _ if somebody is from South India or not, because they would have troubles saying this [...]. (URmRa) int.

(29) BSmGu: Yeah, so, for some of the [Southern] states, they don't take a pause, or some of the states they don't pronounce /a/ properly, not properly, but. GR: Can you give me some examples? BSmGu: Yeah, so you can say, like, we use 'at all' [ætɔːl] so they use 'at all' [ætːɑl]. int.

(30) Ah, like the words such as 'nothing', like they, like, they usually have a very, like not very but more like a strong 'th' sound, and also, like South India, they usually (pauses) When they say words like 'yellow', which was not there in your recordings, but when they speak words like 'yellow' and stuff, they usually say, like they usually do not (pauses) produce the /w/ sound, so it becomes something like 'ello', so, yeah. (DLfMan) int.

(31) They pronounce certain things in a very typical manner, so I think, I forgot what I wrote down about it, but there was, like, these one or two distinctive things which define how they would say, for example, in one of the things, they said, they wouldn't say 'Khiljis' [ˈkhildʒiz], but say [ˈkildʒi], 'cause the [k] the [h] sound, doesn't come very well, yah. (MGfUt) int.

(32) South India is made up out, of a lot of states and I think each state has a different (pauses) identifying feature when they pronounce English, for example, in Bangalore because it's so metropolitan. People have a very (pauses) they have a posh, but slight drawl. but a posh accent, whereas in, in Kerala, (pauses) they have (pauses) they have more of a glide, because that's how Malayalam is, and they also have a strong (pauses) alveolar sound like /d/, so (pause) I mean they don't even say 'Malayalam' [malˈjɑːləm], it's [malˈjɑːɭəm] (pauses) so, and in Tamil Nadu, again, it's different and it's more, it's more guttural, because Tamil is, like, that and then in Telangana and Andhra Pradesh it's even more different because it's an even bigger metropolitan (pauses) state because of the IT industries, so their English is very fast, very, like, not correct punctuation, very, like, unpunctuated because they talk, they have a habit of talking so fast, and Telugu is also a very fast language. So, I think all these, like, I don't think that one accent would be enough to classify all of South India as one big lots, so. (SLfUP) int.

By and large, all the examples above deal with correctness. URmRa, for instance, notes that Southern Indians "find it hard to say [d] and they end up saying [ɖ]". The substitution of the voiced alveolar stop with the voiced retroflex stop, in fact, is a classic feature of many Southern IndE accents (Sailaja 2012). As URmRa rightly states, this "comes naturally from their mother tongue" since many Dravidian languages such as Kannada, Tamil and Telugu have a two-way contrast between plain and murmured (breathy voice). The doctrine of correctness is implied in URmRa's statements according to which they "find it hard" and "they would have troubles" mastering alveolar sounds. The ensuing example is no exception. BSmGu claims that the pronunciation of Southern IndE speakers is far from 'standard' English, especially with respect to the realisation of the near-open front unrounded vowel which tends to be substituted with the open front unrounded one in liaison sound changes ("they don't pronounce /a/ properly"). However, it is interesting to delve into the presuppositions that lie behind such 'allegations'. The variety with which BSmGU is comparing Southern IndE is not standard BrE or standard IndE, but, rather, Northern IndE ("*we* use 'at all' [ætɔːl] so *they* use 'at all' [æt:ɑl]"). The unasserted beliefs behind such statements are that (i) Northern IndE is 'more' correct than Southern IndE and that (ii) Southern IndE speakers are unable to master certain (standard) sounds. On the whole, all such folk linguistic data point to the same observation and come to the same conclusion, i.e., segmental variation almost exclusively deals with correctness.

According to Niedzielski and Preston (2003:266), "the primacy of 'word' as the folk linguistic object par excellence, and discussions of word meanings [...] are common". As the frequency of segments in Tab. 5.2.1 shows, for the community members, lexicon and syntax are not common triggers in perceived accent/dialect recognition. With respect to the assessment of Southern IndE accents/varieties according to the Northern informants, the qualitative content analysis of Survey II,I and the sociolinguistic interviews identify only one instance of their 'folk grammaticality':

(33) I think it's natural for them, there's nothing wrong in having that accent but at the same time it's very hard for us, I mean, people who are not from South India, to actually understand what are they saying most of the times. 'Cause, for instance, (pauses) like, in general English, whenever we address a friend, so it's either like 'dude' or (pauses) yeah, it's 'dude' most of the times, but for them it's 'macha' (laughs). So 'macha' is their 'dude' in English, 'macha' or 'maga', so, at first, it's quite challenging for us to understand, but once you know that, those words and the way they speak it's okay. (SSmUt) int.

The example above sheds light on how the folk most frequently see words as 'classifiable', that is, belonging to certain groupings and on how these classifications bear heavily on social characteristics rather than strictly linguistic ones. While suprasegmental variation is linked with indexicality and segmental variation with correctness, lexical variation is connected with intelligibility ("it's very hard for us, I mean, people who are not from South India, to actually understand what are they saying most of the times"). SSmUt believes that the Northern IndE varieties and the Southern IndE ones are not always mutually intelligible. Moreover, Southern IndE varieties are less universally intelligible: while Northern speakers commonly use the informal AmE noun 'dude' to address their peers, Southern speakers make use of the variants of 'macha'/'maga'. The presupposition behind SSmUt's claims is that Northern IndE varieties are, in comparison, more universally intelligible since they have acquired a more global slang, which can be potentially understood by both native and non-native English speakers. However, for the present analysis, it is not possible to assess any further claim with respect to intelligibility because of lack of data. Intelligibility will be addressed in more detail in Sections 5.2.2.1 and 5.2.2.2 where the qualitative content analysis reveals a more direct connection with the informants' own way of speaking.

The analysis of the above-mentioned examples is consistent with the idea that Northern informants have a high level of consciousness of phonological and phonetic variables with respect to Southern IndE accents/varieties. Interestingly, the results substantiate the quantitative ones outlined above, according to which Northern Indian students seemingly have stereotypical views of Southern IndE accents and speakers (cf. Section 5.1.3.4).

The present section will be dedicated to Southern perceptions of Northern IndE varieties. As briefly discussed above, the main aim of the first part of module II of the sociolinguistic interview is to elicit information about the folk belief of the community according to which Southern Indians have a distinctive way of speaking English. Thus, the majority of questions have been designed to investigate this claim. Some questions, however, have been dedicated to Northern IndE speech in order to get a broader perspective on the assessment of IndE varieties within the student community. In consequence, the following question aims to shed light on the topic: "How about, in comparison to say, Northern India? (int. II.7)". As with the earlier examples, the present ones show metalanguage response to Northern IndE accents/varieties from the point of view of the Southern participants.

A first glance at the instances below suggests that the Southern informants perceive less variation in Northern IndE accents compared to their Northern counterparts, which translates into the recognition of a single monolithic Northern IndE accent/variety:

(34) I'm not sure, but the Northern states' (pauses) Indian accent is maybe a bit rough and a bit tough, and they don't give pauses a lot. (PPmKa) int.
(35) Ah, the Northern Indian accent (pauses) I somehow associate it with more with either if, if they know it, I feel it's fake, pretentious or something like that, if they don't know it, it's completely rural, it's what I always have in my head, and I've seen it that way too, and especially with Gujjus, Gujaratis, they, they have a very strong accent, just what I feel in comparison with the entire North and (pauses) this is actually true when you listen to the Indian Prime Minister. He has a very strong Gujju accent and the Central India, yeah, again, I would say they don't know the pronunciation of a lot of words, so (pauses) it could be that it's either wrong or they're just reading the letters together [...] (ASfKe) int.

In referring to a rather fixed and defined Northern IndE accent/variety, the Southern speakers generally agree with some Northern informants who mainly associate Northern India with Hindi (cf. GSmDe above). Yet, unlike the Northern participants, they very seldom acknowledge sociolinguistic internal variation, with the exception of some accents/varieties which tend to be perceptually more relevant than others, i.e., Bengali English and Gujarati English ("especially with Gujjus, Gujaratis, they, they have a very strong accent, just what I feel in comparison with the entire North"):

(36) They [Southern speakers] don't speak like North Indians and this, I think that Hindi, from, when I categorise I feel like this Hindi, Marathi, Gujarati, Bengali, all sound very similar to me, because I would categorise as one, because it sounds very similar, so (pauses) they have a spe _ something in common, that is what, that is not there in South Indians, that's how I can understand they're from South India. (JGMfKe) int.

What emerges from the example above is that, with some due exceptions, all Northern IndE accents sound "very similar" and would be subsequently "categorise[d] as one". Furthermore, JGMfKe is eager to note that this accent homogeneity "is not there in South Indians"; their accent distinctiveness is what allows her to differentiate among Southern IndE accents ("that's how I can understand they're from South India"). In consequence, the lack of such internal heterogeneity in Northern IndE accents prevents her from recognising beyond the Northern level. On the whole, the majority of Southern informants confirm JGMfKe's stance and, when asked to describe the Northern IndE speech, they provide very basic metalanguage comments:

(37) I think that they [Southern speakers] speak a little bit fluently and (pauses) they're good _ they use good pronunciation of words. Not like people from the North. (SAmKa) int.

(38) The Northerners, as I said, from what I have observed, they drag the words, sort of. And it's (pauses) *how would I say?* It's (pauses) it's okay, it's like a common Northern accent, there's nothing I hate about it. It's, it's understandable, so to say. (AHfKa) int.

In comparison, the two examples below suggest that the folk do not seem to reflect a high level of metalinguistic awareness as was the case with the Northern informants. Overall, their metalanguage comments reflect both the 'continuous segmentability' and 'relative presuppositionality' conditions expressed by Silverstein (1981). The Southern participants definitely perceive clear-cut differences between Northern and Southern IndE accents/varieties and are aware of alleged first-language influence on Northern IndE accents/varieties. Yet, in contrast to their Northern counterparts, they seem to be either less receptive to language variation or less able to comment upon it. Needless to say, there are some exceptions. The qualitative content analysis reveals that half of the Southern informants seem to reflect even Silverstein's (1981) fourth condition, i.e., 'decontextualised deducibility'. The following instance is one such example:

(39) [...] the other thing was the common words of 'only' which I always kind of see and check wha _ how they are doing and if they pronounce it as a North or South Indian and (pauses) yeah, it's the cut, spacing between words, how, how arrogant or polite they are with the words and, yeah. (ASfKe) int.

The capacity of description of specific cues which help in the discrimination of Northern vs. Southern IndE accents/varieties is an example of what Labov (1994; 1972a) describes as markers. As with the Northern sample, Southern participants tend to differentiate mainly on a phonological basis. ASfKe notes that "the cut, [the] spacing between words" is the main cue/clue for accent identification, which may be related to a particular 'tone':

(40) Tone, I think mostly people from the North they didn't have any kind of tone towards, just not _ like the rhythm, so that difference. (NKSfTN) int.

Non-functional suprasegmental features including stress, intonation and word juncture are, however, mentioned very seldom compared to Southern IndE accents. This may lend credence to and further substantiate the community's commonly held folk belief that it is the Southern in-group showing particular distinctiveness of speech, and not the Northern one. However, some interesting metalanguage comments reflecting 'metapragmatic transparency' have been observed in relation to segmental variation. As with Northern comments of Southern IndEs, two further positions are at stake: Ladefoged's (1975) 'ease of articulation' and 'perceptual separation', which seem to be encoded into the doctrine of 'correctness':

(41) Yeah, because the North, I think they have a very strong native language, the accent, the words that they use especially, or these vowels, it's not 'Indian' they say _ they use 'ye' 'yee' or something like that. That is completely different, that changes the way they pronounce the words. (NKSfTN) int.

(42) Yeah, and (pauses) also I would say that /b/ also. I mean, I wouldn't say India [ˈɪndɪə] I would say India [ˈɪnˈdɪɑː] that is from, it, that [a:] but North Indians would say India [ˈɪndɪə], which is written exactly India [ˈɪndɪə] (laughs). But I wouldn't say that, it's kind of (laughs) those things. It's subtle I would say. For me, it is subtle. [...] They have their mother tongue influence, but still I cannot articulate them. I can't tell on them, yeah, you can.

But (pauses) I am generally, I would see the Eastern part, like the Bengali or this part, they would just, they would, they would, they have a more of a [o:] kind of thing. I don't know if it is right, but. (ARmKe) int.

(43) VSmTN: Okay, some of the clues would be, for example, in the South we don't (pauses) give a big stress on letters, consonants like /h/, /j/ (pauses) say, for example, the word is 'thing' [ˈθɪŋ] and there would, there would be a most stress on [ˈθhɪŋ], so they have extra /h/ sound. GR: In the South? VSmTN: In the North, because we do, we do, we (pauses) we don't prefer using those such hard words, hard letters actually. So, in Hindi, by, by nature they have got this (pauses) say, for example, if I have to say 'car' [ˈkɑː] in, in, in my language, I just have one 'car' [ˈkɑː]. I mean, it's easy for me to (pauses) interpret and you not speaks, but in Hindi it's, it's kind of different, they have got [k], [gh], [k], [gh] and all, so it's like they have these letters influence in (pauses) in English obviously. So when they write just /k/ in English, so it could be any [k], [gh], [k], [gh] (pauses), could be any /k/ out of those letters in Hindi. So, I personally believe people who have a bigger stress on these specific consonants are from North. [...] As I said you earlier, it's with the stress on specific consonants that they use. For example, people from Kerala and (pauses) West Bengal, they have a really unique, I would say, really very unique, really easily identify these guys. For example, from Kerala people have a really a nasal (pauses) sound for vowels (pauses) and because West Bengal people they don't have the letter /v/ in Bengali, so they tend to pronounce /v/ as /b/, so for example if I'm called 'Varoon' [vaˈrun] in, in my language, so, they call 'Varoon' [baˈrun] in Bengali. int.

While some metalanguage comments above show that the folk implicitly acknowledge a superordinate Northern IndE variety/accent which is predominantly influenced by Hindi and which subsequently levels all the other regional varieties, some others shed light on the peculiarity of specific ethnic varieties. VSmTN, for instance, points to the glaring distinctiveness of Bengali English ("[...] people from [...] (pauses) West Bengal, they have a really unique, I would say, really very unique, really easily identify these guys") and to one of the most common features of the variety, i.e., the substitution of the voiced labiodental fricative with the voiced bilabial stop ("so they tend to pronounce /v/ as /b/, so for example if I'm called 'Varoon' [vaˈrun] in, in my language, so, they call 'Varoon' [baˈrun] in Bengali"). The recognition of the substitution of a homorganic stop for the fricative and its subsequent capacity of imitation is a valuable example of 'metapragmatic transparency' (Silverstein 1981) and of a stereotype

(Labov 1994, 1972a) since it constitutes the higher degree of consciousness of variables according to the folk theory of language. Likewise, VSmTN notes an alleged over-aspiration of the voiceless glottal fricative in the word 'think', which happens to be a peculiarity of Northern IndE speakers.

On the whole, the qualitative content analysis of the assessment of Northern IndE accents/varieties from the point of view of Southern informants emphasises two major points: (i) Northern IndE accents/varieties are perceived as more homogeneous and compact systems in comparison to Southern IndE ones and (ii) the Southern informants show lower levels of metalinguistic awareness as compared to their Northern counterparts. Whether the latter characteristic is due to their being less receptive to language variation or less able to comment upon is difficult to say. However, the first option seems to be less plausible than the second one. An intuitive account for this result is that Southern speakers are more used to different local languages and cultures. While Northern Indians generally use Hindi as a common *lingua franca*, Southern speakers use English. While it should go without saying that extralinguistic factors including the degree of exposure to different Indian accents/varieties most certainly play a pivotal role in folk scrutiny, what appears to be a paradox at a first glance may be justified by the very same explanation provided above. Being more open to different languages, varieties and, subsequently, accents, Southern Indians should be more receptive to and more aware of language variation. As a matter of fact, they observe more internal variation in their own varieties than in Northern ones and seem to provide much more sophisticated metalanguage comments about them than their Northern counterparts (cf. Section 5.2.2.1). This position should lend credence to the folk belief according to which Southern IndE accents/varieties are truly perceived as more heterogeneous than Northern ones. Hence the Southerners' response to Northern IndE accents/varieties is simply evidence of the degree of such perceived distinctiveness. Section 5.2.2.1 will provide more detail on the topic since it will compare the metalanguage comments of both ethnic groups with respect to their own varieties/accents.

5.2.1.1.3 Affective, Conative and Identity-related Attitudes

As discussed in Section 2.5, the exploration of language attitudes in the present study is based on a threefold attitude concept in which the cognitive, affective and conative components interact to form a super-attitude towards different attitude objects. While Section 5.2.1.1.1 investigates the cognitive component, the present section will analyse the affective, conative and identity-related ones. The following questions are to elicit these attitudes towards local speech:

- *Do you think it is good to have an accent? Why or why not? (II.1.7)*
- *In your opinion, is it necessary to speak with a local accent to 'belong'? (II.1.13)*
- *Do you like the way people from the South of India sound? What do you like about it? What don't you like about it? (int. II.6)*
- *A (if the speaker is from the South) Has anyone ever told you that you sound like a Southern Indian? Did you (would you) take it as a compliment? B (if the speaker is from the North) If you told someone that he sounded like he came from Southern India, would you mean it as a compliment? (int. II.8)*

II.1.7 seeks to verify how respondents defined the importance of having an accent – in the most general terms and whatever accent it is. II.1.13 is a general conative question aiming at both investigating whether informants value a local accent in order to establish and maintain group identity and at eliciting additional information on indexicality. Questions int. II.6 and int. II.8 have been asked during the interview. Their aim is to shed light on the affective attitudinal dimension: through int. II.6, the respondents have been asked to comment on how much they like the way people from Southern India talk and what features they like and dislike most. Int. II.8 seeks to investigate the emotional values projected onto the attitude object in relation to the consideration of Southern IndE local speech as pleasant or unpleasant or, most importantly, as correct or not.

The qualitative content analysis shows that the respondents tend to fall into two main groups, depending on their answers to int. II.1.7: one in favour of having an accent and the other showing neutral or negative attitudes towards it. While no extralinguistic variable seems to have a significant impact on the group, each entry (n = 60) reveals interesting metalanguage responses. The examples below are prototypical comments on the topic:

(44) I feel one can not not have an accent...the question is which accent is perceived as NOT having one? (SSmMa) surv.

(45) Yes it is. Because everywhere there's a stigma about how one speaks. This was especially prominent in India when they make fun of you when you don't speak quite clearly in English. This is reflective of whether or not you went to a private or public school. English is more a classifier of your class or status in society than just a language. (SDfKa) surv.

(46) I think accents are very interesting and they are an important part of the identities of people. Your accent gives you a sense of belonging in the world, but for some, it also becomes a reason to be 'left behind'. The fact that perceptions are sometimes linked with an accent or the lack of it, especially in India, can become a reason for professional success or failure.

'Accent training' at call centres and language schools feeds into insecurities about accents. I would say it is 'natural' to have an accent, and not a question of whether it is good or not. (MGfUt) surv.

SSmMa is among the very few participants to provide a sophisticated metalanguage comment on accents in general. Not only does she point to a universal linguistic truth which often tends to be misinterpreted by laypeople, i.e., the impossibility of not having an accent, but she puts under close scrutiny the role of standard vs. vernacular varieties and the difference between native and non-native accents by asking, in turn, the most interesting question the Indian community has asked so far: "[...] which accent is perceived as NOT having one?". Her comment is a counterargument to the majority of folk responses to accent awareness according to which having an accent equals having a strong or peculiar one and most often implies negative covert attitudes. In acknowledging that there must be some accents which are perceived "as NOT having one", SSmMa recognises that languages shape societal behaviour. In other words, she provides a more general claim to the current Indian sociolinguistic situation that SDfKa and MGfUt comment upon. In arguing that "everywhere there's a stigma about how one speaks" and that "[t]his [is] especially prominent in India when they make fun of you when you don't speak quite clearly in English", SDfKa is indexing the educational disadvantage of attending a state school or a vernacular-medium one, where English is neither properly taught nor the medium of instruction. Her final statement ("English is more a classifier of your class or status in society than just a language") is reminiscent of Kachru's ([1990] 1986:1) famous comparison between English and Aladdin's lamp:

[i]n comparison with other languages of wider communication, knowing English is like possessing the fabled Aladdin's lamp, which permits one to open, as it were, the linguistic gates to international business, technology, science, and travel. In short, English provides linguistic power.

Power refers to the control of knowledge and to the prestige a language acquires as a result of its use in certain important domains. In other words, the more prestigious a domain, the more powerful a language. This is something with which even MGfUt agrees ("[t]he fact that perceptions are sometimes linked with an accent or the lack of it, especially in India, can become a reason for professional success or failure"). In addressing the function of accent training centres, she points to the way these companies use accents as gatekeeper devices in the attribution of global social authority to native speakers and argues that they are the prime examples of how standard language ideology is institutionalised in a global context (Regnoli 2019b). Finally, she is eager to note that " it is 'natural' to have an accent, and not a question of whether it is good or not". Moreover, (45) and (46) shed light on the role of intelligibility and on the ensuing (false) firm belief in correctness. As Chand (2009:400) points out: "[s]peakers from nonstandard dialects are judged against ideologically enforced and constantly reified norms, and structural differences [...] are understood as errors that cause miscommunications and poor service". Unlike the examples above, some other informants point to the emergence of miscommunication and intelligibility issues linked to having an accent:

(47) It is good to have an accent (because I like how it defines me as Bihari) but sometimes when I am with colleagues I don't use it because they don't understand it. (SPfBi) surv.
(48) I don't think to have an accent matters much as long as your communication (pronunciation) of certain words is clearly understandable. (SAmKa) surv.
(49) No. I feel the grammar is more important than the accent for clear and better understanding. (NKSfTN) surv.
(50) It depends on what kind of people you're dealing with. It's not about having an accent but to be clear, I don't think you need to have an accent if you're clear, so it's not necessary. (PGfMa) surv.

The unasserted beliefs which arise from the examples above may be summarised as follows: (i) accents are something that only non-native speakers have and (ii) there are some domains in which – and some participants with whom – it is better to avoid having an accent. It is important to mention, however, that such comments constitute only a moderate portion of the community and that more than 50 % of the sample hold positive attitudes towards having an accent. The following instances are such examples:

(51) I agree to the above statement that it is good to have an accent as it can be a way to identify people around us and since an accent also becomes a part of a person's personality. (AVmDe) surv.
(52) I think it's good to have an accent but it should be understandable to people from different countries. Having an accent identifies you to be a part of the country you come from. (DTfUt) surv.
(53) It's sometimes good because it helps to identify from which place a particular person comes from, without asking him/her. (JGMfKe) surv.
(54) Yes. Because it represents your culture. (BJmGu) surv.
(55) Yes, it is good to have an accent. It differentiates you from the others. (SMfMa) surv.

The examples above show that, on the whole, both the Northern and Southern informants generally agree on the interrelation between having an accent and sociocultural belonging. AVmDe, for instance, notes the perks of having an accent in the following statements; "it can be a way to identify people around us", and it "becomes a part of a person's personality". JGMfKe, on the other hand, is eager to note that, through accents, it is possible to identify the place of origin of somebody without the need of asking them. These answers partially anticipate some conative attitudes towards local speech addressing the relation between accent, belonging and indexicality, which have been obtained from II.1.13 ("In your opinion, is it necessary to speak with a local accent to 'belong'?").

The qualitative content analysis shows that the informants form three subgroups: those who (i) agree with the question, hence, have positive conative attitudes towards local speech; (ii) have neutral conative attitudes and (iii) disagree. The distribution patterns uncover that more than 50 % of community members have positive conative attitudes towards local speech:

(56) Yes, I feel it is something that defines you, gives the basic sense of belonging to something and somewhere. (ABmDe) surv.
(57) I think so. With my boyfriend, for instance, my English is more Indian. It just makes you feel very at home. (VJRfKa) surv.
(58) To some extent yes. Local people will be more happier and tend to help you more. (SSmKa) surv.
(59) Yes, there are a lot of segregations in India. It may be easier to jell with people from the same community or the same state if you share the same accent. (URmRa) surv.
(60) I think Yes because if 4 people in a group of 5 speak in one accent and suddenly another guy says the same word in another accent, people would react differently. They might laugh or tease you for being very different. (SLmKa) surv.

The above-mentioned examples shed light on the close relation between having a local accent and belonging somewhere. While SSmKa points to the willingness of local people "to help you more" when speaking with a local accent, VJRfKa implicitly relates local accentedness with private life domains which tend to be related to the affective dimension ("[w]ith my boyfriend, for instance, my English is more Indian. It just makes you feel very at home"). On the other hand, URmRa and SLmKa acknowledge the usefulness of speaking with a local accent in order to "jell with people from the same community or the same state" since "there are a lot of segregations in India". Yet, local accentedness and accent segregation appear to be two sides of the same coin ("[t]hey [people coming from a different in-group] might laugh or tease you for being very different"). While speaking with a local accent is generally perceived positively since it produces individuality and uniqueness, it is also a sign of the sensible divide between Northern and Southern India:

(61) In India, there has been a remarkable divide because of the North-Indian and South-Indian accent in speaking English. Therefore, accent may not always instill a sense of belonging. I have observed how people with no accent or unascertainable accents, tend to get along with everyone. Moreover, the concept of belongingness through a local accent, may not even be very dominating, in India. Especially because English is a foreign language. (DSfWB) surv.

DSfWB is eager to note that "accent [in English] may not always instill a sense of belonging" in India and, thus, speaking with "no accent" or "unascertainable accents" may be a better solution in order to "get along with everyone". While the folk place much importance on the perception of identity through their English accents, DSfWB argues that this question should not "even be very dominating in India [e]specially because English is a foreign language". In recurring to the 'us' vs. 'them' sociolinguistic conceptualisation which differentiates native and non-native speakers, DSfWB implicitly reflects and fosters 'the ideology of nativeness' (Shuck 2004) which constructs the categories of 'native English speakers' as contiguous with British or Americans and 'non-native English speakers' as contiguous with foreigners (cf. Section 5.2.2.2).

The subgroup of participants showing neutral conative attitudes towards local speech acknowledge, nevertheless, the perks of having a local accent. However, unlike the first subgroup, they do not perceive accent as a strict necessity. While SSmMa considers it "an added support", SMfMa adds an affective component to her conative attitude ("it connects people with you"). Finally, APmTN associates local speech with (lack) of correctness. The presupposition behind his statement substantiates earlier issues covered by question II.1.7, i.e., the emergence of miscommunication and intelligibility problems linked with having an accent:

(62) Not a necessary but sure an added support. (SSmMa) surv.

(63) It is not necessary, but better to speak with a local accent as it connects people with you. (SMfMa) surv.

(64) Its not necessary. I feel its important to be natural and try to change pronunciation when its beyond understandable. (APmTN) surv.

The third subgroup disagrees with the question and holds negative conative attitudes towards local speech. On the whole, they constitute about 20 % of the sample and, as was the case with the neutral subgroup above, they 'fall' into the doctrine of correctness. The major difference, however, lies in their preference for non-accentedness or neutral accentedness (cf. Section 5.2.2.2). Section 5.1.3.1 above shed light of the folk's general abstraction of a standard language, i.e., non-accent, which tends to be interpreted collectively as "an idea of the mind rather than a reality" (Milroy 1991:22). This abstraction produces a series of social and regional associations which, as is the case with the present subgroup, relate to intelligibility and miscommunication issues. The following examples sum up this position:

(65) No, I don't think so because the main important thing is, we convey the meaning. If I had the accent in me, people might recognise where I'm from and if they don't like it, they might exclude me. (PVfKa) surv.
(66) No. I strongly oppose it. a neutral accent is good but sometimes when the locals don't understand, we can switch to the local accent for some words. (VSmTN) surv.
(67) In my opinion, No. For me, it is more important to have a common content to speak about rather than the accent to belong per se. But I have seen people from South India place a lot of importance on languages. (SHfUP) surv.

Affective attitudes have been investigated during the interview. Participants have been asked to comment on whether they like the way people from Southern India sound in English and what features they like and dislike most (int. II.6). The qualitative content analysis shows a clear-cut distinction in the distribution pattern of the answers provided. *Ethnicity* proves to be an important variable to take into account with respect to the affective attitudinal dimension although the quantitative analysis does not provide any significant result (cf. Sections 5.1.3.1 and 5.1.3.2). While the results from the Accent Identification Task were consistent with the idea that the Northern informants seem to have stereotypical views about themselves and the South and that students coming from the South have by and large taken over the stereotypes of the Northerners about themselves, the qualitative content analysis reveals a much more complex pattern. In both the Northern and the Southern subgroups, the informants have two divergent opinions with respect to local Southern IndE speech: they both like it and dislike it, and, in doing so, they always have strong attitudes towards it. As a matter of fact, overt folk metalanguage almost always fails to share any common ground with covert metalanguage comments for most different and obvious reasons – the most important one being the following: when feeling 'threatened', the folk tend to either lie or state the obvious. Several informants, and especially the Northern ones, felt visibly uncomfortable when faced with this question and almost always reacted with long pauses, uncontrolled laughter, 'no comments' and general statements about their impossibility to judge local speech. The following instances from the Northern sample are such examples:

(68) (pauses) It's (pauses) (laughs) like, if they have a really strong accent, the I, I don't really like, yeah. (DLfMan) int.

(69) GR: That's interesting. Do you like the way people from the South of India sound in English?
JGfMa: (pauses) it's fine, yeah. It is understandable, so it's fine.
GR: And is there something that you don't like?
JGfMa: No, I cannot comment on that. int.

(70) (pauses) Yes, I mean, everyone has their own accents, so you really can't judge people by that. (KGfPu) int.

Their reticence to comment upon an innocently curious question shows that local accentedness has a strong social and cultural stigma not only in India but also within the student community – as, after all, many informants acknowledge in some examples analysed earlier ("In India, there has been a remarkable divide because of the North-Indian and South-Indian accent in speaking English"). Such reticence, however, has been somehow expected, hence question II.8 was designed with the main purpose of shedding light on the topic (cf. below).

However, the majority of metalanguage comments is either related to unintelligibility and miscommunication problems – which seemingly derive from accent 'heaviness' – and, thus, to negative affective attitudes, or to questions of indexicality, which are reflected in accent distinctiveness and uniqueness. Metalanguage response to the former is expressed in the examples below:

(71) (pauses) Yeah, I don't have problem as far as it's, like, understandable, I think, it's fine, but some of the people you cannot understand, like, even for me sometimes it's difficult to understand if they are speaking in English. (DTfUt) int.

(72) Not always (laughs) sometimes when it's very strong and the accent is very strong I find it irritating sometimes because I've also lived in the Southern part and sometimes, sometimes I've just avoided interacting with, you know, the people who had very strong accents because half the time I had to, you know, listen very carefully what they were trying to say. (SDfMP) int.

(73) AVmDe: (laughs) No, a big no (laughs).
GR: What don't you like about it?
AVmDe: I mean, it's so. Sometimes it's not so understandable and they put in all their local accents and everything and they pull it out to you. int.

(74) GR: Do you like the way people from the South of India sound in English?
JDfMa: No. GR: Why not?
JDfMa: Because they are this, mix the mother tongue with that English, and it sound like they're emphasise something very strongly on that thing, and I, sometimes I really feel fake when they speak something different and they want to say something different. int.

What emerges from these interview extracts is that, on the whole, local Southern IndE speech is perceived as "difficult to understand", "strong" and, at times, "irritating". While SDfMP is eager to say that sometimes she has avoided interacting with Southern speakers with strong accents because she had to put too much effort in understanding their speech, AVmDe bluntly confesses that it is because of their local distinctiveness that he does not like how they sound ("no, a big no (laughs)"). While for some community members local distinctiveness is a flaw, some others consider it a quality. The following examples inform on positive affective attitudes towards Southern IndE local speech:

(75) It's different from (pauses) other accents, so I think, at times, if you can recognise a person by the accent. It's, it's a good thing (laughs) (pauses) So, like, it becomes easy to approach that person, like, for instance, if I know the person through the accent, like, everything you know from the first time and it's through the accent that she comes from or he comes from, let's say, Maharashtra. So, I would have, I would know how to approach, you know, a Maharashtrian, that may be different from approaching, let's say, a person from a different state. (GSmDe) int.

(76) I do. Personally, I find it quite fascinating (laughs). And also, they're also, like, more clear in their speech versus, maybe, someone from the East or maybe even the North or something, so, yeah. And also, I've had certain South Indian friends, so it's, it's just sounds good to me maybe (laughs). (MGfUt) int.

(77) RFmMa: I guess it is very pleasant to hear, so.
GR: And what do you like about it?
RFmMa: It is very sweet and (pauses) it is soft, so if you compare my voice with them, you can spot the difference that is very sweet, soft. People will (pauses) prefer hearing them then me because is very rough and rigid, but their voice is very sweet and nice to hear.
GR: Is there something you don't like about how they speak?
RFmMa: (pauses) Okay, I can say the pronunciation, some words, but it does, okay that (pauses) it happens, they, they mi #_# they might have some flaws in it, but I guess they are more positive in it. int.

Indexical aspects of Southern IndE local speech seem to point to an opinion extremely divergent from the one discussed above. According to this Northern subgroup, Southern IndE accents are pleasant and soft. Moreover, since they are easy to recognise, they allow for a better and much friendlier approach to the locals ("So, like, it becomes easy to approach that person, like, for instance, if I know the person through the accent").

In acknowledging that each accent carries its own specific features, the Northern sample embraces the complexity of accent variation to the fullest, ultimately engaging in metalanguage content showing high levels of metapragmatic transparency. While the former group shows more negative attitudes towards local speech, the latter acknowledges its perks over its flaws ("they might have some flaws in it, but I guess they are more positive in it"). Overall, while this result is partially consistent with the findings of the Accent Identification Task, i.e., that Northern speakers tend to have stereotypical views about Southern IndE accents, discourse concerning the former having positive attitudes towards Southern IndE accents is present as well and is fundamental to be addressed for the overall picture. With respect to the attitudes of Southern speakers towards local Southern IndE speech – as in Section 5.2.1.1.2 – their metalanguage comments will be analysed in Section 5.2.2.1, which will be dedicated to the assessment of how informants perceive their own speech.

Overt stigmatisation of local Southern IndE speech is further investigated in question int. II.8: "(if the speaker is from the South) Has anyone ever told you that you sound like a Southern Indian? Did you (would you) take it as a compliment?"; (if the speaker is from the North) If you told someone that he sounded like he came from Southern India, would you mean it as a compliment?". As can be seen, the question changes depending on the ethnicity of the informants. It seeks to investigate the affective dimension of the attitude object in relation to the consideration of Southern IndE local speech as pleasant or unpleasant or, most importantly, as right or wrong. The present section will present the results of the Northern sample. Southern metalanguage commentary will be investigated in Section 5.2.2.1.

The initial reticence of some Northern informants to comment on Southern IndE accents/varieties was absorbed by neutral attitudes towards local speech:

(78) I mean, it would be something very neutral. I mean, if that person sounded like a South Indian, Southern Indian guy, then I would say that 'you're from South India'. I mean it's nothing to take it on heart (pauses) and be offended. (AVmDe) int.

(79) (pauses) I think I would not really mean, like, anything bad for this because that's how they, their language, their language influence their accent, so I would just mean it as a fact, and not as a compliment or not something to, that I don't like it, because I also have, like, South Indian friends, so, it's nothing that I would, like, not like the people from the South or something. (DTfUt) int.
(80) Ah, no I wouldn't mean it as a compliment, but I wouldn't mean it as an insult either. Like, it would just mean, like, a feature of that person. (SSfWB) int.
(81) No, it's just some geographical distinction, but they are still equal to us, so I don't distinguish from, with, with the location. (ASmMP) int.

The qualitative content analysis shows that, overall, neutral affective attitudes towards Southern IndE local speech are either related to geographical discrimination ("it's just some geographical distinction") or indexicality ("it would just mean, like, a feature of that person"; "that's how they, their language, their language influence their accent, so I would just mean it as a fact"). Moreover, Northern metalanguage comments sound conciliatory and apologetic, as if the informants feel the need to justify their commenting on the matter ("they are *still* equal to us", emphasis G.R.). What emerges from the examples above is that the Northern participants are always cautious in their replies and prefer more neutral stances in order not to 'offend' the Southern Indian community. However, it is worth mentioning that 30 % of the sample have positive attitudes towards Southern IndE accents/varieties:

(82) I think I will say it as a compliment. (BJmGu) int.
(83) If I were to tell someone? I think it will be a friendly gesture, compliment, yeah. (GSmDe) int.
(84) Yeah, I mean, they have a good grip on language. Maybe their accent is not that understandable, but they have a good grip on the language. (MGofUt) int.
(85) Oh, they are very proud of being South Indians. South Indians are very proud of their language, their state, their culture, so. (SDfMP) int.

The examples above show that, although Northern informants argue that they "will say it as a compliment", they do not express strong positive attitudes towards local Southern IndE speech. As a matter of fact, they do not explicitly agree on either its pleasantness or its correctness. MGofUt, for instance, points to the correctness of their grammar and the unintelligibility of their accents (cf. Section 5.2.2.2) while SDfMP anticipates the possible reaction of Southern speakers and does not provide any meaningful insight into her opinion of local Southern IndE speech. On the contrary, 10 % of the community members show strong negative attitudes towards Southern IndE accents/varieties, thus confirming their overt stigmatisation of local speech:

(86) Actually, I would not mean it as a compliment, because in general, the stereotype of that is that, South Indian English, is that (pauses) I mean, that's a stereotype in itself, South Indian English equals to wrong. So I wouldn't say it directly, but I would try to ask where they're from, maybe I've been to that place, but I would never say that to someone. (SLfUP) int.

(87) SPfBi: (pauses) No (laughs) We generally just do it to tease them (laughs).
GR: Yeah, tell me more about that.
SPfBi: Yeah. 'You have a typical South Indian accent', yeah, we, we just tell them that. int.

Northern informants belonging to this subgroup show a high level of metalinguistic awareness since the social and regional connotations of both Northern and Southern local IndE speeches seem to be part of common knowledge. In particular, the discussion raised by SLfUP is an account of the social stereotypes surrounding Southern IndEs and of related standard language ideologies. This participant is, in fact, eager to note that she "would not mean it as a compliment, because in general, the stereotype of that is that, *South Indian English [...] that' s a stereotype in itself, South Indian English equals to wrong* (emphasis, G.R.). In arguing that Southern IndE is a stereotype in itself and, according to popular opinion, it 'equals to wrong', she seems to reflect the 'perceptual separation' position expressed by Ladefoged (1975), which would appear to be a presupposition about the quality of the 'standard'. Her unasserted beliefs about Southern IndE local speech point to the following folk assessment: even if not perceived as the 'standard', Northern IndE varieties/accents are the ones closer to it. Her unapologetic behaviour, however, is attenuated by her intention not to comment with any Southern Indian about their origins since most probably, they may not take it the right way either.

Overt stigmatisation of Southern IndE speech is, again, apparent in metalanguage response concerning a possible reaction of Southern speakers to Northerners' enquiries regarding their place of origin. The qualitative content analysis shows two massively disproportional distribution patterns: the predominant one consists of those informants hypothesising a negative reaction from the Southern counterparts and the other one, of those who speculate on a positive reaction. The following examples indicate the prototype of metalanguage comments speculating on the former:

(88) I mean, depending on the person, though. But if I was, it was me, I would feel it a bit not complimented though. Something negative. (BsmGu) int.

(89) DSfWB: [...] the way things are in India right now, especially giving the hostels scenes that I have witnessed, people get pissed, they get offended, you know? like _
GR: I mean if you say that they're from the South of India?
DSfWB: If you say that 'you sound South Indians' I mean it's a matter of fact, but then it, I mean, especially when it comes from a North Indian, it's more derogatory because people of it perceive things like that, they are, and it's, it's true, people, like, North India _ I mean I would say up to Madhya Pradesh I would count as North India _ they all make fun of South Indians, I mean, it's clear, yeah, so that. int.

(90) (pauses) Yeah, I can say (pauses) the person can (pauses) like it in a way that he is, I can understand the different accents but sometimes people also think that 'why do you always have to discriminate between North and South India?', so that can also be a problem (KGfPu). int.

In their discussion of Southerners' reactions, these respondents are particularly concerned with a number of social as well as linguistic matters. The North vs. South divide is expressed strongly and reveals a deep folk disparity between the presupposition that Northern IndE speakers feel that their local speech is somewhat superior on the one hand and the emphasis on the lack of correctness of Southern IndE accents on the other. For many, this folk perception of superiority is very explicit:

(91) TDfMa: Depends, South Indians would definitely not like it.
GR: Why?
TDfMa: Because I think they get offended by it, and I guess it's, it's a joke between, again, the North and the South and the North Indians keep saying 'oh, you're from South, so the way you speak is from _ the way you look or the way you speak is also' _ I mean, they just mark as a South Indian which I think is, is mean, yeah.

(92) Ah, no generally people get offended by that, I don't know why because they, it is a generalised idea that Northern people always just dis _ disrespect Southern people (laughs) because they always feel superior than themselves and (pauses) they always say, like, "Yeah, you do not know, like, you pronounce every word wrong and every pronunciation is, like, 'uh↓ da↑ da↓ da↑'" and, so, this is how it goes, but, more or less it is not a compliment. It is more or less offense, I think, yeah. (ATmDe)

Although very few community members belonging to the Northern sample, i.e., 10 %, have strong negative attitudes towards Southern IndE local speech, as can be seen from the examples above, there are many folk opinions 'back home' which attribute global social authority to Northern IndE accents/varieties. These opinions reverberate overseas but are generally taken for what they are: stereotypes. Moreover, whether the informants agree with them or not, it is worth anticipating that sustained contact with other varieties or dialects usually raises the level of overt and covert social consciousness of regional variants (Labov 1972a). Subsequently, despite perceived differences in the degree of standardness of IndE varieties within the Indian subcontinent, the ensuing consequences of dialect stabilisation allow for a higher level of awareness of language variation. Among speakers of different dialects, extended exposure can either cause the adoption of new features or "be strongly constrained by the degree to which [they] create positive or negative allegiances across groups" (Sharma 2005:8). Although the question will be addressed in more detail in Section 5.2.2, here it is to be pointed out that the sociolinguistic situation of the student community reflects the latter process since the persistent contact among Northern and Southern members allows for a clearer picture of those North vs. South language ideologies 'back home' and for the subsequent modifications/accommodations of their sociolinguistic behaviour depending of the amount of time they have lived in Heidelberg (cf. Section 5.1.3.4).

With respect to the subgroup of informants who speculate on the positive reaction of Southern speakers, the code system indicates only two instances:

(93) [...] it depends on the South Indian because many of them they get _ I mean, they don't get offended that's what I've observed, because I've many friends from South India (SSmUt). int.

(94) Ah, so far I've said this to two people, and none of them took it in a very negative manner. They took it quite well, and (pauses) I think it might be my way of saying it, because I didn't say it in a compliment way or neither, like, 'hey, I'm judging you're from South India'. It's just a fact, putting out a fact (NPfMP). int.

This result is self-explanatory since it points to the fact that only 6 % of the Northern sample believe in a potential positive reaction of Southern speakers with regard to the perception of their local speech. On the whole, this finding suggests that the Northern community is well aware of the North/South sociolinguistic divide and of the perceived ethnicity-based intrinsic superiority of Northern IndE accents/varieties. Moreover, they seem to predict a rather univocal negative reaction from their counterparts. However, Southern perceptions and presuppositions may be completely different and account for the relativity of such ideological resources (cf. section below). In recurring to the response of a Northern participant to int. II.8, the following example might be the key to the investigation of Southern folk perceptions:

(95) Because I feel that in general all the Indians are pretty sensitive about the culture and their languages and I, I feel that in particular in South India it's more of their (pauses) a question of their identity and if you comment on and say something 'okay, you sound like this' and as (pauses) offensive comment, I think they would not like it. Because they are a bit more sensitive towards how (pauses) seriously they take to their languages, so. (SHfUP). int.

5.2.1.2 Ethnic and Pan-Indian Identities: Integrative and Dissociative Attitudes

Group identity is an important factor in the definition of social groups, values and evaluations. Likewise, language plays a major role in the definition of group identity. Section 2.4 emphasises how different symbolic values are attached to different linguistic forms and how, to some extent, language creates identity. Thus, the choice of a certain language or variety can deliberately express a particular affiliation to or distance from a certain group. Moreover, an individual's identity is a complex construct and is always related to different group identities. Depending on the sociocultural and linguistic situation, different aspects of one's identity are brought to the fore. This social categorisation, in the words of Tajfel (1978:61–2),

> refers to the ordering of social environment in terms of groupings of persons in a manner which makes sense to the individual" and "helps to structure the environment according to certain general cognitive principles.

In this sense, identities are dynamic and subjective, i.e., they are simultaneously defined by group membership and the individual's self-perception. They are formed and developed through different processes of social comparison, the most important ones being 'identification' and 'demarcation' (Tajfel 1981). While the first process refers to the way individuals identify with a group, the second one corresponds to the way in, and the extent to, which they separate from the other group members or out-groups. Both processes find expression in integrative and dissociative attitude orientations (Schlieben-Lange 1991). More specifically, the integrative attitude orientation is concerned with the attachment to or solidarity with a group, its language and its culture while the dissociative one deals with a wish to be different from the group. These orientations depend on perspective: with regard to the present context, a positive integrative attitude towards a pan-Indian identity can be seen as reflecting a dissociative attitude towards Northern and Southern ethnic ones, especially in diasporic contexts. However, this may not be the case since informants may hold a positive attitude towards their own local identities (embodied in their L1 and/or in their local IndE languages) and yet have a positive integrative orientation towards their more general pan-Indian one.

The cluster analysis and bubble matrix for the dependent variable *identity development* show that 67 % of the sample generally agree on their native language being the one they most strongly identify with, while the remaining 33 % consider English their identity language (cf. Section 5.1.2.2 and Fig. 5.1.6). While there is no significant difference in *gender* and *time spent in Heidelberg*, *ethnicity* prove to be an interesting extralinguistic variable. 40 % of the respondents who associate with English come from Southern India vs. 60 % from the North. This result is partially confirmed by many of the examples discussed in Section 5.2.1.1.3 which point to the strong attachment of Southern speakers to their local languages and cultures according to the Northern sample. Sections 5.2.1.1.3 and 5.2.1.1.1 have indirectly shed some light on the positive and negative attitudes of the community members towards their group counterparts. However, they have not provided any insight into the informants' attitudes towards their in-group. The present section aims to analyse the integrative and dissociative attitudes of Northern and Southern participants towards their in-groups in order to anticipate the discussion of the speakers' awareness of local speech, which will be commented on in the following section.

Because everyone wants to hold positive attitudes towards their in-group, a negative evaluation of the in-group by the sociocultural environment may create conflict. Section 5.2.1.1.3 emphasises the perceived attitude of superiority of some Northern speakers towards their Southern counterparts and their overall negative evaluation with respect to accent variation. In other words, the section sheds light on the folk's perception of a seemingly superior group, i.e., the Northern one, and an inferior one, i.e., the Southern community. However, it does not go into the attitudes of the participants towards their own vernacular. Two questions from the interview schedule have been designed to enquire after the informants' integrative and dissociative attitudes towards their local speech:

- *Do you like the way people from the South of India sound? What do you like about it? What don't you like about it? (int. II.6)*
- *A (if the speaker is from the South) Has anyone ever told you that you sound like a Southern Indian? Did you (would you) take it as a compliment? B (if the*

speaker is from the North) If you told someone that he sounded like he came from Southern India, would you mean it as a compliment? (int. II.8)

While Section 5.2.1.1.3 analyses the Northern perspective on Southern local speech, the present section seeks to verify both Northern and Southern participants' attachment to/detachment from their language in-group. The qualitative content analysis shows that 85 % of the Southern participants hold positive associative attitudes towards their own vernacular:

(96) I have always taken it as a compliment because I felt that I stand out. (ASfKe) int.
(97) I think they're distinct, that's what I like about them, that they're different. (MMfKa) int.
(98) Yeah, I mean (pauses) everybody has a signature, a signature when they say things, and I think it's pretty good. (SLmKa) int.
(99) I get to know things from them, in their accent, so (pauses) what I thought was only limited language as where they're in India, but when I met with them, I would, I was able to explore many things. (SPmKa) int.
(100) (pauses) They has, they have not (pauses) not trying to imitate someone, so they are being their own, so it's (pauses) what I like about that, that's it. (SVmKa) int.
(101) [...] we can learn a little bit about their cultures through these things, because why they are pronouncing these ways it comes basically from the (pauses) how, how they are brought up and how those cultural things also (pauses) that matters because the cultural language, we always do mix up this English with the local language, so this, the influence of the local language will be there on the English that we speak, that's what I feel. (PNmKe) int.

The examples above reflect the folk's indexical component of accent variation, which may be summarised in the following statement: 'I like how we sound because we are different'. The 'signature' of the Southern informants allows them not only to 'stand out', but also to 'get to know many things' about themselves. In other words, their local speech is indexical of their culture as well as their identities and they are proud of its tangible 'audibility'. Contrary to the Northern informants – who perceive Southern IndE local speech as rough and, at times, unintelligible, the Southern ones consider their accents 'pleasant', 'polite' and generally 'clear'. The examples below inform on their positive integrative attitudes towards their own vernaculars and on the 'sociolinguistic competition' with their Northern counterparts:

(102) They sound more (pauses) straightforward, present and polite basically. (VSmTN) int.

(103) GR: What do you like about it?
MNmKa: The way they speak out, the pronunciation, like, it makes me, like, yes, I'm like them, the way they communicate, the way they speak out. int.

(104) Yeah, some people speak very fluently English because (pauses) South Indian, in South India people are more educated and there is a high literacy rate in South India, so mostly, as per my observations, South Indians speak (pauses) somewhat fluent English compared to North regions. It's totally like it. (DVfAP) int.

(105) [...] it's just easy to understand what they speak, I think they are more clear in _ when they speak, I can understand them very clearly. They don't have different way of using the word or something, so whatever they speak is straight and it's very easy to understand it, so. (NKSfTN) int.

(106) Yeah, I think South _ yeah, I think, I think people are more educated so compared to North India. It's, it's a decent accent, we, we can communicate. People are, I think, confident because they get the confidence (pauses) so I think the, I think education place a lot of role in their accent, see, they are, if they _ if they have lived in different, different, they have lived outside their hometown, I think people are more comfortable English. They are stay only in their hometown; they they are not very comfortable with English. But what I feel is eventually people don't get adjusted to English. (KDmKe) int.

In providing a description of Southern IndE varieties/accents, the Southern informants have a tendency to compare themselves with Northern ones. In doing so, they generally distinguish Northern poorer speech as a result of greater educational disadvantage. It is not surprising, perhaps, to find that, according to the Southern sample, Northern IndE accents are strong. An interesting theme emerges here when KDmKe notes, however briefly, that "people don't get adjusted to English". The implication is that, despite their level of education, they cannot suddenly accommodate their speech. The interrelation between local speech and education is crucial even in the metalanguage content of Northern informants discussed in Sections 5.2.1.1.2 and 5.2.1.1.3. Overall, the community members agree on the greater educational settings of Southern India, but while Northern informants do not see any meaningful relation between accent and education, Southern speakers ascribe their higher literacy rates to the straightforwardness, clarity and politeness of their local accents.

Dissociative attitudes towards Southerners' own vernaculars are rare and add up to 15 % of the speakers. They are elicited through the "What don't you like about it?" part of int. II.6. When present, however, these attitudes resemble those held by the Northern community and are related to issues of unintelligibility and lack of correctness:

(107) There's nothing that I hate about it. Maybe if I find it hard to understand, that's when I get nervous and, yeah. (APmTN) int.

(108) Sometimes it feels a very _ feels very rural (pauses) their _ they actually know good English but just because of their accent they come across as people who are not very well educated, some, that _ that does not reflect correctly on them, so I think (pauses) people can improve their accents though (pauses) yeah, and not come across as bad, as who they are actually. (VJRfKa) int.

(109) Yeah, of course, the influence of mother tongue, because sometimes it's so weird, the, they are changing the entire word itself, so you will hear, like, an entirely different word, sometime. (SSmKe) int.

Despite the massively disproportional distribution pattern, the Southerners' dissociative attitudes towards local speech seem to substantiate content-wise the findings discussed in the quantitative section, according to which the Southern informants have seemingly taken over the stereotypes of the Northerners about themselves (cf. Sections 5.1.3.4 and 5.2.2).

With respect to the Northern community, likewise, 65 % of the sample hold associative attitudes towards their own vernacular. The following examples shed light on the attachment to their language in-group and their positive opinions of local speech:

(110) Northern Indian people are very more friendly than Southern people, they are not stubborn. Southern people are very stubborn regarding their languages. Northern people are very chill person [...] Northern _ English spoken in the North side is usually light. (JGfMa) int.

(111) Yeah, it's quite clear and although it's quite diverse, I mean it's a mixed bag of a lot of things, but, yeah, I, I find that (pauses) Northern English accent is quite clear. (AVmDe) int.

(112) Right, so I feel in (pauses) North India the accent is not so strong [...] there is a certain tone they have, that is true, but then what they are saying _ you can actually ascertain what they are saying or then you can figure out, you know? (DSfWB) int.

(113) Yeah, North Indian accents are pretty much clear and they _ that is not too much influence of their mother tongue because in the North part of India, Hindi is the only, like, mother tongue is there. There are no regions _ much regional languages and everybody is familiar with Hindi, so they don't have any different accents, but in the Southern part the influence of mother tongue is too much, so. (MGofUt) int.

(114) So, yeah, the Northern Indian accents, I think, they are more understandable than the person having, like, a strong South Indian accent. (DTfUt) int.

What emerges from these folk metalanguage comments is that, overall, the Northern informants think that their accents are much clearer than the Southern ones. As was the case with their counterparts, they seem to employ strategies of sociolinguistic competition when describing their own vernaculars. An intuitive way of accounting for this result is that both groups are very well aware of the North/South sociolinguistic divide and linguistic power imbalance, hence of the conflict of interest between their respective in-groups. Interestingly, the perceived attitude of superiority of some Northern speakers, raised and discussed in Section 5.2.1.1.3, seems to be confirmed by further metalanguage comments on the topic:

(115) For me it's, like, a standard English accent, I would say [...] (SHfUP) int.

(116) They sound normal (laughs). (PGfMa) int.

In recurring to Ladefoged's (1975) 'perceptual separation' position, the folk encode their metalanguage comments into their doctrine of correctness by overtly stating that Northern IndE local speech "it's, like, a standard English accent". (116) seems to presuppose the quality of the 'standard'. This phenomenon sheds light on the fact that the Northern folk appear to believe that pronouncing the standard variety is tied to ethnicity. Moreover, by considering their own vernacular a 'standard', they support Kroch's (1978:18) position according to which the elite dialect "[...] characteristically resists normal processes of phonetic conditioning (both articulatory and perceptual) that the speech of non-elite strata regularly undergoes". Interestingly, however, both communities rely on the doctrine of correctness in the description of their local speech. Yet, while the Southern informants relate this to their fluency and higher educational rates ("South Indians speak (pauses) somewhat fluent English compared to North regions"), their Northern counterparts explicitly connect it to their accent.

Discourse regarding dissociative attitudes towards local speech exists concurrently. Surprisingly, as compared to the Southern sample, a higher percentage of the Northern one (35 %) holds negative attitudes towards their own vernacular:

(117) North India, I feel, is a bit more loud, it's more rough and sometimes it's, it's impolite. (TDfMa) int.
(118) So, North Indians are the quite rough, I mean, they are clean, no doubt, but they are not that particular in armor [i.e., harmony], they're not that clear with the grammar but they somehow, they, they, I mean, they can speak English, yeah. (BSmGu) int.
(119) But with the North India, like the differences the North India, they really separate the word, they try to pronounce everything like even the silent word, they try to pronounce it. Like, they, every word is a different for they, there's no flow. (BJmGu) int.
(120) Ah, Northern India. Oh, so people in North, they generally speak broken English (pauses) but (pauses) and also people in Northern India, they speak a lof of #_# they make a lot of errors while speaking because they're not very educated compared to the Southern. (SSfWB) int.
(121) (pauses) With English, okay, so, yeah, so North India will be having (pauses) how do you call it? not very good, they're not very good in English even if they are decently educated, but compared to that South Indians, most of them will be able to communicate in English. It's one thing. (SPfBi) int.

The examples above substantiate the results from the previous discussion according to which Northern participants relate their standardness to their accent and not to their grammar. Moreover, they emphasise that both communities agree with each other with respect to their own areas of language 'specialisation', so to say. As a matter of fact, they both seem to attribute accent standardness to Northern IndE local speech and lexico-syntactical accuracy to Southern IndE varieties.

On the whole, the results are consistent with the idea that both ethnic communities hold positive integrative attitudes towards their own vernaculars. Their local speech not only indexes locally situated ethnic identities, but it is perceived as an individual identity-affirmation (cf. Section 5.2.2). The general feeling is that the Southern informants tend to be prouder of their own languages and IndE varieties, which allow them to express their identities and cultures to the fullest. While this 'Southern pride' is pinpointed by some Northern participants as well, the latter do not seem to share the same enthusiasm with regard to their local speech. The speakers' constant need of renegotiating the 'problem of ethnicity' (Jayaram 2004) is resolved in their willingness to shed their regional, linguistic and ethnic identities, sometimes in deference to their more general pan-Indian one. In this sense, "a person may be Bengali [or] Indian" (Friesen/Kearns 2008:225) depending on specific sociocultural and linguistic circumstances. While the community members generally adopt their ethnic identities and cling to their distinctiveness within their community of practice, they tend to adopt their pan-Indian identity in their everyday lives:

(122) I think it's the overall identity for me, yeah, so I would never say that 'No, I'm from Uttarakhand, you're from South' it's always, like, we're Indians, that's the most important thing (laughs), I mean, that's who I am. (SSmUt) int.

(123) SSfWB: When I was in India, it was more important to be a Bengali (smiles), but ever since I moved here, I think it's more important to be an Indian, then.
GR: Why was it more important to be a Bengali?
SSfWB: Because in India I was only interacting with Indians, here I, I don't interact with Indians at all (pauses) I barely have an Indian friend here. So, for me, it's more important to be an Indian because as a community nobody would know Bengal, Bengalis, but as an Indian people would know me, so. int.

(124) I don't want to be distinguished between North Indian and a South Indian. I just want to be recognised as an Indian, which would be better, I think. (SSmKa) int.

It is worth mentioning that while most topics are implicit in the design of the questionnaire and of the interview task, discourse regarding a pan-Indian identity is covered quantitatively only, through question I.3.5 ("The use of my background languages is a strong part of my identity in Heidelberg as well as among other Indians"), which is discussed in Section 5.1.2.2. However, one advantage of the qualitative design is that recurrent issues may be incorporated into the interpretation of the results although they had not been foreseen in the design of the questionnaire. The instances above are one such example: while the interview task has not been designed to shed light on the topic, some informants have felt the need to address the issue nevertheless. SSfWB, for instance, notes that in a country where people know neither West Bengal or Bengalis, but would recognise all ethnic identities as one, being a Bengali and acting as one is only possible in India. As SSfWB confesses, she does not have many multiplex relations within her community of practice ("here I, I don't interact with Indians at all (pauses) I barely have an Indian friend here"). As a matter of fact, she is a highly unintegrated member according to the network-strength scale (cf. Section 5.1.1.4 and Tab. 5.1.5). Nevertheless, with some due exceptions, the majority of the informants display their local and situated ethnic identities within their community of practice. It is only here, in fact, that "the kaleidoscope of ethnic identities acquires sociolinguistic significance" (Regnoli 2019c:176).

5.2.2 Diaspora Consciousness

The present section sheds light on the reasons why and the extent to which perceived differences in accent variation matter in the Heidelberg Indian student community. In investigating folk awareness concerning the idiolects of the informants and in relating them to their broader in-group local speech – which has just been discussed – the aim of the final part of the present thesis is to draw attention to how diaspora consciousness shapes ideologies of nativeness, network bonds and transnational ties. Sociolinguistically related concerns about the role of English in the diaspora have heightened the need for further investigation concerning the extent to which linguistic differences inform our understanding of community structures, attitudinal orientations and identity development (Hundt/Sharma 2014).

The concept of diaspora *as* consciousness puts great emphasis on identity and examines "a particular kind of awareness said to be generated among contemporary transnational communities" (Vertoveč 1999:285). This 'social reproduction' (Friesen/Kearns 2008) involves dual or even multiple identities in which "many ethnic associations have been formed to facilitate the maintenance of a specific Indian regional culture [...] At the same time, there is a strong imperative to establishing a pan-Indian identity" (Friesen/Kearns 2008:222). This constant need of renegotiating the 'problem of ethnicity' (Jayaram 2004) is often resolved in the willingness of the diasporic subjects to shed their regional, linguistic and/or ethnic identities depending on the contingent circumstances (cf. Section 5.2.1.2). In transient multilingual speech communities, "be[ing] a Bengali [or] an Indian" (Friesen/Kearns 2008:220) is generally characterised by a certain fluidity in terms of the norms that guide speakers' interactions both within and outside their community of practice. This happens mainly because these relatively short-lived contexts usually share different ideological patterns compared to more stable speech communities. Subsequently, such shared assumptions cannot be assumed *a priori* in transient multilingual communities and, thus, need to be investigated in more depth. The Heidelberg Indian student community proves to be no exception, and the folk belief that the community holds, i.e., that South Indians have a distinctive speech in English constitutes its most important component.

The present section will inform on the grass roots triggering the informants' attitudes towards accent variation as discussed in Section 5.2.1. In doing so, it will take a step back and start from the investigation of the speakers' perceptions of their own idiolects (cf. Section 5.2.2.1) in relation to their global standard language ideologies and the resulting myth of non-accent or neutral accent (cf. Section 5.2.2.2). Finally, an analysis of the informants' network affiliations and transnational ties will account for the importance of the transient aspect of the Heidelberg Indian student community (cf. Section 5.2.2.3).

5.2.2.1 Accent Awareness

Section 5.1.1.2 shed light on how the favourable environment of the university town of Heidelberg contributes to developing an overt consciousness of English accent variation among the members of the Indian student community. Section 5.2.1.1 shows that, with the exception of one Southern female informant who has been living in Heidelberg for less than a year, all community members agree on the existence of different Indian accents of English (cf. Tab. 5.2.2). The mere acknowledgement and occurrence of some IndE varieties which have distinctive features is enough to count as a 'performance' of them and qualifies any use of them as a likely trigger of metalanguage response. As a matter of fact, II.1.10 enabled the participants to provide an accurate classification of local speech. In order to elicit metalanguage awareness concerning the speakers' idiolects and their subsequent affiliations to those in-groups as pointed out by their earlier classification of local speech, the following questions have been asked:

- *How do you label your own spoken variety of English? (I.II.5)*
- *Do you think you have an accent? (II.I.2)*
- *If yes, what accent to do you think you have? (II.I.3)*
- *In your opinion, is your accent different from the accent of nearby towns and cities, or of other parts of India? Can you think of any specific ways in which it is different? For instance, are there different words and/or words which are pronounced differently? (II.I.4)*
- *I am prepared to spend money on taking courses to improve my accent (II.I.9)*

I.II.5 seeks to verify how respondents identify their own spoken variety of English in order to compare the results with I.II.2 ('General preference for models of English') and to make more general claims about underlying standard language ideologies and ideologies of nativeness (cf. Section 5.2.2.2). II.1.2 is the first question of Survey II.1, designed with the precise function of an 'icebreaker' in the discussion of accent and identity. II.1.3 and II.1.4 seek to investigate how the informants define their own accents in order to establish and maintain group identity. Finally, through II.I.9 respondents have been asked to place themselves on a scale from 1 to 5 on how much they were willing to spend money to improve their accent. II.I.9 has a rating scale from 'very" to 'rather not'. The aim was to check the consistency of the affective and dissociative attitudes towards local speech discussed in Section 5.2.1.2.

The distribution pattern of Tab. 5.2.3 reveals that both the males and the Northern part of the community, as well as those who have been living in Heidelberg for considerable time have the most favourable attitudes towards 'Indian English' as their linguistic identity marker. On the other hand, women, Southern speakers and newcomers self-label their own spoken variety of English as a 'mixture' of BrE, AmE and IndE. Although no extralinguistic variable reach significance, *ethnicity* is, again, an interesting correlate to discuss.

Tab. 5.2.3 Self-labelling of speakers' variety of English according to the community, gender, ethnicity and time spent in Heidelberg

How do you label your own spoken variety of English? (I.II.5)	**N**		**%**	
'Mixture' of all three	24		40	
Indian English	23		38	
'Good' English	8		13	
Unsure	3		5	
British English	2		3	
Total	60		99	
(a) according to gender	Male		Female	
	N	%	N	%
'Mixture' of all three	10	33	14	47
Indian English	15	50	8	27
'Good' English	4	13	4	13
Unsure	1	3	2	7
British English	0	0	2	7
Total	30	99	30	101
(b) according to ethnicity	North		South	
	N	%	N	%
'Mixture' of all three	12	35	12	46
Indian English	13	38	10	38
'Good' English	4	12	4	15
Unsure	3	9	0	0
British English	2	6	0	0
Total	34	100	26	99
(c) according to time spent in Heidelberg	0.1–1		1.1–5	
	N	%	N	%
'Mixture' of all three	16	41	8	38
Indian English	14	36	9	43
'Good' English	6	15	2	10
Unsure	1	3	2	10
British English	2	5	0	0
Total	39	100	21	101

It is striking that the Southern informants answer more positively to '"Mixture' of three since 'Indian English' seems a more appropriate answer in view of their positive associative attitudes to local speech (cf. Section 5.2.1.2). This might be due to a higher awareness of their social category (superior education/graduate students) which directly reverberates the alleged North vs. South educational divide discussed above. Moreover, only Northern informants answer neutrally (9 %) and attribute global social authority to their own spoken English by labelling it 'British English' (6 %). Despite the low percentage, however, this result substantiates earlier folk commentary according to which Northern spoken English is perceived as constituting a standard accent of English.

On the whole, the informants acknowledge (cf. Tab. 5.2.3a) that education – achieved mostly in private and English-medium schools – has played a central role in their accent 'upgrade' ('Mixture' of all three; 40 %). Most importantly, attitudes are positive in attributing locality and pan-ethnic features to the speakers' own spoken variety of English ('Indian English'; 38 %). To detect their own (level of) accent awareness and to check the consistency of the answers provided in I.II.5, metalanguage response was looked at more closely through II.I.2 and II.I.3.

Tab. 5.2.4 Own accent awareness according to the community, gender, ethnicity and time spent in Heidelberg

Do you think you have an accent? (II.I.2)	**N**		**%**	
Yes	41		68	
No	3		5	
Unsure	16		27	
Total	60		100	
(a) according to gender	Male		Female	
	N	%	N	%
Yes	24	80	17	57
No	2	7	1	3
Unsure	4	13	12	40
Total	30	100	30	100
(b) according to ethnicity	North		South	
	N	%	N	%
Yes	22	65	19	73
No	3	9	0	0
Unsure	9	26	7	27
Total	34	100	26	100
(c) according to time spent in Heidelberg	0.1–1		1.1–5	
	N	%	N	%
Yes	26	67	15	71
No	2	5	1	5
Unsure	11	28	5	24
Total	39	100	21	100

68 % of the informants agree on having an accent in English. Notably, men, Southern informants and community members who have been living in Heidelberg for considerable time are more strongly aware than their respective counterparts (cf. Tab. 5.2.4). While *ethnicity* is the most interesting variable to look at with respect to speakers' self-labelling of their spoken variety of English (cf. Tab. 5.2.3c), *gender* (cf.Tab. 5.2.3b) plays a crucial role in the informants' accent awareness. Considering their even ratio, it is striking how disproportional the distribution pattern of the variable is. While 80 % of men are aware of having an accent, only 57 % of women agree with it. Subsequently, women tend to be more unsure than men in this respect (40 % vs. 13 %).

At a first glance, this result is surprising in that women generally show more awareness of prestige norms in both their speech and their attitudes towards it (Wolfram/Fasold 1974). Moreover, it does not seem to confirm earlier findings according to which they are the ones exhibiting stronger attitudes than men with respect to IndE accent variation (cf. Section 5.1.3.4). While they generally show strong positive attitudes towards Northern IndE accents and react strongly negatively towards Southern IndE ones, they seem to hold rather neutral ones towards whether they have an accent themselves. However, a more in-depth investigation reveals that many community members hold a strong preference for non-accentedness or neutral accentedness (cf. Sections 5.2.1.1.2 and 5.2.2.2). Thus, acknowledging the presence of whatever accent in their English – which they tend to equate with non-standardness – might be a challenging task, especially for women who generally show lower rates of stigmatised vernacular variants and higher rates of prestige forms (Trudgill 1983). In this sense, women's neutral stances towards having an accent are justified by the not-so-implicit meaning that some community members attribute to having an accent, i.e., non-standardness (cf. Section 5.2.2.2).

With respect to the other extralinguistic variables, *ethnicity* and *time spent in Heidelberg* show a fairly proportional distribution pattern indicating that the majority of the informants acknowledge the presence of an 'accent' in their English. Question II.I.3 seeks to verify the speakers' first impressions of their 'having an accent' through the elicitation of metalanguage comments concerning what type of accent they think they have. The qualitative content analysis shows that, overall, three main sub-codes constitute the core of the answers provided: (i) an Indian accent; (ii) a mixture; (iii) uncertainty. As can be seen, such sub-codes substantiate the informants' reactions to II.I.2. As far as (i) is concerned, different subcategories shed light on just as many reasons why the participants consider their accents Indian. The examples given here are general statements regarding the nature of the accent in question:

(125) I think I have an Indian English accent because it is not comparable to British and American English Accent. It has some cultural touch. (KGfPu) surv.

(126) I think I have an Indian accent. This is because I have grown up in India and have learnt this language from other fellow Indians who themselves had this accent. And I have lived among people having the same accent. Hence, I think this might be the reason. (MMfKa) surv.

(127) Indian. I pronunce the words with a strongly and with sharp cuts. I often mis-pronunce too when it comes to new words. I think this is mainly because I grew up in an environment where correct pronunciation was not a necessity. People understood what I wanted to say and vice-versa. (ASfKe) surv.

(128) I am trying to improve my accent (from Indian English) and I don't know how far I have come with pronounciation with some words. (BSmGu) surv.

What emerges from these examples is that speakers clearly relate the acquisition of an Indian accent to their (Indian) surroundings. MMfKa, for instance, notes that she believes in her having an Indian accent "because [she has] grown up in India and ha[s] learnt this language from other fellow Indians who themselves had this accent". Moreover, she points to her extended exposure to "people having the same accent", which inevitably causes the adoption of typical local IndE features. On the other hand, ASfKe and BSmGU relate their Indian accents to mispronunciation problems and point to the fact that they "grew up in an environment where correct pronunciation was not a necessity" and intelligibility was never a problem. The presupposition behind such comments reflects Ladefoged's (1975) 'perceptual separation' position and is encoded in the doctrine of correctness. In other words, both ASfKe and BSmGU are making an implicit reference to the fact that their accents are Indian, *therefore*, they lack 'correct' pronunciation. Similar presuppositions are observed in relation to the lack of interaction with L1 English speakers:

(129) I have a Indian accent. This could be attributed to the fact that, I have never interacted with a native speaker in my life. The English that I was taught was with accent as well. This could be the reason. (APmTN) surv.

(130) Indian accent because I used to speak with other Indians and we learn from each other I have had limited opportunities to speak with native English speakers while I was in India. (KMmKe) surv.

The examples above foster some ideologies of nativeness (Shuck 2004, cf. Section 5.2.2.2). Here, APmTN and KMmKE are downgrading the quality of their accents by reflecting the presupposition that they are Indian *because of* some lack of 'improvement' deriving from no mutual interactions with L1 English speakers.

Several community members acknowledge culture-specific and ethnic Indian accents locally situated as strong identity markers. While some shed light on specific regional accents ("I have malayali accent"; "Accent of a Marathi person speaking English"), others refer to broader ethnic ones ("General North Indian urban accent") and make an implicit reference to urban standardness:

(131) I have malayali accent. But not the typical malayali accent. (JGMfKe) surv.

(132) General North Indian urban accent. From my experience with Indians from most parts of India I feel my accent is similar to theirs. (HTmUP) surv.

(133) Accent of a Marathi person speaking English, because Marathi-speaking people tend to enunciate every pronounciation and tend to emphasize a few sounds. (RMfMa) surv.

Network affiliations both within and outside the Indian student community are fundamental in raising the level of overt consciousness. (134) and (135) shed light on the above-mentioned phenomenon of 'diaspora consciousness' (Vertovec̆ 1999), i.e., a particular kind of awareness generated among contemporary transnational communities, and on how daily interactions with German and international people have helped shape informants' accent awareness:

(134) Indian, because my foreign friends here in Heidelberg agreed upon it. (ASmMP) surv.

(135) I think have an Indian accent because when I interact with people here in Heidelberg, I realise that the Germans can easily identify my nationality while on the other side the Indians living here can easily identify me as a north Indian that's because of my pronunciation and my way of stressing on words in a sentence when I speak.. So, I think I have an Indian accent and also I have grown up using this language all the times with Indians and I think I picked up the Indian accent. (AVmDe) surv.

The examples substantiate earlier findings according to which the majority of the informants are more prone to display their ethnic identities within their community of practice while they prefer to assume a more general pan-Indian one outside. AVmDe summarises this position when he states that "Germans can easily identify my nationality while on the other side the Indians living here can easily identify me as a north Indian that's because of my pronunciation and my way of stressing on words in a sentence when I speak". As pointed out in Section 5.2.1.2, ethnic identities acquire sociolinguistic significance only within their network since in a country where people know neither West Bengal nor Bengalis, they would recognise all ethnic identities as one.

Diaspora consciousness is the main theme of the second sub-code, which constitutes the speakers' perceptions of their own accents as a 'mixture'. The qualitative content analysis shows an interesting distribution pattern in the answers provided: while the majority of the informants perceive their own accents as a 'mixture' of IndE, BrE and AmE, some others rely on a 'miscellany' of L1 varieties of English and local speech:

(136) I think I have a mixture of Punjabi and American accents. Because I was grown up in a Punjabi family. And especially, my father has a very very strong Punjabi accent while speaking English. I think I got most of it from him. And I love watching American sitcoms and movies so that's how I learnt it, maybe. (GSmDe) surv.

(137) A mixture of Indian, British, American. Because, I grew up watching a lot of American movies, while at school, I had Indian teachers who taught using British English. (DLfMan) surv.

While both examples suggest an increasing influence of AmE, which derives principally from mainstream movies and tv-series, GSmDe's metalanguage comment sheds light on the perceived influence of Punjabi into his English accent, which is connected to his ethnic family background. However, the majority of the informants make a direct reference to their diaspora consciousness in deriving their accent 'mixture' peculiarity from out-group folk metalanguage commentary:

(138) A mixture of Indian and British accent. Its because of many of my international friends have told me. (DTfUt) surv.

(139) My brother and I studied in Christian schools back in India where they're extremely particular about pronounciation. They focused on British English so I say some words how they're pronounced in the British way, but due to exposure to American TV shows and movies, my friends and I developed an accent more leaning towards the American. My accent is therefore a mix of all, and also contains the Indian southern accent. In Heidelberg, the American is more pronounced when speaking to native speakers of English or German or international. It becomes more Indianised when I speak to Indian family or friends. (SDfKa) surv.

(140) Because I have seen a lot of American shows and I have stayed in the UK for more than a year I guess both the accents have influenced me. (JGfMa) surv.

The examples above not only emphasise how language is a constant topic of discussion for laypeople (already in Niedzielski/Preston 2003) but also how powerful others' descriptions of one's own accents can be for self-definition. DTfUt, for instance, relies on how her international friends defines her accent unconditionally ("as a mixture of Indian and British") and does not seem to question their perceptions. SDfKa, on the contrary, provides a deeper metalinguistic interpretation of her mixed accent relying on early educational experiences first (embodied in BrE), then on popular global culture (AmE) and, finally, on local and cultural practices (Southern IndE local speech). Her diaspora consciousness reveals a type of awareness in her willingness to accommodate to "native speakers of English or German or international [people]" by "leaning towards the American", which, in her opinion, is more intelligible and minimises miscommunication problems.

Finally, the third sub-code highlighted by the qualitative content analysis reveals some uncertainty with respect to the speakers' indexical type of accent:

(141) I am unsure of whether or not I have an accent is because I generally tend to adopt variegated approach to pronunciation of words – some words follow the British pronunciation style and some others, American. While speaking, I use what naturally comes to me. Hence, I may or may not have an accent. (DSfWB) surv.

(142) Personally, I do not think that I have an accent, but other people have told me that I have an accent. I am unsure what to make of that comment especially since I consider English my mother tongue, and it's a language that I have spoken throughout my life. (SLfUP) surv.

Two positions are embodied in the examples above: the informants who are unsure of their accents (i) generally describe them as a 'mixture' of different ones, and (ii) they have neutral conative attitudes towards accents in general. Moreover, DSfWB and SLfUP seem to reflect the 'ideology of nativeness' as expressed by Shuck (2004) since they both rely on standard English (in its forms of BrE and AmE) when describing their accents but fail to mention a possible Indian influence on them (cf. Section 5.2.2.2).

On the whole, regardless of their gender, ethnicity or time spent in Heidelberg, the community members show a high level of awareness in the descriptions of their own accents and emphasise some major aspects of language contact and language variation and change. Most importantly, they claim that they make very frequent use of accommodation processes outside of their networks by adjusting their accents, styles and/or other aspects of language according to the speech style and the level of English of the other participants in order to avoid possible misunderstandings or miscommunication problems. Here, accommodation most often takes the form of convergence, i.e., when a speaker chooses a language or a variety (as with SDfKa above, who uses AmE) that seems to fit the style of the other speaker in order to signal social proximity. The example below summarises this position:

(143) Sometimes I have a very Indian accent, especially when I'm talking to other Indians. I naturally tend to pronounce my consonants harder and roll my r's more. I consciously change my enunciation when speaking to non-Indians, making myself clearer in order to be better understood. I am unsure of how to define my accent, as some people tell me I have an Indian accent, while others say that it's not typically 'Indian'. (MGfUt) surv.

Question II.I.4 ("In your opinion, is your accent different from the accent of nearby towns and cities, or of other parts of India? Can you think of any specific ways in which it is different? For instance, are there different words and/or words which are pronounced differently?") seeks to provide linguistic support to II.I.3 by investigating what linguistic features the informants rely on in order to establish and maintain group identity. The qualitative content analysis reveals that phonetics and phonology are, once again, the major categories the community members rely on. As in Section 5.2.1.1.2, the informants do not discuss phonology qua phonology (Niedzielski/Preston 2003:261), but rather reveal their beliefs about the phonetic features that, in the perception of their own accents, are salient to accent variation and discrimination. The examples below provide some insight into some general phonetic features of the participants:

(144) My accent is not different from the nearby cities, but it is different from other parts of India. The way I pronounce the letters M,L,S,Y etc. is different than the way south Indians do it. I cannot roll my accent as much as they can do it. (SMfMa) surv.

(145) Yes, it is. We have a strong accent at the end of a sentence. Sometimes the statements that we make seem like questions and some of the words are vague. (OFmTN) surv.

While SMfMa is pointing to some features of her own accent, OFmTN notes that "we" (presumably the Southern Indians) make use of a rising intonation at the end of the sentence with the direct consequence of "mak[ing] [it] seem like questions". In referring to *their* accents, rather than to *his* accent only, OFmTN is both establishing and maintaining group identity, ultimately extending local features to his accent as well.

Another way of establishing group identity is to describe what is perceived as a common and salient feature of one's state of origin and make it indirectly one's own. (146) and (147) are such examples:

(146) Yes. Every state in India seems to have a different English accent. For example, the word film is pronounced as filum in Karnataka because the locals merge the local language (kannada) and English together. (RDfKa) surv.

(147) Yes it is way much different that english pronounced in Punjab and Southern part of India. For example, if the word is Petrol, then a punjabi accent suggest, Ptrol whereas a southern accent goes like Peterol. (ATmDe) surv.

Interestingly, both speakers hint at the same linguistic process taking place in the same dialect area, South India. The process in question is vowel epenthesis, i.e., the insertion or development of a vowel in the body of a word, and apparently characterises Southern IndE accents (according to ATmDe, a Northern participant) and Kannada English (according to RDfKa, a Southern participant). While RDfKa provides the example of 'film' which tends to be pronounced as 'filum' by Kannadigas, ATmDe compares the Punjabi pronunciation of 'petrol' – which seems to undergo the opposite linguistic process, i.e., elision – with the Southern IndE one 'peterol'. These examples are important for two main interrelated reasons: (i) they suggest that vowel epenthesis is a regularly acknowledged linguistic process happening in Southern IndE local speech and is evaluated uniformly by the community members and that (ii) the speakers' high level of awareness of this phenomenon makes it a 'stereotype' in Labovian terms since its social and regional connotations have become part of common knowledge.

The last question aiming to shed light on the participants' perceptions of their own accents is II.I.9. Respondents have been asked to place themselves on a scale from 1 to 5 on how much they were willing to spend money to improve their accent. II.I.9 has a rating scale from 'very' to 'rather not'. The overall results according to the extralinguistic variables selected are shown in Tab. 5.2.5.

Tab. 5.2.5 Own accent improvement according to the community, gender, ethnicity and time spent in Heidelberg

I am prepared to spend money on taking courses to improve my accent (II.I.9)	**N**		**%**	
Very	1		2	
Somewhat	5		8	
Neutral	5		8	
Not very	8		13	
Rather not	41		68	
Total	60		99	
(a) according to gender	Male		Female	
	N	%	N	%
Very	1	3	0	0
Somewhat	2	7	3	10
Neutral	3	10	2	7
Not very	5	17	3	10
Rather not	19	63	22	73
Total	30	100	30	100
(b) according to ethnicity	North		South	
	N	%	N	%
Very	1	3	0	0
Somewhat	2	6	3	12
Neutral	1	3	4	15
Not very	4	12	4	15
Rather not	26	76	15	58
Total	34	100	26	100
(c) according to time spent in Heidelberg	0.1–1		1.1–5	
	N	%	N	%
Very	1	3	0	0
Somewhat	4	10	1	5
Neutral	2	5	3	14
Not very	4	10	4	19
Rather not	28	72	13	62
Total	39	100	21	100

At a first glance, the fairly linear distribution patterns of all extralinguistic variables uncover that 68 % of the informants do not agree with the affective statement above. While only 8 % hold neutral attitudes towards accent improvement, an exiguous 2 % is willing to spend money on taking courses to improve their accent. The latter group consists of one informant only, i.e., AVmDe, a male student from Northern India who has been living in Heidelberg for less than a year. However, although not statistically significant, the distribution patterns of *ethnicity* show some interesting results worth discussing. While the Northern informants follow the general trend described above – with the only exception of AVmDe – their Southern counterparts seem to be more inclined towards accent improvement. Although 58 % of the sample disagree with the statement, 12 % are somewhat prepared to spend money on taking courses to improve their accent, and 15 % have neutral affective attitudes towards it.

These results are in line with earlier findings according to which Northern Indian students have stereotypical views about themselves while Southern informants have by and large taken over the stereotypes of the Northerners about themselves and, subsequently, are more inclined towards accent improvement (cf. Sections 5.1.3.4 and 5.2.1.1).

5.2.2.2 Ideologies of Nativeness and the 'Neutral' Accent

Sections 5.1.3.1 and 5.2.1.1.2 shed light on the assessment of IndE accents within the Heidelberg Indian student community from a folk perspective. Thus far, it has been set forth that their evaluation and stereotyping emphasise how IndE accents are functionally variable – one of the functions of variation being to convey social, ethnic and geographical meaning. Moreover, the analysis of metalanguage comment has highlighted the informants' general high level of awareness of accent variation. Interestingly, the qualitative content analysis has shown how, although accents have been perceived as "loose bundles of prosodic and segmental features distributed over geographic and/or social space" (Lippi-Green 1997:42), the concepts of standard language and its corollary, non-accent, immediately follow the folk discussion on IndE accents.

A working definition of standard language and non-accent as they are used in the present thesis follows Lippi-Green (1997:41), who defines non-accent as "a collectively held ideal, which brings with it a series of social and regional associations". According to Milroy and Milroy (1991:22–3), the concept of standard language need not be understood as any actual language, but as "an idea in the mind rather than a reality – a set of abstract norms to which actual usage may conform to a greater or lesser extent".

Non-accent is a major issue for many members of the Heidelberg Indian student community. As already mentioned above, the presuppositions behind speakers' willingness to acquire a neutral accent, or a non-accent, so to say, derive from Shuck's (2004) 'ideology of nativeness'. In order to delve into the sociocultural mechanisms that guide speakers in their willingness of acquiring a non-accent or a neutral accent, individual assessments will be presented and discussed from two perspectives. The first one will analyse the informants' general preferences for models of English in different domains. The second one will investigate the individuals' stances towards their own accents with respect to accent 'pride' and accent embarrassment. The analysis of both perspectives will be framed within the ideologies of nativeness and standard language.

Table 5.2.6 provides an indication of the informants' attitudes towards different models of English according to preference. The results suggest that IndE is positively connotated (43 %). This comes as no surprise since 38 % of the population self-label their own spoken variety of English as Indian (cf. Tab. 5.2.3). Likewise, BrE holds a similar position: 42 % of the sample prefer it to other varieties of English.

Tab. 5.2.6 General preference for models of English

General preference for models of English (I.II.2)	N	%
Indian English	26	43
British English	25	42
American English	5	8
Unsure	4	7
Total	60	100

Question I.II.3 has been designed to investigate whether and to what extent standard ideologies play a crucial role in the community. Specifically, it seeks to verify which varieties of English have acquired global social authority in the educational domain. Table 5.2.7 shows the faculty preferences for models of instruction according to the community members. It is not surprising that 55 % of the sample considers BrE the most eligible variety (already in Regnoli 2016; Kachru 1976). However, before drawing any far-reaching conclusions, one must note that the positive attitude towards BrE may simply be accounted for in historical terms. BrE provides a perceived norm to follow though localised non-native varieties have always been 'detrimental'. This somewhat predicts the general positive attitudes towards IndE reported in Tab. 5.2.6. While the preference for BrE may be explained in historical terms, that of AmE – which has been selected by 18 % of the sample – may be framed within a more globally prestigious perspective.

Tab. 5.2.7 Faculty preference for models of instruction

Faculty preference for models of instruction (I.II.3)	N	%
British English	33	55
American English	11	18
Unsure	10	17
Indian English	6	10
Total	60	100

However, global social authority is relative and unequal (Blommaert 2003), and the evaluation of particular language practices and varieties hinges upon the devaluation of others (Chand 2009). This unequal power relationship is often responsible for the abandonment of practices considered to hold low social value in favour of globally prestigious ones. While this is not always the case within the Indian student community, the qualitative content analysis of Survey II,I and the sociolinguistic interviews uncover some interesting folk comment which relates to the ideology of nativeness. According to Wassink and Curzan (2004:175) "these belief systems which often reinforce the [perceived] dominance of the standard, provide a (if not the) lens through which speakers interpret and understand the language variation that they encounter". Here, a direct ideological link exists between 'nonstandard' speech and unintelligibility (cf. Sections 5.2.1.1.2 and 5.2.1.1.3).

The following questions have been designed to elicit such metalanguage comment:

- *Are you proud of your accent or would you rather not have any accent at all? (II.I.5)*
- *Would you prefer to have a different accent? If so, which one? Why? (II.I.6)*
- *Have you ever felt embarrassed about your accent? When? Why? (II.I.8)*
- *Have you ever tried to change anything about the way you talk? What? (int. II.11)*
- *Well, if you could change the way you talk, what would you change? (int. II.14)*

While II.1.5 seeks to verify how the respondents define the importance of their own local IndE accents, II.I.6 aims to determine the informants' dissociative attitudes towards their accents. II.I.8 has been designed to check the consistency of the answers provided in II.I.5. Int. II.11 and II.14 have been asked during the interview when the respondents were to talk about their accents, related aspects they have modified (or tried to) and the ones they still want to change. The aim is to determine the ideologies of the participants about standardness.

Tab. 5.2.8 Accent pride according to the community, gender, ethnicity and time spent in Heidelberg

Are you proud of your accent or would you rather not have any accent at all? (II.I.5)	**N**		**%**	
Yes	35		58	
No	13		22	
Unsure/Neutral	12		20	
Total	60		100	
(a) according to gender	Male		Female	
	N	%	N	%
Yes	15	50	20	67
No	9	30	4	13
Unsure/Neutral	6	20	6	20
Total	30	100	30	100
(b) according to ethnicity	North		South	
	N	%	N	%
Yes	22	65	13	50
No	5	15	8	31
Unsure/Neutral	7	21	5	19
Total	34	101	26	100
(c) according to time spent in Heidelberg	0.1–1		1.1–5	
	N	%	N	%
Yes	23	59	12	57
No	8	21	5	24
Unsure/Neutral	8	21	4	19
Total	39	101	21	100

Table 5.2.8 shows the percentage of responses to II.I.5. The results indicate that 58 % of the sample are proud of their accents and would not want to change it. Considering that the majority of the informants call their own accents Indian (cf. Section 5.2.2.2), it is important to observe how they value them and what they may represent, i.e., their ethnic origins, education and any other relevant social aspect of their upbringing and life experiences. Another 20 % of the informants show neutral attitudes towards accents in general, hence they do not hold them in high regard. An interesting subgroup is the one holding dissociative attitudes towards their own accents. 22 % of the sample are not proud of their accents and would rather change it.

A close look at the figures suggests an interesting correlation of extralinguistic variables. While time *spent in Heidelberg* reveals that newcomers (21 %) are less proud of their accents than members who have been living in Heidelberg for some time (24 %), *gender* and *ethnicity* show that men and Southern speakers are the ones who tend to be more inclined towards accent improvement.

This finding is in line with further results discussed in the sections above, i.e., Southern Indians are the least proud members of the community with respect to their accents and are most willing to spend money on taking courses to improve it. On the other hand, men constitute 30 % of the informants who are not proud of their accents. Here, again, this result substantiates earlier claims that men are more inclined towards accent improvement.

The monoglot standard ideology interprets dialects as being unequal, with a 'single' standard and multiple 'nonstandard' dialects (Silverstein 1996). In conjunction with Shuck's (2004) already cited 'ideology of nativeness', this hegemonic ideology is intertwined with sociolinguistic conceptualisations of 'us' versus 'them', questions of (un)intelligibility and subsequent commodification of a 'standard' (Blommaert 2003). Dominant ideologies are perpetuated through speakers' interactions with in-group members versus others and allow for presumed social differences such as education or intelligence to be fronted as explanations of linguistic variation (Silverstein 1996). In so far as we "perceive variation in the speech of others and [...] use it to structure our knowledge about that person" (Lippi-Green 1997:30), dominant ideologies tend to be naturalised and reified.

Although only a discrete minority of the community members reflect the 'ideology of nativeness', it is nevertheless fundamental to gain insight into the topic and draw some conclusions in relation to the Indian student community as a whole. Questions II.I.6 – int. II.14 described above will be analysed dependently and concurrently in order to shed new light on both the monoglot standard ideology (Silverstein 1996) and the 'ideology of nativeness' (Shuck 2004).

The qualitative content analysis shows that, when questioning their own accents, the informants either refer to BrE or to 'non-accent' or neutral accent. The attitudes of the community towards BrE are positive and mostly related to the participants' willingness to acquire its accent:

(148) Like, instead of learning the Indian (pause) accent I would, I would prefer, like, British accent, to follow the British accent, yeah. (RNmKa) int.

(149) I mean, I would love to be, love to learn the accent, the British accent. I mean, [...] I find very fascinating the way they speak and the way they sound and the way they eat words and all, ya. (AVmDe) int.

(150) I don't know I just like the British accent so (laughs) maybe I will probably learn how to speak in the British accent so that's just my personal preference. (NKsfTN) int.

(151) If I could completely change the way I talk, I would prefer the British accent (smiles) because I'm so fascinated by it [...]. (SSfWB) int.

(152) JGMfKe: [...] I love British accents so I, I, something I personally want to do is I would like to do some Erasmus to English speaking countries so that I can really have this _ I really like this British accent.
GR: What do you like about it?
JGMfKe: It's so beautiful, it's, like, that's the _ I feel, like, that's it's the original way, version of English, so (pauses) I think that's what everyone want [...]. int.

What emerges from these examples is that, on the whole, speakers are 'fascinated' by the BrE accent. Whether they want to replace their way of speaking with another ("If I could completely change the way I talk, I would prefer the British accent") or they would like to add a new phonology ("Like, instead of learning the Indian (pause) accent I would, I would prefer, like, British accent"), the informants are reflecting Shuck's (2004) 'ideology of nativeness' in their construction of the category of native speaker of English as contiguous with British. JGMfKe, in particular, points to the beauty of the BrE accent and directly relates it to the "original [...] version of English" she aspires to get. She continues by noting that "I think that's what everyone want[s]". The unasserted beliefs which underlie the above-mentioned statements reflect the global 'liabilities' and pejorative links associated with IndE. Here, a direct ideological link exists between 'non-native English speakers' as contiguous with 'foreigners' – what the speakers in the examples above consider themselves to be – 'non-standard' speech and (un)intelligibility. If knowing English in India is like possessing the fabled Aladdin's lamp (Kachru [1986] 1990), acquiring the BrE accent (and sometimes the AmE one) equals having a high social status. The following examples contribute to a more comprehensive account of the topic:

(153) Sometimes in India it is also matter of prestige and status if you speak very, I mean, if you are speaking UK accent, then people see you as (pauses) you know, have a good status (pauses). If you are not able to match the UK status or US status, then you are usually _ there are stereotypes which usually consider you to be a middle-class, you know, thing. (PPmKa) int.

(154) The, the strict, like, the formal English or the, the proper English or the Queen's English or the accents within English itself. Like I said, I, I don't like American English as much as British English because that's what we were taught, so that sort of go, gets into your head as well, that certain Englishes are better than the other Englishes [...]. (SDfKa) int.

(155) Because I think (pauses) English is a language when you speak you felt, feel very proud or privileged, so that's why they (pauses) they make it

_ to make it sound more good they build up this kind of accent [BrE]. (PGfMa) int.

The presuppositions behind such folk comment have much to do with the concept of 'governmentality' as proposed by Foucault (1991). He explains how language practices in school regulate the ways in which language is used and establish language hierarchies in which some languages are more valued than others. As a matter of fact, SDfKa is overtly pointing at "what we were taught" in schools and acknowledges that "that sort of [...] gets into your head as well, that certain Englishes are better than the other Englishes". Such hegemonic practices ensure that people acquiesce to invisible cultural power and inevitably consider BrE the only possible norm to follow. However, discourse positioning itself as a counterargument to such hegemonic practices exists concurrently. The example below sheds light on how TDfMa – a female Maharashtrian student who has been living in Heidelberg for less than a year – after living in the UK for some time and being "very mesmerised by the British accent", tried to acquire some of its pronunciations but later decided to abandon them "because that's not how I have been born and brought up":

(156) TDfMa: Yes, as I, I think I've mentioned in the survey as well, when I was younger and I was in the UK I was very mesmerised by the British accent, and I tried to speak _ I tried to, you know, pronounce the way they would (pauses) pronounce things, and that in a way resulted in me having an accent and when, consciously or unconsciously I realised that I had an accent, I had to stop myself from, you know, (pauses) using it or talking the way they were talking because that's not how I have been born and brought up. So, when I went back to India, I could see that there was a difference, and I had to work hard to bring it back to normal stage. Even sometimes when I have to talk to people who don't understand my accent, I have to maybe stress on certain words, or I might (pauses) I might just modulate the way I'm saying a word, yeah [...].
GR: And, what about your attitude towards it now?
TDfMa: Oh, no, now I frown upon it, I, I, I might make fun of it, when people try and imbibe a certain kind of accent [...]. int.

(156) defines the attitudes of the majority of the community members: while they acknowledge the intrinsic standardness of BrE, they nevertheless value their own local IndE accents and do not consider them as inferior in any way. On the contrary, they help them define their ethnicity and their identities and changing them would mean to eradicate their Indian and regional distinctiveness (cf. Section 5.2.1.2).

The corollary of standard language is non-accent. In conjunction with the monoglot standard ideology (Silverstein 1996) and the 'ideology of nativeness' (Shuck 2004), non-accentedness or neutral accentedness reflects the folk's idea that "if we try hard enough, we can acquire a perfect language, one which is clean, pure, free of variation" (Lippi-Green 1997:45). Thus, language which is not perfect does not have to be accepted. The community members who have this sociolinguistic abstraction in mind constitute 20 % of the total sample. This rather small group is structured as follows: 50 % are women, 67 % come from Southern India and another 67 % are constituted by newcomers. While these percentages come as no surprise, it is interesting to note that according to these informants, it is possible to substitute their phonology (their accents) for another, hence to neutralise their accents "*consistently and in a permanent way*" (Lippi Green 1997:45; emphasis in the original). The examples below show interesting metalanguage insight on the topic:

(157) I am (laughs) I am somebody who thinks that we should all approach or improve towards a neutral accent at some point of time, so. I would be (pauses) I'm okay with anybody who speaks in any accents as long as I can understand, but personally I think that, that everybody should try to get to a neutral state if not British, I thought impossible but neutral state or tend to a neutral state would be (pauses) more good. (ARmKe) int.

(158) (pauses) Okay, there is one actual accent that everyone should follow, but unfortunately, they don't, because of the influence from mother tongues. I think one, one has to stick to this neutral accent, what it, how it has to be, so we should definitely try to come out of this influence of the mother tongues and trying to speak one neutral accent, one unique accent. That's close to the native accents (laughs). (VSmTN) int.

(159) NPfMP: I mean I believe that you should have a neutral accent, okay, so not the British.
GR: Why?
NPfMP: Again, so, I won't say British accent is good, American accent is good. I would say, a person should have a neutral accent because it's, it's more (pauses) because it's more (pauses) clear in that way to the people around you [...]. int.

What emerges from these examples is that there seems to be agreement on what non-accent (or neutral accent) is. On the whole, it is a "unique accent [t]hat [i]s close to the native accents", but not quite. Ideally, this "neutral state" allows for more clarity and is understood globally since it does not index any social or ethnic identity. Moreover, it should be something towards which everyone should lean, hence it should be valued as positively as BrE, possibly better ("I think that, that everybody should try to get to a neutral state if not British, I thought impossible but neutral state or tend to a neutral state would be (pauses) more good"). Finally, after its acquisition, one should use it "*consistently and in a permanent way*" (Lippi Green 1997:45; emphasis in the original), thus, one should not downgrade to local speech norms ("I think one [...] has to stick to this neutral accent, [...] how it has to be, so we should definitely try to come out of this influence of the mother tongues"). The example below shows VSmTN's metalanguage response to neutral accentedness:

(160) VSmTN: (pauses) I personally have a neutral accent, I believe (pauses) I would not stick to British accent or I could not, like, stick to American accent, but I wanted to always have a neutral one. If I have to change something in me, in my accent (pauses) there are few words I might still sound Indian or the typical Indian accent might be few words.
GR: So, you would like to get rid of your Indian accent _
VSmTN: Yeah. It's not about I want to get rid of the Indian accent and become a proper British accent speaker or an American accent speaker, but I wanted to be, to always stay in a neutral one where people cannot identify me, a Britishers or an American or (pauses) Indian. int.

VSmTN is eager to note how not everyone wants to be put on the map, so to say, and, at times, it may feel compelling to move away from one's own background when speaking. Neutral accentedness, in his opinion, may help avoid the 'indexical' problem and position the speaker in a "neutral state" which irremediably brings neutral attitudes towards the speakers themselves. This prompts the following consideration: "[i]f a person is very dedicated, works hard, and has good guidance, it may be possible to fool some of the people some of the time. The question is, *of whom do we require this trick, and why?*" (Lippi-Green 1997:51; emphasis in the original).

The examples above emphasise how, for some community members, changing their way of talking is tantamount to acquiring a BrE accent or a neutral one. However, the majority of the informants argue that they will never change their accent. While some would correct their pronunciation and/or grammar, some others would work on their fluency or on the acquisition of new words:

(161) Yeah because I sometime, I, like, I have this slippery tongue to I didn't pro _ some the words that I can't pronounce so well, so then there are people who tried to improve, like, correct me. So, I'm happy about it, that they are making me better. (PGfMa) int.

(162) Yeah. I've always tried to improve my (pauses) grammar _ I think it's not that good and (pauses) I'm pretty happy with my accent. (MGofUt) int.
(163) Let's say, I would like to involve a lot more words in my vocabulary and this helps me be concise with my emotions. So, I, I lack a lot of emotional words. I use repetitively 'very': 'I was very happy, very good, very whatever' and for this I think it requires some efforts or reading a lot of novels and I can maybe, if I have time then I will do it. (ASmMP) int.
(164) Yes, I mean (pauses) sometimes I think I'll miss my fluency in English, that I need to practice well and, yeah, if I practice that good, then everything will be fine. (DVfAP) int.

The present section has been dedicated to an exiguous number of community members who generally have negative affective attitudes towards their local IndE speech and seem to reflect hegemonic language practices in the form of the monoglot standard ideology (Silverstein 1996), the 'ideology of nativeness' (Shuck 2004) and non-accentedness or neutral-accentedness (Lippi-Green 1997). Although such ideologies do not 'tell the story' of the entire community, they are still part of it. In addressing issues of 'standard' and 'nonstandard' speech, native English speakers and non-native English speakers, such perspectives may help understand the community's internal sociolinguistic conceptualisation of 'us' versus 'them' which seems to dominate the North versus South linguistic discourse (cf. Section 5.2.1.1). In light of these considerations, such ideologies may help interpret the quality of network affiliations and distance as well as transnational ties within the Indian student community.

5.2.2.3 Network Affiliations and Transnational Ties

Section 5.1.1.4 emphasises the importance of a network approach for the present case study since it provides a set of procedures which enable a study of a small community where speakers cannot be discriminated in terms of any kind of social class index. The network-strength scale reported above indicates that network relations are dense and multiplex (cf. Tab. 5.1.5). Considering that one of the main consequences of extreme density is homogeneity of norms and values (Milroy 1980), it comes as no surprise that the community members generally hold similar attitudes with respect to IndE accent variation (cf. Section 5.1.3.1). Besides, the density and the multiplexity of the network support the speakers' first languages resisting institutional pressures to language shift. Unlike in stable communities, network ties very seldom weaken in transient multilingual ones. In such contexts, minority languages usually resist institutional pressures to language shift because the close-knit, dense and multiplex affiliations are supported by its transiency. As a matter of fact, these relatively short-lived contexts promote language maintenance practices – manifest in the stable and continuous use of the speakers' L1s – which, in turn, structure internal network subgroups based on ethnicity (cf. Section 5.2.1.2).

In light of these findings, the present section aims to emphasise how the network constructs itself, especially around the Heidelberg Indian student association (HISA). Module III of the interview task, 'Heidelberg and Networking' has been designed to elicit the informants' attitudes towards other community members and HISA as well as to monitor their transnational activities. Specifically, the following questions have been asked:

- *Do you know many Indians residing in Heidelberg? (int. III.4)*
- *Why, do you think, Indians come to Heidelberg? (int. III.5)*
- *Did you make friends with some of them here? (int. III.6)*
- *Are there some that you see almost every day? (Get ethnicity, age, first language) (int. III.7)*
- *Where do you guys hang out around here? (int. III.8)*
- *What do you usually do together? (int. III.9)*
- *Do you know HISA? Do you usually go to its cultural events? What do you think of it? (int. III.10)*
- *What are your plans for the future? Are you planning to go back to India at some point in your life? (int. III.11)*

While the answers provided in questions int. III.4, int. III.6 – int III.10 have been used to devise the network-strength scale (cf. Tab. 5.1.5 in Section 5.1.1.4), and hence, will not be directly investigated here (with the only exception of int. III.10), int. III.5 seeks to verify how respondents define the importance of having an Indian community in Heidelberg. Int. III.6 – int. III.9 aim to determine the informants' in-group affiliations and distance, while int. III.10 has been designed to elicit their commitment to the only Indian association in Heidelberg. Finally, int. III.11 aims to shed some light on the informants' transnational activities and their transient condition.

The qualitative content analysis shows that participants generally consider the Indian student migration to Heidelberg as a mass phenomenon resulting from the excellent education and research opportunities that the university town provides (cf. Section 3.2.1):

(165) To Heidelberg? I (pauses), I don't know (pauses) Because it's, it, it offers, like, wide ranges of opportunities, I think, compared to where I lived before. For example, when I was in Düsseldorf, I didn't see any Indians at

all at the University. And here, it's comparatively really a lot. So, I would say this has more (pauses) it's famous, for one thing, and second thing is, for example, maybe it has programmes that have been in English for so long that people know about the place. That matters a lot, I think. (AHfKA) int.

(166) I think for better (pauses) job perspectives and also like here the education is one of the best in the world and also not that expensive and to (pauses) have an education over others in India, people choose to come here. Although they have to, you know, adapt to other culture, another country, and learn the language. But yeah, Indians, in this case, Indians are very versatile. (AVmDe) int.

(167) (pauses) Of course the name, Heidelberg University itself, better education, of course free, better, and good exposure for competing and master from a foreign country especially, like, in Germany, UK or US and if you're going back to India, you will get a better job. (SSmKe) int.

These examples inform on the highly competitive and international university environment Heidelberg offers. Moreover, in comparing Heidelberg to Düsseldorf, AHfKa notes that she "didn't see any Indians at all at the University" there, and, most probably, because Heidelberg "has programmes that have been in English for so long that people know about [it]". The Heidelberg university environment has allowed many community members to make friends with their peers. As a matter of fact, the implicational ordering of the network-strength scale emphasises how the attendance of the same faculty with at least two more Indian students is the prime condition to be satisfied. In other words, their relationships with other university colleagues are the most significant network criteria. It is from the laboratories and the university classes that the network constructs itself. The following examples shed new light on the topic:

(168) [...] from my Institute, yeah, because my supervisor has two students, and both of us are Indians, so, (pauses) from my Institute I know at least around five, six people who are Indians. (ASfKe) int.

(169) So, most of them are also doing their Ph.D. because it's the easiest to meet those people because they are also in the University and sometimes you just meet them in some courses or something and they are like, in the age group between, I would say, 25 to 32, 33, like, the same age group kind of. Yeah, most, like, some are post-docs now because they finished their Ph.Ds. and now, they are post-docs, and they are, some of them are from North, some from West, some from South, so, yeah (pauses) and

also from East, actually. I have a friend, so it's from everywhere (laughs). (DTfUt) int.

(170) (pauses) With my Indian friends I, I go to class with'em (laughs), either we cook together, we make some nice spicy Indian food, yeah, and we go to the, we go shopping together, go to the city centre, go to the Neckar river (pauses) and drink beers (laughs) and go party in the night, yeah [...]. (OFmTN) int.

What emerges from these descriptions is that the informants tend to first make friends with other Indian students at the university because "it's the easiest" way and then strengthen the quality of their network bonds by spending their free time with them either cooking Indian food, partying or shopping. In doing so, not only do their network bonds become stronger, but they also become multiplex. The success of the friend-of-a-friend approach used to find and interview informants on voluntary basis confirms and suggests that the individual network positions of the respondents and their overall network flows are sufficiently dense and multiplex. As a matter of fact, the participants rather frequently refer to some other Indian friends they know I interviewed previously during interview sessions.

After their proximity to more than five Indians students and their willingness to spend their free time with other Indian friends, the last criterion which the participants deem important for the network structure of their community is their regular participation in Indian associations in Germany and, particularly, in HISA. The qualitative content analysis shows that almost every community member knows of the association. While only 38 % of the informants regularly participate in their events and start-up competitions (cf. Tab. 5.1.5), more than 85 % of the sample look forward to taking part in future events. The examples below show some of the informants' most strongly positive attitudes towards HISA:

(171) It's really _ it's great actually that we have such a (pauses) such an organisation. I (pauses) I don't know how this is going to reach them, like, I really want more students to come forward and join this organisation and (pauses) because it really helps you connect _ stay connected to your culture, I mean, it's difficult for a person coming for a short term after staying for so long in a specific environment and culture _ practicing a specific culture to suddenly change (pauses) to a new culture and practice, so, you will take time and 'til then I think it's a great idea to stay connected with your roots. And also, I, I mean, also because you enjoy it and, so it's great that we have such an (pauses) organisation and yeah. If somehow

a message the students could be passed, that more people could _ more students should come forward and (pauses) get in this organisation. It would be great (laughs). (TKfMa) int.

(172) I think it's nice that we, we, we have the freedom to form such groups and (pauses) pass, I mean (pauses) to exchange our cultures within our community also with other people outside of the community, but I think although it's good that we have this community, they should be more open to having non-Indians also be part of it if they want to be part of it and not be, like, 'okay, this is a closed community, we don't want others around us'. I don't think HISA is that way, they're pretty multicultural, so I think it's cool (laughs). (VJRfKa) int.

(173) Ah, it's great because (pauses) I think there're a lot of things which, through HISA, they keep a lot of events and everything due to which a lot of people from, you get to know a lot of other Indians and plus to these events you can get a lot of people from other countries to showcase your culture, in a way. Which you cannot do single-handedly. Suppose you want to play Holi, or there's something like that, then you, you can, you can't play alone Holi, you need a people, look out for people to enjoy more and (pauses) Diwali or something like that, so it's a great way of getting (pauses) people from your own country as well as so in the power of your community to the world, of how united you stand, and united you are (pauses). That way you can make a huge difference and use impact on the word. (MMfKa) int.[91]

Overall, these descriptions emphasise the strong impact that HISA has on the everyday lives of the community members since it "helps [...] stay connected

91 *Holi* is an ancient Hindu festival also known as the Indian 'festival of spring' or 'festival of colours'. It signifies the arrival of spring, the end of winter, and the blossoming of love. The festival also celebrates the beginning of a good spring harvest season. It lasts for a night and a day, starting on the evening of the *Purnima* (Full Moon day) falling in the 'Vikram Samvat' Calendar, in the Hindu calendar month of *Phalgun* which falls around middle of March in the Gregorian one. *Diwali*, *Deepavali* or *Dipavali* is also known as the 'festival of lights', during which temples, homes, and shops are brightly illuminated. It is celebrated by Hindus, Jains, Sikhs and some Buddhists and symbolises the spiritual victory of light over darkness, good over evil and knowledge over ignorance. Light is a metaphor for knowledge and consciousness. The rituals usually last five days and climax on the third day coinciding with the darkest night of the Hindu lunisolar month *Kartika*. In the Gregorian calendar, the festival generally falls between mid-October and mid-November. For a more detailed account cf. Sharma (2008).

to [the Indian] culture" by organising festivals and cultural events. Moreover, it provides valuable support on different topics through different social media and, in being "pretty multicultural", it allows everyone to join their events in order to bridge the gap between the local communities. Most importantly, it connects India to Germany through border-crossing connections.

Much sociolinguistic research has shed light on transnationalism as a valuable phenomenon allowing to rethink certain traditional notions of social structure (Sharma 2014). Some of its proponents have observed that

> [s]omething like a transnational public sphere has certainly rendered any strictly bounded sense of community or locality obsolete. At the same time, it has enabled the creation of forms of solidarity and identity that do not rest on an appropriation of space where contiguity and face-to-face contact are paramount (Gupta/Ferguson 1992:9).

However, this 'dismantling' of community does not seem to apply to multilingual speech communities and, particularly, to the transient Heidelberg Indian student community. 90 % of the community members plan to return to India and settle down, thus, they try to keep their long-distance and border crossing connections during their temporary stay in Heidelberg. The remaining 10 % seem to be undecided. However, the qualitative content analysis shows that the majority of the participants have come to Germany in the first place in order to get an education which will allow for better work opportunities back home:

(174) I mean, eventually I do wanna go back, I don't _ lots of people wanna come here, settle down or I don't know, I mean. Even when I miss home, like here people, people miss people, I miss Delhi, I would definitely attach to Delhi and settle, the culture, the language, the food, everything. For me Delhi is something else, so yeah, Delhi for me is another person that I miss in some ways, so yeah. (ABmDe) int.

(175) Actually, I would like to explore the world a little bit more. I, I don't mind travelling to other places in Europe or even go all the way across the world, to New Zealand, maybe, to work, but eventually I do wanna go back to India because I want to teach not really in the big cities or so, but more in the rural India because I think that's where the help is really needed, so in the long run that's my plan. (VJRfKa) int.

(176) Yeah, like, not in the short term but like in long term if I consider, maybe after around 5 to 10 years I have plans to go back to India and get things done there, because yeah obviously my family is leaving there and it's always that in emergency situations if I want to go from different country it's very hard to travel [...]. (PVfKa) int.

What emerges from these three examples is that, on the whole, the community is resolved on first getting an internship and a post in Germany for 5 to 10 years and then on returning to India financially independent, economically stable and with a well-paid and secured position. However, discourse concerning indecision is also present:

(177) I haven't really decided on th _ that's a good question. I haven't really given enough thought to that, but yeah, sure, it's, it crosses my mind. I have nothing for or against going back to India, so I'm more than happy to go back to my own country with my _ the people I mean, I've grown up with. But sure, I mean, for me priority one is opportunities which is my field is quite limited back home, so yeah. I mean, let's see wherever my passion and the field drives me. (SSmMa) int.

(178) I don't think in the near future I'm going back to India. Probably, if I ever want to, maybe it's after ten years or so. First, I would like to get some job where, which challenges my abilities and then at the same time it's interest _ easy enough that I'm not completely stressed out and after gaining sufficient experience I can go back to India on a job profile which suits my abilities. (ASmMP) int.

(177) and (178) reflect an inherent desire of the participants to return home ("so I'm more than happy to go back to my own country with my _ the people I mean, I've grown up with"). At the same time, however, their future job position may hinder their plans ("for me priority one is opportunities which is my field is quite limited back home"; "after gaining sufficient experience I can go back to India on a job profile which suits my abilities").

The qualitative content analysis reveals that whether they plan to settle down in India or somewhere else, the informants are well aware of their temporary migration condition. Most importantly, sustained contact with other community members shows that questions of kinship and in-group allegiances seem to exceed North/South linguistic power imbalances in light of the transient aspect of the community. Their cultural affiliations tend to overrule linguistic and ideological matters and to result in dense and multiplex network bonds. These ties appear to be fundamental for these speakers since questions of in-group affiliations play a major role in the shaping and the performance of their identities, which are at times ethnic, at times pan-Indian.

6 Summary and Conclusion

The main aims of the present study have been: (i) to investigate how the members of the Heidelberg Indian student speech community perceive different IndE accents; (ii) to analyse whether differences in L2 phonological characteristics index local and situated ethnic identities; (iii) to shed light on the way in which different IndE accents affect the language consciousness, attitudes and behaviour of the participants.

IndE is among the most longstanding varieties of New Englishes and is characterised by having its own phonological, grammatical, lexical and discourse features which are, overall, mutually intelligible between IndE speakers (Sailaja 2012; Kachru 1983). English is an associate official language in India. In the literature, it is referred to as a complex (Schneider 2007), indigenised (Kachru [1986] 1990, 1983) and transplanted (Wiltshire/Harnsberger 2006) variety owing to the influence of the indigenous languages spoken in the subcontinent, the development of its own phonological system and its use as a *lingua franca* both within and outside the subcontinent.

The context under investigation is very interesting with respect to the community focus of the present work. Traditionally, Heidelberg is a non-anglophone setting, hence English does not hold any official status. However, the prestigious university environment and its correlated degree of internationalisation allows for the language to be the second *lingua franca* of the town. This rather favourable situation contributes to the development of an overt consciousness of English accent variation among the community members. English stochastically dominates German, Hindi and the speakers' mother tongues in their everyday interactions in different domains, i.e., it is the language spoken most frequently within and outside the community.

Yet, the main key features that distinguish diasporas from individual migrants are (i) the members' ability to create groupness and (ii) their awareness of their origins and roots. With respect to (i), in order to investigate the effects of interpersonal relationships on language variation and language perception, a network strength scale has assessed the participants' network characteristics with reference to those different relationships within their community which emerged during the fieldwork as significant to them according to four main criteria: (i) same faculty as at least two more Indian students; (ii) proximity to more than five Indian students; (iii) free time spent with other Indian students; and (iv) regular participation in Indian associations in Germany, particularly in HISA. The

Guttman Coefficient of Reproducibility and the Rasch Scalability Coefficient revealed that network density and multiplexity are statistically significant. The comparison of the sociometric status of the community members with their integration indices shows a significant correspondence for the highly integrated members since they top the scale for integration just as they do for status. In other words, while highly integrated members constitute the ego of the first order network zone, unintegrated ones occupy the more peripheral area of the network. Interestingly, the content of the links emphasises that the members integrated most constitute the linguistically influential peer group of the community.

The second main feature that contributes to the differentiation of diasporas from individual migrants is their awareness of their origins. While this is usually heightened by transnational activities and retained in memories, food and other artefacts of the community's cultural life, it is also generally mirrored in specific attitudes towards observed linguistic practice. Hierarchical/agglomerative cluster analysis has shown a strong correlation between the respondents' high level of identity and language consciousness as well as their overt attitudes towards accent and belonging as well as indexicality. To gain insight into what the anthropologist Steven Vertovеč (1999) defines as 'diaspora consciousness' and into the identity development of the community members, the clustering procedure accounts for the pivotal role that the respondents' mother tongues play in their everyday lives in Heidelberg. The reported results indicate that sociolinguistic practices (such as language transmission) and social relationships (such as in-group network ties and affiliations) affect the process of language maintenance and shift in the transient student community.

The pilot study conducted in 2016 argues that the community members have a commonly held folk belief that Southern Indians speak English with a distinctive accent. Their English has often been termed 'funny', 'stereotypical' and 'highly influenced by their L1s', in contrast to the English of Northerners, which has commonly been described as 'smoother' and 'thick' (Regnoli 2016). What has emerged from the pre-investigation is that the speakers' perceptions of accent variation seem to concern a North to South distinction rather than a state-to-state one. In order to test this folk belief, the participants' evaluations of four Northern and four Southern stimuli have been tested with the help of Likert-scale ratings of reliability, readiness-for-action, intellectuality and amiability traits. Mann Whitney has revealed statistically significant differences in the extralinguistic variables selected between the subgroups and has indicated fine-grained differences in the ratings of Northern and Southern IndE accents, with the Northern IndE guises getting better ratings than the Southern ones. The cluster analysis of the data supports these findings. The reported results show that the respondents' norm-orientation is unidimensional since Northern varieties serve as a superordinate norm in the migrant community. As expected from the pilot study, the lack of significance in the reactions of the Northern and the Southern participants is somewhat disappointing since it indexes the linguistic power of the majority, i.e., the Northern Indians, whose views have gradually been accepted and copied by the minorities, i.e., the Southern part of the community. The Northern Indian participants have stereotypical views about themselves and the South. However, the Southern participants do not openly compensate the perceived lack of their intellectual qualities by judging themselves more polite, friendly, etc. Interestingly, Wilcoxon signed-rank and Bonferroni show that the accent perceptions of both the Northern sample and the Southern one are aligned with the ethnicity of the guises and reach significance for most attitude scales.

A further step in the data analysis has been to associate the covert attitudes of the participants with the alleged origin of the stimuli in order to elicit their metalinguistic awareness in second language acquisition. The reported results show that the Northern IndE accents are detected more easily than the Southern ones. These perceived differences, in addition to supporting earlier results, indicate that the speakers differentiate the guises on a binary level (North vs. South) rather than on a state-to-state one. The implicational analysis of the data supports this finding. Moreover, the results shed light on a higher awareness of perception with respect to Southern IndE accents. Although their location has only been partly recognised or, at times, not recognised at all, the Southern stimuli have been identified easily according to precise phonetic realisations which seemingly index specific accents of Southern IndE. The extralinguistic variables *gender*, *ethnicity* and *time spent in Heidelberg* reveal interesting insights as well. While the male students have been more accurate in discriminating the guises, a division surfaces among the two subgroups: the male speakers recognise the Southern stimuli better and the female ones do so with the Northern ones. Their recognition of Northern guises over Southern ones sheds light on their already ascertained higher awareness of perception and production of prestige norms, thus supporting earlier research on the topic and earlier claims according to which Northern IndE varieties serve as the superordinate norms in the student community. With respect to *ethnicity*, the results suggest that the participants from either the same state of the guises or their same ethnic locations are more accurate in accent discrimination, i.e., the Northern informants recognise the Norther guises better and the Southern participants do so with the Southern ones. *Time spent in Heidelberg* reveals that the newcomers are better at recognising the guises whereas those who have been living in Heidelberg longer have a tendency to mark Northern vs. Southern differences more strongly.

Correlation analysis has aimed to establish if there are possible connections between how the participants react towards accent variation and whether this is due to their gender, ethnicity, length of stay in Heidelberg or their network in-group affiliations. Spearman-Rho rank and Pearson's product-moment coefficient's correlation reveal that the correlations between *time spent in Heidelberg*, network density and accent recognition are statistically significant. While the association between time spent in Heidelberg and accent recognition is weak negative, i.e., the less time the participants have been spending in Heidelberg, the better they are at recognising the guises, the one between network density and accent recognition is weak positive, i.e., the more integrated participants are better at recognising the guises.

As to the parameters the participants rely on in accent identification, a close look at the Bonferroni-corrected results shows that (i) some informants have higher standards than others with respect to accent variation, and (ii) some find the differences between the Northern and the Southern stimuli more striking than others. To do so, the Likert-scale values have been arranged according to similarities and differences. The results substantiate earlier claims according to which the female sample has higher standards than the male one. The latter, however, appears more unified in its ratings, i.e., the male participants handle the Likert scales rather similarly. Again, this finding concurs with earlier ones, characterising men as stylistically less flexible than women and with a tendency to develop narrower linguistic repertoires. With regard to *ethnicity*, the Northern participants have more unified views about IndE accents. The ratings of the Southern ones shed light on the degree to which they perceive the Northern/Southern accent differences, which appear as massively demarcated and leaning towards the preference for Northern IndE accents. In consequence, the Southern informants exhibit stronger language attitudes towards accent variation, especially with respect to the readiness-for-action trait <accent improvement>. These findings support the Bonferroni statistical analyses discussed above. *Time spent in Heidelberg* sheds light on the newcomers constituting the more homogeneous sample. However, a closer examination of the data reveals that the longer the Northern informants have been living in Heidelberg (and, hypothetically, have met other Indian ethnicities), the more the differences increase. This is most probably due to their assimilation into the German/international environment of Heidelberg. This finding is in line with earlier claims that the Northern participants have stereotypical views about themselves and the South and seems to confirm and strengthen the stereotype. On the other hand, the longer the

Southerners have been living in Heidelberg and have had contacts with Northern speakers, the lesser the stereotypes and the more liberated from their former prejudices they get. In other words, while Northern stereotypes increase with time spent in Heidelberg, Southern ones decrease.

Arranging the Likert scale values of the Accent Identification Task according to their similarities and differences has allowed for a deeper understanding of the structure of the community and has revealed some 'anomalous' individuals within the Northern sample: SSmMa, a male speaker from Haryana, and BSmGu, a male speaker from Gujarat. Following earlier description of such cases, it has been possible to group these individuals in two broad categories: 'oddballs', i.e., the subgroup whose attitudes mark them as non-conformists both linguistically and socially, and 'insiders', i.e., the subgroup that appears to be marked by extreme conformity. SSmMa falls into the oddball category of an 'interloper', i.e., someone who has moved from one dialect area to another and whose abilities to master the new dialect depend partly upon his age. His sociolinguistic position in the community as an integrated member justifies this categorisation and, although he favours Southern IndE accents in all attitude traits, he defines himself as "negatively biased" towards them. On the other hand, BSmGu is an insider. His ratings from all attitude traits are fairly typical, yet significantly in favour of the Northern IndE guises. Although he is highly integrated in the student network, he is not among the members acknowledged most. His reactions towards ethnicity-clusterd stimuli justify this categorisation since his elusiveness appears to arise from his very normalcy.

In order to shed light on the social stereotypes and overt attitudes of the participants towards accent variation in India, the 'draw-a-map' task has been used. The results were presented and discussed in two subsections. The first one deals with the *perception* of accent variation, i.e., the elicitation of the speakers' overt stigmatisation and stereotypes of IndE accents. The second one considers its *production*, i.e., the correlation between covert attitudes and accent variation. With respect to the first one, a computer-determined mental map reveals seven macro-areas in which English is spoken differently: (i) Northernmost IndE; (ii) Delhi IndE; (iii) Northern IndE; (iv) North-western IndE; (v) North-eastern IndE; (vi) Central IndE; and (vii) Southern IndE. The adjectives that the participants provide to describe each area suggest that their perceptions of IndE accents and dialects are descriptors of (i) the social status of the people who speak them, e.g., 'educated', 'multicultural, 'posh'; (ii) their alleged personal qualities, e.g., 'lazy'; (iii) their ethnicities, e.g., 'Chinese', and (iv) their religious affiliations, e.g., 'Muslim'. The composite map shows seven transitional speech areas approximating the dialect or informal end of the continuum as low-prestige IndE and those closer to the national 'standard' or formal end as high-prestige IndE. Overall, Northernmost IndE, Northern IndE and North-eastern IndE are connotated negatively, while the dialect areas of Delhi English, North-western IndE, Central IndE and some parts of Southern IndE are seen positively. This happens because these varieties have been associated with different levels of prestige depending on their status in society. In consequence, this degree of prestige is invariably passed onto and associated with the speaker. The seemingly contradictory perception of Southern IndE accents as carrying both positive and negative connotations is due to a clear-cut difference that the respondents make between heavily accented speech and syntactic (in)accuracy. While this has been investigated elsewhere (Regnoli 2019b), it is important to mention that, although Southern IndE accents are often perceived as 'sharp' and 'rough', the general trend is to attribute to Southern Indians a higher competence in, and command of, English than to their Northern counterparts, either with reference to the higher literacy rate of major Southern states or to the status of the language as the *lingua franca* of the different Dravidian languages of the speech area.

The discussion of the assignment of the guises to the site they are perceived to belong on the blank map points to a general conclusion common to all the guises selected as well as the participants. However transitional the IndE landscape appear to be, there are folk conceptions such as 'Northern IndE', 'Southern IndE' etc. which cannot remain unnoticed, whatever reservations dialectologists might have about boundaries. Though this conclusion can potentially be extended to all the IndE accents selected for the present study, there are some which are less identifiable than others. The analysis of the results from the Likert-scales has suggested that Southern IndE accents are the least recognised ones. The cognitive map task substantiates these findings and adds a new perspective to the topic: the higher the recognition, the less fuzzy the boundaries. In other words, the informants harbour more precise ideas about dialect boundaries when the guise is from Northern India. The present findings justify the folk belief of the community, i.e., that Southern Indians have a distinctive accent when speaking English, to the extent that social stereotypes play a fundamental role in accent recognition.

The topics for the qualitative part have been prepared and analysed by applying a revised form of the qualitative content analysis developed by Mayring (2014). The qualitative data analysis software MAXQDA was used in the organisation and the structuring of the data following a bottom-up approach. All the sub-codes detected cluster into two main topics: indexicality and metalinguistic awareness. The qualitative analysis of the data supports the results of the quantitative one and provides a more comprehensive account of the speakers' classifications of local speech and their assessments of IndE varieties. All the community members agree on the existence of different IndE accents and differentiate them on a North vs. South basis first, and then, depending on their degrees of interactions with different IndE speakers and exposures to different IndE accents, they operationalise differences on a more local/ethnic level.

The conversational data emphasise the major role that ethnicity plays for the community members mainly with respect to education and indexicality. The quantitative analysis has shown that the informants almost always attribute a Northern ethnicity to those Southern guises they perceive to be less educated by locating them in some of the poorest states of Northern India. The qualitative content one reveals that the North vs. South distinction is far more complex in terms of educational practices since many Southern states, e.g., Kerala and Karnataka, have the highest literacy rates. According to the majority of the informants, education does play a role in accent variation but its main trigger is ethnicity. By pointing to the undoubted multiculturalism of the South – which is due to the coexistence of many local languages and which subsequently results in people willing to send their children to English-medium schools, the community members implicitly equal English and higher education. This unasserted belief is implicit in what Shuck (2004) postulates as the 'ideology of nativeness', which constructs the categories of 'native English speaker' as contiguous with British or American, and 'non-native English speakers' as contiguous with foreigner.

Apart from education, a further sociolinguistic factor linked to ethnicity is indexicality. The qualitative content analysis has shown that all community members agree on a distinctive speech characteristing Southern IndE accents/varieties, which, in turn, index a particular 'folk object', i.e., Southern IndE speakers and their 'normal' language behaviour. Moreover, the folk shed new light on two other factors: (i) there are as many Southern IndE accents/varieties as there as Southern languages, and (ii) there is considerable variation even within one dialect/accent. Moreover, idiolects are to be taken into account as well. The fact that the informants are able to provide such sophisticated metalanguage detail substantiates earlier claims which emphasise their high level of awareness towards IndE varieties despite their gender, ethnicity and time spent in Heidelberg. The reported results suggest that phonology is the main linguistic category to be addressed with regard to language variation. According to the community members, the particular 'tone' and singsong accent characteristic of Southern IndE accents might be due to non-functional suprasegmental features including stress, intonation and word juncture, as well as segmental ones. Here, a curious division surfaces: while variation in intonation and rhythmic correlates is tolerated and, at times, acclaimed for its indexical force of distinctiveness and uniqueness, variation in segmental phonology does not seem to be accepted. It is often encoded into the doctrine of 'correctness' which shows that Northern IndE accents are perceived to be 'more' correct than Southern IndE ones. This result substantiates earlier claims.

With respect to the investigation of the affective, conative and identity-related attitudes of the community members, the qualitative content analysis has revealed that the respondents fall into two main groups: one in favour of having an accent and the other showing neutral or negative attitudes towards it. Overall, while more than 50 % of the sample hold positive attitudes towards having an accent and connect it with indexicality, a moderate portion of the community thinks that: (i) accents are something that only non-native speakers have and (ii) there are some domains in which – and some participants with whom – it is better to avoid having an accent. The reported results account for the perceived attitude of superiority of some Northern speakers towards their Southern counterparts and their overall negative evaluations with respect to accent variation. In other words, they shed light on the folk's perception of a seemingly superior group, i.e., the Northern ono, and an inferior one, embodied by the Southern community.

In order to go into the attitudes of the participants towards their own vernacular, integrative and dissociative attitudes have been investigated with respect to in-group identity. The Southern sample considers its accents 'pleasant', 'polite' and generally 'clear'. Unlike their Northern counterparts who perceive Southern IndE local speech as 'rough' and, at times, 'unintelligible', Southern Indians perceive their local speech as indexical of their cultures as well as their identities. The qualitative content analysis reveals that dissociative attitudes towards the Southerners' own vernacular are rare, adding up to 15 % of the speakers. When present, however, these attitudes resemble those held by the Northern community and are related to issues of unintelligibility and lack of correctness. Despite the massively disproportional distribution pattern, the dissociative attitudes of the Southern sample towards local speech seem to substantiate content-wise the findings discussed in the quantitative section, according to which the Southern informants have seemingly taken over the stereotypes of the Northerners about themselves.

With respect to the Northern community, 65 % of the sample hold associative attitudes towards their own vernacular and perceive their accents to be much clearer than Southern ones and more standard-like. Interestingly, both communities rely on the doctrine of correctness in the description of their local speech. Yet, while the Southern informants relate this to their fluency and higher educational rates, their Northern counterparts explicitly connect it to their accent. Discourse regarding dissociative attitudes towards local speech exists concurrently. Surprisingly, as compared to the Southern sample, a higher percentage of the Northern one (35 %) hold negative attitudes towards their own vernacular. This result substantiates the findings from the discussion according to which the Northern participants relate their standardness to their accent and not to their grammar.

On the whole, the results are consistent with the idea that ethnic communities hold positive integrative attitudes towards their own vernaculars. Their local speech not only indexes locally situated ethnic identities, but it is perceived as an individual identity-affirmation. The general feeling is that the Southern informants are prouder of their own languages and IndE varieties, which allow them to express their identities and cultures to the fullest. While this 'Southern pride' is pinpointed by some Northern informants as well, the latter do not seem to share the same enthusiasm with regard to their local speech.

The speakers' constant need of renegotiating the 'problem of ethnicity' (Jayaram 2004) is resolved in their willingness to shed their regional, linguistic and ethnic identities, sometimes in deference to their more general pan-Indian one. In this sense, "a person may be Bengali [or] Indian" (Friesen/Kearns 2008:225) depending on specific sociocultural and linguistic circumstances. While the community members generally adopt their ethnic identities and cling to their distinctiveness within their community of practice, they adopt their pan-Indian identity in their everyday lives (cf. Section 5.2.2.3).

The present study has provided the first detailed account of the language attitudes and ethnic identities of a transient community of Indian university students located in Heidelberg, Germany and has contributed to the research on the following areas of investigation: (i) Indian diasporic communities located in non-anglophone settings; (ii) transient multilingual speech communities and (iii) folk linguistics and perceptual dialectology. Through a series of questionnaires, accent identification tasks and semi-structured recorded interviews, the perceptions of several IndE migrant varieties have been investigated to provide and expand the understanding of IndE internal variation, neglected in earlier experimental research. The role of ELF in the Indian diaspora in Germany, language attitudes and ethnic identities from the perspective of folk linguistics, perceptual dialectology and network structure in transient multilingual communities have been among the aspects researched the least.

The mixed-method approach designed *ad hoc* to suit the needs of the present context has enabled the determination of accurate folk perceptions regarding

IndE accent variation on the basis of those sociolinguistic variables relevant for the community under investigation. Moreover, it has for the first time added a detailed description of the mapping of perceptual landscapes in IndE – a method which is almost always neglected in perceptual studies on New Englishes. The findings of the Accent Identification Task, substantiated by those of the implicational analysis, the correlation one and the cognitive map task, suggest that methodology triangulation is effective and produces valid, replicable and reliable results. The eight stimuli selected for mapping accent perceptions and attitudes to variation are responsible for the observed effects, i.e., that Northern IndEs have higher ratings than Southern ones, and refer to the consistency of the measurements.

The study has primarily extended the knowledge of the role of English in the Indian diaspora in Germany. Indian migration to Germany is momentous (Aksakal 2019; Burkhart *et al.* 2017), yet there is a considerable lack of research on Indian speech communities. Although small, the Heidelberg Indian student community is a fully established group whose fluidity in terms of linguistic norms entails a constant (re)negotiation of language choice and the social meaning associated with different ways of speaking. Their "ethnograph[ies] of speaking" (Hymes 1964) have been investigated through the theoretical framework of transient multilingual speech communities, i.e., social configurations in which people from diverse sociocultural and linguistic backgrounds come together for a limited period of time around specific shared activities (Mortensen/Fabricius 2014). The results show that the transient character of the community is a valuable sociolinguistic factor in the fostering of in-group affiliations and distance and that the constant need of the community members to renegotiate their identities is indexed in their willingness (or not) to shed their regional, linguistic and ethnic identities in deference to their pan-Indian ones depending on the fluid sociolinguistic circumstances of the community.

The present study has also provided the first perceptual map of India showing aggregated English dialect areas, thus contributing to language attitude research in New Englishes, which often fails to use mixed methods and the mapping of perceptual landscapes. The 'draw-a-map' task proved to be an effective method to elicit dialect consciousness and to ascertain whether accent variation has salience for the community. Moreover, it shed new light on the social stereotypes of the participants, emphasising their use of a similar cognitive template for area identifications despite their gender, ethnicity or time spent in Heidelberg.

More generally, the study has contributed to the research on folk linguistics and has provided further evidence that in the world outside linguistics, people who are not engaged in any study of language talk about it nevertheless and offer insightful comments on language variation and change which deserve careful consideration.

Despite the contribution this study makes to the field of IndE, the results indicate a number of possibilities for future research. One of the ongoing debates on IndE concerns its conceptualisation as the linguistic epicentre of English for South Asia (Gries/Bernaisch 2016; Hoffmann *et al.* 2011).[92] Although legitimate concerns over the status of English in India and the standardisation of such a variety have often been raised (Calabrese/Russo 2018; Dasgupta 1993; Krishnaswamy/Burde 1998), very little attention has been given to migrant pluricentrism. The results from the present study suggest that Southern IndE varieties are perceived as non-dominating varieties (NDVs) of (i) the nationally pluricentric variety of IndE and (ii) the internationally recognised pluricentric language of English. Moreover, Northern IndE varieties serve as a superordinate norm in the migrant community. Building on the present findings, more experimental research is needed to delineate the underpinnings of IndE migrant pluricentricity involving multiple IndE varieties.

The production experiments of the present study do not include an investigation of the phonological aspects of the IndE varieties selected for the Accent Identification Task. Conclusions about the perceptions of accent variation have been reached on the basis of folk metalanguage comments and only partially on segmental and suprasegmental linguistic analyses. Future finer phonological analyses will inform on the degree to which folk perceptions share a common ground with ascertained linguistic facts. In particular, research on intonational phonology, speech rhythm and other stress correlates (Cumming 2010; Fuchs 2016; He 2012) will shed new light on the folk belief of the community members and account for the acquisition of L1 transfer, ultimately contributing to the underresearched area of IndE acoustic phonology.

92 Gerhard Leitner (1992:225) defines as 'epicentres' those native varieties of English other than BrE and AmE that have also developed into norm-producing secondary centres with their own endo-normative standards, often serving as models for neighbouring Englishes. Australian English is one such example. Leitner suggests that besides L1 varieties, institutionalised L2 varieties of English such as IndE can develop into new epicentres as well. For a more comprehensive account of the developmental stages in the formation of English epicentres cf. Leitner (2010).

7 Bibliography

Abbuhl, R., S. Gass and A. Mackey. 2013. "Experimental research design". In R. J. Podesva and D. Sharma, eds, *Research Methods in Linguistics*. Cambridge: Cambridge University Press, 116–31.

Agheyisi, R. and J. Fishman. 1970. "Language attitude studies: A brief survey of methodological approaches". *Anthropological Linguistics* 12: 137–57.

Ajzen, I. 1988. *Attitudes, Personality and Behaviour*. Milton Keynes: Open University Press.

Aksakal, M. 2019. "International migration and place-based inequalities. The case of high-skilled migration and student mobility to eastern Germany". In S. I. Rajan, ed., *India Migration Report 2019. Diaspora in Europe*. New Delhi: Routledge, 1–15.

Alam, F. and J. Stuart-Smith. 2014. "Identity, ethnicity and fine phonetic detail. An acoustic phonetic analysis of syllable-initial /t/ in Glaswegian girls of Pakistani heritage". In M. Hundt and D. Sharma, eds, *English in the Indian Diaspora*. Amsterdam: Benjamins, 29–53.

Allen, H. and M. D. Linn. 1986. *Dialect and Language Variation*. Orlando, FL: Academic Press.

Allport, G. W. 1935. "Attitudes". In C. M. Murchison, ed., *A Handbook of Social Psychology*. Worcester, MA: Clark University Press, 789–844.

Anderwald, L. 2017. "World Englishes and Dialectology". In M. Filppula *et al.*, eds, *The Oxford Handbook of World Englishes*. Oxford: Oxford University Press, 252–71.

Angouri, J. 2010. "Quantitative, qualitative or both? Combining methods in linguistic research". In L. Litosseliti, ed., *Research Methods in Linguistics*. London: Falmer Press, 241–57.

Anisfeld, E. and W. E. Lambert. 1964. "Evaluational reactions of bilingual and monolingual children to spoken languages". *The Journal of Abnormal and Social Psychology* 69: 89–97.

Arvaniti, A. 2009. "Rhythm, timing and the timing of rhythm". *Phonetica* 66: 46–63.

Baayen, R. H. 2013. "Multivariate statistics". In R. J. Podesva and D. Sharma, eds, *Research Methods in Linguistics*. Cambridge: Cambridge University Press, 337–72.

Baker, C. 1992. *Attitudes and Language*. Clevedon: Multilingual Matters. BAMF = Bundesamt für Migration und Flüchtlinge. <https://www.bamf.de> (last accessed: 04/07/2019).

Bansal, R. K. 1978. *Introductions to English Language Teaching, Vol. 2. Phonetics and Spoken English*. Delhi: Oxford University Press.

Bansal, R. K. and J. B. Harrison. [1972] 1994. *Spoken English. A Manual of Speech and Phonetics*. London: Sangam.

Barz, R. K. and J. Siegel. 1988. *Language Transplanted: The Development of Overseas Hindi*. Wiesbaden: Harrassowitz.

Bayly, S. 2001. *Caste, Society and Politics in India from the Eighteen Century to the Modern Age*. Cambridge: Cambridge University Press.

Beine, M., A. Boucher, B. Burgoon, M. Crock, J. Gest, M. Hiscox and E. Thielemann. 2016. "Comparing immigration policies: An overview from the IMPALA database". *International Migration Review* 50: 827–63.

Beinhoff, B. 2013. *Perceiving Identity through Accent. Attitudes Towards Non-native Speakers and Their Accents in English*. Oxford: Peter Lang.

Bell, A. 2001. "Back in style: Reworking audience design". In P. Eckert and J. R. Rickford, eds, *Style and Sociolinguistic Variation*. New York: Cambridge University Press, 139–69.

Bernstein, B. 1971. *Class, Codes and Control, Vol. 1. Theoretical Studies towards a Sociology of Language*. London: Routledge.

Berruto, G. 2000. *Fondamenti di Sociolinguistica*. Roma-Bari: Laterza.

Bettoni, C. 2006. *Usare un'altra lingua. Guida alla pragmatica interculturale*. Roma-Bari: Laterza.

Bex, T. 1999. "Representations of English in twentieth-century Britain: Fowler, Gowers and Partridge". In T. Bex and R. J. Watts, eds, *Standard English. The Widening Debate*. London: Routledge, 89–109.

Bhardwaj, M. R. 1995. *Colloquial Punjabi*. London: Routledge.

Bhatia, S. 2007. *American Karma: Race, Culture and Identity in the Indian Diaspora*. New York, NY: New York University Press.

Bhatia, T. 1993. *Punjabi*. London: Routledge.

Bhatt, R. M. 2017. "World Englishes and language ideologies". In M. Filppula *et al.*, eds, 291–311.

Bloomfield, L. 1933. *Language*. New York: Holt.

Bloomfield, L. 1944. "Secondary and tertiary responses to language", *Language* 20:45–55 (reprinted in C. F. Hockett, ed., 1970, *A Leonard Bloomfield Anthology*. Bloomington and London: Indiana University Press, 413–25).

Blommaert, J. 2003. "Commentary: A sociolinguistics of globalization". *Journal of Sociolinguistics* 7: 607–23.

Blommaert, J. and D. Jie. 2010. *Ethnographic Fieldwork: A Beginner's Guide*. Clevedon: Multilingual Matters.

Boas, F. 1917. "Introduction". *International Journal of American Linguistics* 1: 1–18.

Boersma, P. 1998. *Functional Phonology. Formalizing the Interactions between Articulatory and Perceptual Drives*. The Hague: Holland Academic Graphics.

Boissevain, J. 1974. *Friends of Friends: Networks, Manipulators and Coalitions*. Oxford: Blackwell.

Boissevain, J. and J. C. Mitchell. eds. 1973. *Network Analysis: Studies in Human Interaction*. The Hague: Mouton.

Bourdieu, P. 1991. *Language and Symbolic Power*. Cambridge, MA: Harvard University Press.

Briggs, C. 1986. *Learning How to Ask: A Sociolinguistic Appraisal of the Role of the Interview in Social Science Research*. Cambridge: Cambridge University Press.

Bucholtz, M. 1999. "'Why be normal?': Language and identity practices in a community of nerd girls'. *Language in Society* 28: 203–23.

Bucholtz, M. and K. Hall. 2004. "Language and Identity". In A. Duranti, ed., *A Companion to Linguistic Anthropology*. Oxford: Blackwell, 369–94.

Buchstaller, I. and G. Khattab. 2013. "Population samples". In R. J. Podesva and D. Sharma, eds, 74–95.

Burkhart, S., N. Chehab-van den Assem, K. Essig, J. Grützmacher, U. Heublein, L. Jechel, S. Kammüller and J. Kercher. 2017. *Wissenschaft Weltoffen. Daten und Fakten zur Internationalität von Studium und Forschung in Deutchland*. Bielefeld: Wbv.

Burton, F. 1978. *The Politics of Legitimacy: Struggles in a Belfast Community*. London: Routledge.

Bussmann, H. 1996. *Routledge Dictionary of Language and* Linguistics, G. P. Trauth and K. Kazzazi, trans. and eds, London: Routledge.

Butsch, C. 2017. "The 'Indian diaspora' in Germany: Emerging networks and new homes". *Diaspora Studies* 1: 1–22.

Calabrese, R. and K. E. Russo. 2018. "A diachronic analysis of multiword constructions in Indian English and Australian Aboriginal English". In R. Muhr and B. Meisnitzer, eds, *Pluricentric Languages and Non-Dominant*

Varieties Worldwide: New Pluricentric Languages – Old Problems. Bern: Lang, 137–56.

Campbell-Kibler, K. 2010 "Sociolinguistics and perception". *Language and Linguistics Compass* 4: 377–89.

Carr, P. 1999. *English Phonetics and Phonology*. Oxford: Blackwell.

Carrie, E. and R. Drummond. 2016. *Posh, Artsy, Rough, Country and Working-class: Perceptions of Urban Language Varieties in Manchester*. Conference presentation. University of Murcia, 15/06.

Census of India. 2001. <www.censusindia.gov.in> (last accessed: 23/01/2019).

CGI = Consulate General of India, Munich. 2019. *Bilateral/Economic Relations, Bilateral Brief: Baden Württemberg-India*. <https ://cgimunich.gov.in/pdf/Bilateral_Brief_on_Baden_Wuerttemberg_Jfeb5_2019.pdf> (last accessed: 02/07/2019).

Chambers, J. K. 1995. *Sociolinguistic Theory. Linguistic Variation and its Social Significance*. Oxford: Blackwell (reprinted and revised in 2009).

Chambers, J. K. and P. Trudgill. 2004. *Dialectology*. Cambridge: Cambridge University Press.

Chand, V. 2009. "[v]at is going on? Local and global ideologies about Indian English". *Language in Society* 38: 393–419.

Chand, V. 2010. "Postvocalic (r) in urban Indian English". *English World-Wide* 31: 1–39.

Chanda, R. and D. Mukherjee. 2014. "Investment and skilled mobility linkages between Indian and the EU". In G. Tejada, U. Bhattacharya, B. Khadria and C. Kuptsch, eds, *Indian Skilled Migration and Development: To Europe and Back*. New Delhi: Springer, 47–70.

Chaudhary, S. C. 1989. *Some Aspects and Phonology of Indian English*. Ranchi: Jayaswal Press.

Cheshire, J. 1982. "Linguistic variation and social function". In S. Romaine, ed., *Sociolinguistic Variation in Speech Communities*. London: Edward Arnold, 153–66.

Cheshire, J., V. Edwards, and P. Whittle. 1989. "Urban British dialect grammar: The question of dialect levelling". *English World-Wide* 10: 185–225.

Chomsky, N. 1965. *Aspects of the Theory of Syntax*. Cambridge, MA: The MIT Press.

CIEFL = Central Institute of English and Foreign Languages. 1972. *The Sound System of Indian English Monograph 7*. Hyderabad: CIEFL.

CIM = Centrum für Internationale Migration und Entwicklung. <http://www.cimonline.de> (last accessed: 08/09/2020).

Clarke, S. 1987. "Dialect mixing and linguistic variation in a non-overtly stratified society". In K. M. Denning, S. Inkelas, F. McNair-Knox and J. R. Rickford, eds, *Variation in Language: NWAV-XV at Stanford*. Stanford, CA: Dept. of Linguistics, Stanford University, 74–85.

Cohen, A. [1985] 2001. *Symbolic Construction of Community*. London: Routledge.

Coupland, N. 1990. *English in Wales*. Clevedon: Multilingual Matters.

Coupland, N. and H. Bishop. 2007. "Ideologised values for British accents". *Journal of Sociolinguistics* 11: 74–93.

Coupland, N., A. Williams and P. Garrett. 1999. "'Welshness' and 'Englishness' as attitudinal dimensions of English language". In D. Preston, ed., *Handbook of Perceptual Dialectology, Vol. 1*. Amsterdam: Benjamins, 333–44.

Creswell, J. and V. Plano Clark. 2011. *Designing and Conducting Mixed Methods Research*. Thousand Oaks, CA: Sage.

Crystal, D. 1995. "Documenting rhythmical change". In J. Windsor Lewis, ed., *Studies in General and English Phonetics: Essays in Honour of Professor J. D. O'Connor*. London: Routledge, 174–9.

Crystal, D. 2003. *English as a Global Language*. Cambridge: Cambridge University Press.

Cumming, R. E. 2010. *The language-specific integration of pitch and duration*. Ph.D. dissertation. University of Cambridge.

D'Andrade, R. 1987. "A folk model of the mind". In D. Holland and N. Quinn, eds, *Cultural Models in Language and Thought*. Cambridge: Cambridge University Press, 112–48.

Dasgupta, P. 1993. *The Otherness of English. India's Aunty Tongue Syndrome*. New Delhi: Sage.

Dasgupta, P. 2002. "The presence of English in India at the crossroads". In A. Datta, P. Dasgupta and U. Misra, eds, *English at Crossroads: The Post-Colonial Situation: Kumud Chandra Dutta Memorial Lecture Series, 1997–1998*. Guwahati: Students Stores.

Davis, H. 1999. "Typography, lexicography and the development of the idea of 'Standard English'". In T. Bex and R.J. Watts, eds, *Standard English. The Widening Debate*. London: Routledge, 69–88.

Davis, L. M. 1983. *English Dialectology: An Introduction*. Tuscaloosa, AL: University of Alabama Press.

DeCamp, D. 1971. "Toward a generative analysis of a post-creole speech continuum". In D. Hymes, ed., *Pidginization and Creolization of Languages. Proceedings of a Conference Held at the University of the West Indies Mona, Jamaica, April 1968*. Cambridge: Cambridge University Press, 349–70.

De Decker, P. and J. Nycz. 2011. "For the record: Which digital media can be used for sociophonetic analysis?". *University of Pennsylvania Working Papers in Linguistics* 17: 51–9.

Deprez, K. and Y. Persoons. 1987. "Attitude". In U. Ammon, N. Dittmar and K. Mattheier, eds, *Soziolinguistik – Sociolinguistics: An International Handbook of the Science of Language and Society, Vol.1*. Berlin: de Gruyter, 125–32.

Derwing, T. M. 2003. "What do ESL students say about their accents?". *Canadian Modern Language Review* 59: 547–66.

Desai, A. [1980] 2001. *Clear Light of Day*. London: Vintage.

DESTATIS = Deutsches Statistisches Bundesamt. <https://www.destatis.de> (last accessed: 30/09/2020)

De Vaus, D. A. 2001. *Surveys in Social Research*. London: Routledge.

Dorian, N. C. 1982. "Defining the speech community to include its working margins". In S. Romaine, ed., *Sociolinguistic Variation in Speech Communities*. London: Arnold, 25–33.

Dovidio, J. F., J. C. Brigham, B. T. Johnson and S. L. Gaertner. 1996. "Stereotyping, prejudice, and discrimination: Another look". In C. N. Macrae, C. Stangor and M. Hewstone, eds, *Stereotypes and stereotyping*. New York: Guilford, 276–319.

D'Souza, J. 1997. "Indian English: Some myths, some realities". *English World-Wide* 18: 91–105.

Duranti, A. 1997. *Linguistic Anthropology*. Cambridge: Cambridge University Press.

Duranti, A. ed. 2004. *A Companion to Linguistic Anthropology*. Oxford: Blackwell.

Eagly, A. H. and S. Chaiken. 1993. *The Psychology of Attitudes*. Fort Worth, TX: Harcourt Brace Jovanovich.

Eckert, P. 1989. *Jocks and Burnouts: Social Categories and Identity in the High School*. New York: Teachers College Press.

Eckert, P. 2000. *Linguistic Variation as a Social Practice. The Linguistic Construction of Identity in Belton High*. Malden, MA: Blackwell.

Eckert, P. 2013. "Ethics in linguistic research". In R. J. Podesva and D. Sharma, eds, 11–26.

Eckert, P. and S. McConnel-Ginet. 1992. "Communities of practice: Language, gender, and power all live". In K. Hall, M. Bucholtz and B. Moonwoman, eds, *Locating Power. Proceedings of the 1992 Berkeley Women and Language Conference*. Berkeley: Berkeley Women and Language Group, 89–99.

Eraly, A. 2015. *The Age of Wrath: A History of the Delhi Sultanate*. London: Penguin.

Erickson, F. 1987. "Transformation and school success: The politics and culture of educational achievement". *Anthropology and Education Quarterly* 18: 335–56.

Escudero, P. 2007. "Second-language phonology: The role of perception". In M. C. Pennington, ed., *Phonology in Context*. London: Palgrave Macmillan, 109–34.

Esses, V. M., G. Haddock and M. P. Zanna. 1993. "Values, stereotypes, and emotions as determinants of intergroup attitudes". In D. M. Mackie and D. L. Hamilton, eds, *Affect, Cognition and Stereotyping: Interactive Processes in Group Perception*. New York: Academic Press, 137–66.

Fairbanks, G. 1960. *Voice and Articulation Drill Book*. New York: Harper and Row.

Faist, T., M. Aksakal and L. Schmidt. 2017. *Indian High-skilled Migrants and International Students in Germany: Migrations Behaviours, Intentions and Development Effects*. Gütersloh: Bertelsmann Stiftung.

Fasold, R. W. 1984. *The Sociolinguistics of Society*. Oxford: Blackwell.

Ferguson, Ch. 1959. "Diglossia". *Word* 16: 325–40.

Filppula, M., J. Klemola and D. Sharma. eds. 2017. *The Oxford Handbook of World Englishes*. Oxford: Oxford University Press

Fischer, J. L. 1958. "Social influences on the choice of a linguistic variant". *Word* 14: 47–56.

Fishman, J. A. 1971. *Sociolinguistics*. Rowley, MA: Newbury House.

Flores d'Arcais, G. 1988. "Language perception". In F. J. Newmeyer, ed., *Linguistics: The Cambridge Survey, III. Language: Psychological and Biological Aspects*. Cambridge: Cambridge University Press, 97–123.

Foucault, M. 1991. *Discipline and Punish: The Birth of a Prison*. London: Penguin.

Francis, W. N. 1983. *Dialectology. An Introduction*. London and New York: Longman.

Friesen, W. and R. A. Kearns. 2008. "Indian diaspora in New Zealand: History, identity and cultural landscapes". In P. Raghuram, A. K. Sahoo, B. Maharaj and D. Sangha, eds, *Tracing an Indian Diaspora. Contexts, Memories, Representations*. New Delhi: Sage, 210–36.

Fuchs, R. 2014. "Integrating variability in loudness and duration in a multidimensional model of speech rhythm: Evidence from Indian English and British English". *Speech Prosody* 7: 290–94.

Fuchs, R. 2016. *Speech Rhythm in Varieties of English*. Singapore: Springer.

Gaetanides, S. 2003. "Partizipation von Migranten/innen und ihren Selbstorganisationen". *E&C-Zielgruppenkonferenz Interkulturelle Stadt(teil) politik, Dokumentation der Veranstaltung vom 8. und 9. Dezember 2003 Berlin*, 1–33.

Gardner, R. C. and W. E. Lambert. 1972. *Attitudes and Motivation in Second-Language Learning*. Rowley, MA: Newbury House.

Gargesh, R. 2004. “Indian English: Phonology”. In E. W. Schneider, K. Burridge, B. Kortmann, R. Mesthrie and C. Upton, eds, *A Handbook of Varieties of English, vol. 1*. Berlin: Mouton de Gruyter, 992–1002.

Gargesh, R. 2009. “South Asian Englishes”. In B. B. Kachru, Y. Kachru and G. Nelson, eds, *The Handbook of World Englishes*. Malden, MA: Blackwell, 90–113.

Gargesh, R. and P. Sailaja. 2017. “South Asia.” In M. Filppula *et al.*, eds, 425–47.

Garrett, M. F. 1988. “Processes in language production”. In F. J. Newmeyer, ed., *Linguistics: The Cambridge Survey, III. Language: Psychological and Biological Aspects*. Cambridge: Cambridge University Press, 69–96.

Garrett, P. B. 2004. “Language contact and contact languages”. In A. Duranti, ed., 46–72.

Geertz, C. 1973. “Thick description: Toward an interpretive theory of culture”. In C. Geerz, ed., *The Interpretation of Cultures: Selected Essays*. New York: Basic Books, 3–30.

Giddens, A. 2006. *Sociology*. Cambridge: Polity Press.

Giles, H. 1970. “Evaluative reactions to accents”. *Educational Review* 22: 211–27.

Giles, H. and N. Coupland. 1991. *Language: Context and Consequences*. Milton Keynes: Open University Press.

Giles, H. and P. Johnson. 1981. “The role of language in ethnic group relations”. In J. Turner and H. Giles, eds, *Intergroup Behavior*. Chicago: University of Chicago Press, 199–243.

Gilliéron, J. and E. Edmont. 1902–1912. *Atlas Linguistique de la France*. 13 vols. Paris: Champion.

Glauser, B. 1974. *The Scottish-English Linguistic Border: Lexical Aspects*. Bern: Francke (The Cooper Monographs, 20).

Glauser, B. 1991. “Transition areas versus focal areas in English dialectology”. *English World-Wide* 12: 1–24.

Glauser, B. 1994. “Dialect Maps: Depicting, constructing or distorting linguistic reality”. In G. Melchers and N. L. Johannesson, eds, *Nonstandard Varieties of Language. Papers from the Stockholm Symposium 11–13 April 1991*. Stockholm: Almqvist and Wiksell.

Glauser, B. 2000. “The Scottish/English border in hindsight”. *International Journal of the Sociology of Language* 145: 165–78.

Goel, U. 2002. “Indische Engel in Deutschland”. *Südasien* 22: 61–3.

Goel, U. 2007. “Germany”. In B. V. Lal, ed., *The Encyclopedia of the Indian Diaspora*. Singapore: Didier Millet, 358–60.

Gooden, S., K. A. Drayton and M. Beckham. 2009. "Tone inventories and tune-text alignments: Prosodic variation in 'hybrid' prosodic systems". *Studies in Language* 33: 396–436.

Görlach, M. 1996. "And is it English?". *English World-Wide* 17: 153–74.

Gosalia, S. 2002. "Indische Diaspora und kulturelle Identität". In D. Werner, ed., *2002: Indien – Politik, Wirtschaft, Gesellschaft*. Hamburg: Institut für Asienkunde, 233–45.

Gottschlich, P. 2012. "German case study". *CARIM-India RR 2012/03*. Robert Schuman Centre for Advanced Studies. San Domenico di Fiesole, FI: European University Institute.

Gottschlich, P. 2013. "From Germany to India: The role of NRI and PIO in economic and social development assistance". In T. Y. Tam and M. Rahman, eds, *Diaspora Engagement and Development in South Asia*. London: Palgrave Macmillan, 20–40.

Gould, P. and R. White. 1986. *Mental Maps*. Harmondsworth, Middlesex: Penguin.

Grabe, E. and E. Low. 2002. "Durational variability in speech and the rhythm class hypothesis". *Laboratory Phonology* 7: 515–46.

Gradoll, D. 2003. "The decline of the native speaker". In G. Anderman and M. Rogers, eds, *Translation. Today Trends and Perspectives*. Clevedon: Multilingual Matters, 152–66.

Gries, S. Th. 2013. "Basic significance testing". In R. J. Podesva and D. Sharma, eds, 316–36.

Gries, S. Th. and T. Bernaisch. 2016. "Exploring epicentres empirically. Focus on south Asian Englishes". *English World-Wide* 37: 1–25.

Gumperz, J. J. 1968. "The speech community". *International Encyclopaedia of the Social Sciences, Vol. 9*: 381–6.

Gumperz, J. J. 1971. *Language in Social Groups*. Stanford: Stanford University Press.

Gumperz, J. J. 1972a. "Introduction". In J. J. Gumperz and D. Hymes, eds, *Directions in Sociolinguistics: The Ethnography of Communication*. New York: Holt, Rinehart and Winston, 1–25.

Gumperz, J. J. 1972b. "The speech community". In P. P. Giglioli, eds, *Language and Social Context*. Hamondsworth: Penguin, 219–31.

Gumperz, J. J. 1982. "Social network and language shift". In J. Gumperz, ed., *Discourse Strategies*. Cambridge: Cambridge University Press, 38–58.

Gumperz, J. J. and D. Hymes. 1964. "The ethnography of communication". Special issue of *American Anthropologist* 66.

Gupta, A. and J. Ferguson. 1992. "Beyond culture: Space, identity and the politics of difference". *Cultural Anthropology* 7: 6–23.

Hall, R. A. Jr. 1950. "Obituary of Leonard Bloomfield". *Lingua* 2: 117–23.

Hallet, J. 2010. "Code-switching in diasporic Indian and Jewish English-language media". In R. Facchinetti, D. Crystal and B. Seidlhofer, eds, *From International to Local English-and Back Again*. Bern: Lang, 27–49.

Halliday, M. A. K. 1976. "Anti-Languages". *American Anthropologist* 78: 570–84.

Hamilton, D. L. and J. W. Sherman. 1994. "Stereotypes". In R. S. Wyer and T. K. Srull, eds, *Handbook of Social Cognition: Basic Processes*. Hillsdale, NJ: Erlbaum, 1–68.

Hartley, L. C. 1999. "A view from west: Perceptions of US dialects by Oregon residents". In D. Preston, ed., 315–32.

Hashemi, M. 2012. "Reflections on mixing methods in applied linguistic research". *Applied Linguistics* 33: 206–12.

Hatch, E. and A. Lazaraton. 1991. *The Research Manual. Design and Statistics for Applied Linguistics*. New York, NY: Newbury House Publishers.

Hayhoe, M. and S. Parker. 1994. *Who Owns English?* Milton Keynes: Open University Press.

He, L. 2012. "Syllabic intensity variation as a quantification of speech rhythm: Evidence from both L1 and L2". *Speech Prosody, 6th International Conference*, Shangai, 466–69.

Heselwood, B. and L. McChrystal. 2000. "Gender, accent features and voicing in Panjabi-English bilingual children". *Leeds Working Papers in Linguistics* 8: 45–69.

Hesse-Biber, S. and P. Leavy. 2006. *The Practice of Qualitative Research*. London: Sage.

Hiraga, Y. 2005. "British attitudes towards six varieties of English in the USA and Britain". *World Englishes* 24: 289–308.

HISA = Heidelberg Indian Students' Association. <http://hisaheidelberg.com> (last accessed: 08/07/2019).

Hockett, C. F. 1958. *A Course in Modern Linguistics*. New York: Macmillan.

Hoenigswald, H. 1966. "A proposal for the study of folk-linguistics". In W. Bright, ed., *Proceedings of the UCLA Sociolinguistics Conference*. The Hague: Mouton, 16–26.

Hoffmann, S., M. Hundt and J. Mukherjee. 2011. "Indian English – an emerging epicentre? A pilot study on light verbs in web-derived corpora of South Asian Englishes". *Anglia* 129: 258–80.

Hoffmeyer-Zlotnik, P. and J. Grote. 2019. "Attracting and retaining international students in Germany". *BAMF*, German National Contact Point for the European Migration Network (EMN). *Working paper* 85: 1–85.

Hogg, M. A. and G. M. Vaughan. 2002. *Social Psychology*. London: Prentice Hall.

Holmes, J. 1997. "Setting new standards: Sound changes and gender in New Zealand English". *English World-Wide* 18: 107–42.

Holmes, J. and M. Meyerhoff. 1999. "The community of practice: Theories and methodologies in language and gender research". *Language in Society* 28: 173–83.

Hosali, P. 2005. "Butler English". *English Today* 21: 34–9.

Hudson, R. 1980. *Sociolinguistics*. Cambridge: Cambridge University Press (reprinted and revised in 1996).

Hughes, A., P. Trudgill and D. Watt. 2005. *English Accents and Dialects: An Introduction to Social and Regional Varieties of English in the British Isles*. London: Hodder Arnold.

Hundt, M. 2014. "Zero articles in Indian Englishes: A comparison of primary and secondary diaspora situations". In M. Hundt and D. Sharma, eds, 131–70.

Hundt, M. and D. Sharma. eds. 2014a. *English in the Indian Diaspora*. Amsterdam: Benjamins.

Hundt, M. and D. Sharma. 2014b. "Introduction". In M. Hundt and D. Sharma, eds, 1–8.

Hymes, D. ed. 1964. *Language in Culture and Society. A Reader in Linguistics and Anthropology*. New York: Harper and Row.

Hymes, D. 1972. "On communicative competence". In J. B. Pride and J. Holmes, eds, *Sociolinguistics*. Harmondsworth: Penguin, 269–93.

Hymes, D. 1974. *Foundations in Sociolinguistics: An Ethnographic Approach*. Philadelphia: University of Pennsylvania Press.

ILOSTAT = International Labour Organization database. <https://www.ilo.org> (last accessed: 05/10/2020).

Indian Students in Germany. <http://www.indianstudentsgermany.org> (last accessed: 08/11/2020).

Inoue, F. 1977/8. "Hôgen Imêji no Tahenryô Kaseki" [Multivariate analysis of dialect image] (Part I). *Gengo Seikatsu* 311: 82–91.

Inoue, F. 1995. "Classification of dialects by image. English and Japanese". In W. Viereck, ed., *Verhandlungen des Internationalen Dialektologenkongresses, Bamberg, 29.7–4.8.1990; Proceedings of the International Congress of Dialectologists, Bamberg, July 29–August 4, 1990. Zeitschrift fuür Dialektologie und Linguistik* 75–77. Stuttgart: Franz Steiner, 355–68. (reprinted in D. Preston, ed., 1999, 147–59).

Inoue, F. 1996. "Subjective dialect division in Great Britain". *American Speech* 71: 142–61.

Jackendoff, R. S. 1997. *Consciousness and the Computational Mind.* Cambridge, MA: MIT Press.

Jayaram, N. 2004. *The Indian Diaspora. Dynamics of Migration.* New Delhi: Sage.

Jenkins, J. 2000. *The Phonology of English as an International Language.* Oxford: Oxford University Press.

Jenkins, J. 2007. *English as a Lingua Franca: Attitude and Identity.* Oxford: Oxford University Press.

Jobling, D. and E. J. Snell. 1961. "The use of the coefficient of reproducibility in attitude scaling". *The Incorporated Statistician* 11: 110–8.

Jones, E., T. Oliphant and P. Peterson. 2001. "SciPy: Open source scientific tools for Python". <www.scipy.org> (last accessed: 22/10/2020).

Johnson, D. E. 2013. "Descriptive statistics". In R. J. Podesva and D. Sharma, eds, 288–315.

Johnstone, B. 2000. *Qualitative Methods in Sociolinguistics.* New York, Oxford: Oxford University Press.

Kachru, B. B. 1976. "Models of English for the third world: White man's linguistic burden or language pragmatics?". *TESOL Quarterly* 10: 221–39.

Kachru, B. B. 1983. *The Indianization of English. The English Language in India.* Oxford: Oxford University Press.

Kachru, B. B. 1985. "Standards, codifications and sociolinguistic realism: The English language in the outer circle". In R. Quirk and H. G. Widdowson, eds, *English in the World: Teaching and Learning the Language and Literatures.* Cambridge: Cambridge University Press, 11–30.

Kachru, B. B. [1986] 1990. *The Alchemy of English. The Spread, Functions and Models of Non-native Englishes.* Urbana: University of Illinois Press.

Kachru, B. B. 1994. "English in South Asia". In R. Burchfield, ed., *The Cambridge History of the English Language, Vol. 5. English in Britain and Overseas. Origins and Development.* Cambridge: Cambridge University Press, 497–552.

Kachru, B. B. 2001. "World Englishes and culture wars". In T. C. Kiong, A. Pakir, B. K. Choon and R. B. H. Goh, eds, *Ariels: Departures & Returns: Essays for Edwin Thumboo.* Singapore: Oxford University Press, 392–414.

Kasper, G. 2008. "Data collection in pragmatics research". In H. Spencer-Oatey, ed., *Culturally Speaking: Culture, Communication and Politeness Theory.* London: Continuum, 279–303.

Kellermann, A. 2001. *A New, New English: Language, Politics, and Identity in Gibraltar.* Heidelberg: Heidelberger Schriften zur Sprache und Kultur.

Kerswill, P. and P. Trudgill. 2005. "The birth of new dialects". In P. Auer, F. Hinskens and P. Kerswill, eds, *Dialect Change: Convergence and Divergence in European Languages*. Cambridge: Cambridge University Press, 196–220.

Khadria, B. 2014. "The dichotomy of the skilled and unskilled among non-resident Indians and persons of Indian origin: Bane or boon for development in India?". In G. Tejada, U. Bhattracharya, B. Khadria and C. Kuptsch, eds, *Indian Skilled Migration and Development: To Europe and Back*. New Delhi: Springer, 29–45.

Khubchandani, L. M. 2001. "Language demography and language education." In C. J. Daswani, ed., *Language Education in Multilingual India*. New Delhi, India: UNESCO, 3–47.

Kirkham, S. 2011. "The acoustics of coronal stops in British Asian English". *Proceedings of the 17th ICPhS*. Hong Kong, 1102–5.

Kloss, H. 1977. "Über einige Terminologie-Probleme der interlingualen Soziolinguistik". *Deutsche Sprache* 3: 224–37.

Kolb, H. 2005. "Die Deutsche 'Green Card' ". *Focus Migration* 3: 1–3.

Kremer, L. 1999. "The Netherlands-German national border as a subjective dialect boundary". In D. Preston, ed., 31–6.

Krishnaswamy, N. and A. S. Burde. 1998. *The Politics of Indians' English: Linguistic Colonialism and the Expanding English Empire*. Oxford: Oxford University Press.

Kristensson, G. 1983. "Dialectology and historical linguistics". In M. Davenport, E. Hansen and H. F. Nielson, eds, *Current Topics in English Historical Linguistics: Proceedings of the 2nd International Conference on English Historical Linguistics, Held at Odense University, 13–15 April, 1981*. Odense, University Press, 29–35.

Krivokapić, J. 2013. "Rhythm and convergence between speakers of American and Indian English". *Laboratory Phonology*: 39–65.

Kroch, A. 1978. "Toward a theory of social dialect variation". *Language in Society* 7: 17–36.

Kroskrity, P. 2004. "Language ideologies". In A. Duranti, ed., 496–517.

Kuhl, P. K. and P. Iverson. 1995. "Linguistic experience and the perceptual magnet effect". In W. Strange, ed., *Speech Perception and Linguistic Experience*. Baltimore: York Press, 121–54.

Labov, W. 1966a. *The Social Stratification of English in New York City*. Washington, DC: Center for Applied Linguistics.

Labov, W. 1966b. "The Linguistic variable as a structural unit". *Washington Linguistics Review* 3: 4–22.

Labov, W. 1972a. *Sociolinguistic Patterns*. Pennsylvania: University of Pennsylvania Press.

Labov, W. 1972b. "Some principles of linguistic methodology". *Language in Society* 1: 97–120.

Labov, W. 1972c. *Language in the Inner City: Studies in Black English Vernacular*. Philadelphia: University of Pennsylvania Press.

Labov, W. 1984. "Field methods of the project on linguistic change and variation". In J. Baugh and J. Sherzer, eds, *Language in Use. Readings in Sociolinguistics*. Englewood Cliffs, NJ: Prentice Hall, 28–66.

Labov, W. 1994. *Principles of Linguistic Change, Vol. 1: Internal Factors*. Oxford: Blackwell.

Labov, W. 2001. *Principles of Linguistic Change, Vol. 2: Social Factors*. Oxford: Blackwell.

Ladefoged, P. 1975. *A Course in Phonetics*. New York: Harcourt Brace Jovanovich.

Lal, B. V., P. Reeves and R. Rai. eds. 2006. The *Encyclopedia of the Indian Diaspora*. Singapore: Singapore University Press.

Lambert, W. E. 1967. "A social psychology of bilingualism". *Journal of Social Issues* 23: 91–109.

Lambert, W. E., R. C. Hodgson, R. C. Gardner and S. Fillenbaum. 1960. "Evaluational reactions to spoken languages". *Journal of Abnormal and Social Phychology* 60.1: 44–51.

Lamnek, S. 1995. *Qualitative Sozialforschung. Band I: Methodologie*. Weinheim: Belz.

Lance, D. M. 1999. "Regional variation in subjective dialect divisions in the United States". In D. Preston, ed., 283–314.

Lange, C. 2012. *The Syntax of Spoken Indian English*. Amsterdam: Benjamins.

Lave, J. and E. Wenger. 1991. *Situated Learning: Legitimate Peripheral Participation*. Cambridge: Cambridge University Press.

Leimgruber, J. R. E. and L. Sankaran. 2014. "Imperfectives in Singapore's Indian Community". In M. Hundt and D. Sharma, eds, 105–30.

Leitner, G. 1992. "English as a pluricentric language". In M. Clyne, ed., *Pluricentric Languages: Differing Norms in Different* Nations. Berlin: Mouton de Gruyter, 179–237.

Leitner, G. 2010. "Developmental stages in the formation of epicentres of English". In O. Palusci, ed., *English but Not Quite*. Trento: Tangram, 17–35.

Le Page, R. B. and A. Tabouret-Keller. 1985. *Acts of Identity: Creole-based Approaches to Language and Ethnicity*. Cambridge: Cambridge University Press.

Leung, G. A. 2013. "A synchronic sociophonetic study of monophthongs in Trinidadian English". Ph.D. dissertation. University of Freiburg.

Leung, G. A. and D. Deuber. 2014. "Indo-Trinidadian speech. An investigation into a popular stereotype surrounding pitch". In M. Hundt and D. Sharma, eds, 9–27.

Levon, E. 2013. "Ethnography and recording interaction". In R.J. Podesva and D. Sharma, eds, 195–213.

Li Wei. 1995. "Variations in patterns of language choice and codeswitching by three groups of Chinese/English speakers in Newcastle upon Tyne". *Multilingua* 14: 297–323.

Lippi-Green, R. 1989. "Social network integration and language change in progress in a rural alpine village". *Language in Society* 18: 213–34.

Lippi-Green, R. 1997. *English with an Accent: Language, Ideology, and Discrimination in the United States*. London: Routledge.

Llamas, C. 2000. "Middlesbrough English: convergent and divergent trends in a 'Part of Britain with no identity'". *Leeds Working Papers in Linguistics* 8: 123–48.

Löw-Wiebach, D. 2005. *Language Attitudes and Language Use in Pitmedden (Aberdeenshire)*. Frankfurt: Lang (VarioLingua, 24)

Lütkehaus, L. ed. 2004. *Nirwana in Deutschland: Von Leibniz bis Schopenhauer*. München: Deutscher Taschenbuch.

Malinoswki, B. 1922. *Argonauts of the Western Pacific*. London: Routledge and Kegan Paul.

Mase, Y. 1999a. "Dialect consciousness and dialect divisions: Examples in the Nagano-Gifu Boundary Region". In D. Preston, ed., 71–100.

Mase, Y. 1999b. "On dialect consciousness: Dialect characteristics given by speakers". In D. Preston, ed., 101–14.

Masica, C. P. 1972. *The Sound System of Indian English*. Hyderabad: CIEFL.

Maxwell, O. 2014. "The Intonational phonology of Indian English. An autosegmental-metrical analysis based on Bengali and Kannada English". Ph.D. dissertation. University of Melbourne.

Maxwell, O. and J. Fletcher. 2009. "Acoustic and durational properties of Indian English vowels". *World Englishes* 28: 52–70.

Maxwell, O. 2010. "The acoustic characteristics of diphthongs in Indian English". *World Englishes* 29: 24–44.

Mayer, M. M., S. Yamamura, J. Schneider and A. Müller. 2012. "Immigration of International students from third countries". *BAMF*, German National

Contact Point for the European Migration Network (EMN). *Working paper* 47: 1–85.

Mayring, P. 1992. *Einführung in die qualitative Sozialforschng: Eine Anleitung zu qualitativem Denken*. Weinheim und Basel: Beltz.

Mayring, P. 2014. *Qualitative Inhaltsanalyse: Grundlagen, Techniken, Software* Weinheim und Basel: Beltz (trad. *Qualitative Content Analysis. Theoretical Foundation, Basic Procedures and Software Solution*. Klagenfurt: SSOAR.

McArthur, T. 1992a. "Models of English". *English Today* 32: 12–21.

McArthur, T. 1992b. *The Oxford Companion to the English Language*. Oxford: Oxford University Press.

McKenzie, R. M. 2015. "UK university students' folk perceptions of spoken variation in English: the role of explicit and implicit attitudes". *International Journal of the Sociology of Language* 236: 31–53.

MEA = Ministry of External Affairs, Government of India. <http://mea.gov.in> (last accessed: 01/11/2020).

Mesthrie, R. 1991. *Language in Indenture. A Sociolinguistic History of Bhojpuri-Hindi in South Africa*. Johannesburg: Witwatersrand University Press (reprinted in 1992, London: Routledge).

Mesthrie, R. 1992. *English in Language Shift. The History, Structure, and Sociolinguistics of South African Indian English*. Cambridge: Cambridge University Press.

Mesthrie, R. 2008. "South Asian languages in the second diaspora". In B. B. Kachru, Y. Kachru and S. N. Sridhar, eds, *Language in South Asia*. Cambridge: Cambridge University Press, 497–514.

Mesthrie, R. 2014. "A lesser globalisation: A sociolexical study of Indian Englishes in diaspora, with a primary focus on South Africa". In M. Hundt and D. Sharma, eds, 171–86.

Mesthrie, R. 2017. "World Englishes, second language acquisition, and language contact". In M. Filppula *et al.*, eds, 175–193.

Mesthrie, R. and R. M. Bhatt. 2008. *World Englishes. The Study of New Linguistic Varieties*. Cambridge: Cambridge University Press.

Mesthrie, R. and A. Chevalier. 2014. "Sociophonetics and the Indian diaspora: The NURSE vowel and other selected features in South African Indian English". In M. Hundt and D. Sharma, eds, 85–104.

Meyerhoff, M. 2002. "Communities of practice". In J. K. Chambers, P. Trudgill, and N. Schilling-Estes, eds, *The Handbook of Language Variation and Change*. Oxford: Blackwell, 526–48.

Milroy, J. and L. Milroy. 1985. "Linguistic change, social network and speaker innovation". *Linguistics* 21: 339–84.

Milroy, J. and L. Milroy. –. 1991. *Authority in Language: Investigating Language Prescription and Standardisation*. London: Routledge.

Milroy, L. 1980. *Language and Social Networks*. Oxford: Blackwell.

Milroy, L. 1987. *Observing and Analysing Natural Language*. Oxford: Blackwell.

Milroy, L. and J. Milroy. 1992. "Social networks and social class: Toward an integrated sociolinguistic model. *Language in Society* 21:1–26.

Milroy, L. and M. Gordon. 2003. *Sociolinguistics: Method and Interpretation*. Oxford: Blackwell.

Mohanty, A. K. 2006. "Multilingualism of the unequals and predicaments of education in India: Mother tongue or other tongue?". In O. García, T. Skutnabb-Kangas and M. E. Torres-Guzmán, eds, *Imagining Multilingual Schools: Language in Education and Glocalization*. Clevedon: Multilingual Matters, 262–83.

Mohanty, A. K. 2013. "Multilingual education in India: Overcoming the language barrier and the burden of the double divide." In I. Gogolin, P. Siemund, M. E. Schulz and J. Davydova, eds, *Multilingualism and Language Diversity in Urban Areas: Acquisition, Identities, Space, Education*. Amsterdam: Benjamins, 305–26.

Montaut, A. 2005. "Colonial language classification, postcolonial language movements and the grassroot multilingualism ethos in India". In M. Hasan and A. Roy, eds, *Living Together Separately. On the Historicity of India's Composite Culture*. Amsterdam: Benjamins, 75–106.

Morgan, M. 1994. "The African-American speech community: Reality and sociolinguistics". In M. Morgan, ed., *Language and the Social Construction of Identity in Creole Situations*. Berkeley: Centre for African-American Studies, 121–48.

Morgan, M. 2002. *Language, Discourse and Power in African American Culture*. Cambridge: Cambridge University Press.

Morgan, M. 2004. "Speech Community". In A. Duranti, ed., 3–22.

Morgan, M. 2014. *Speech Communities*. Cambridge: Cambridge University Press.

Mortensen, J. and A. Fabricius. 2014. "Language ideologies in Danish higher education: Exploring student perspectives". In A. K. Hultgren, F. Gregersen and J. Thøgersen, eds, *English in Nordic Universities: Ideologies and Practices*. Amsterdam: Benjamins, 193–223.

Mufwene, S. 2001. *The Ecology of Language Evolution*. Cambridge: Cambridge University Press.

Mugler, F. and J. Tent. 2008. "Fiji English: Morphology and syntax". In K. Burridge and B. Kortmann, eds, *Varieties of English. The Pacific and Australasia.* Canberra: Pacific Linguistics, 95–108.

Mukherjee, J. 2007. "Steady states in the evolution of new Englishes: Present-day Indian English as an equilibrium". *Journal of English Linguistics* 35: 157–87.

Munro, M. J., T. M. Derwing and S. L. Morton. 2006. "The mutual intelligibility of L2 speech". *Studies in Second Language Acquisition* 28: 111–31.

Narang, V., D. Misra and R. Yadav. 2011. "Acoustic space of Indian English vowels". *Journal of the School of Language, Literature & Cultural Studies* 14: n.p.

Neuhauser, S. and A. P. Simpson. 2007. "Imitated or authentic? Listeners' judgements of foreign accents". *Studies in Second Language Acquisition* 28: 111–31.

Niedzielski, N. A. and D. R. Preston. 2003. *Folk Linguistics*. Berlin: de Gruyter.

Nihalani, P., R. K. Tongue and P. Hosali. 1979. *Indian and British English: A Handbook of Usage and Pronunciation*. New Delhi: Oxford University Press.

Nishihara, T. and J. van de Weijer. 2011. "On syllable-timed rhythm and stress-timed rhythm in World Englishes: Revisited". *Bulletin of Miyagi University of Education* 46: 155–63.

NUEPA = National University of Educational Planning and Administration. <www.nuepa.org> (last accessed: 01/11/2020).

Oberkircher, V. 2006."Die deutsche Greencard aus der Sicht indischer IT-Experten". In C. Brosius and U. Goel, eds, *Masala.de: Menschen aus Südasien in Deutschland*. Heidelberg: Draupadi, 161–88.

Oonk, G. 2007. *Global Indian Diasporas: Exploring Trajectories of Migration and Theory*. Amsterdam: Amsterdam University Press.

Orton, A. 2010. *India's Borderland and Disputes: China, Pakistan, Bangladesh, and Nepal.* New Delhi: Epitome Books.

Palstring, V. S. 2015. "Das Potenzial der Migration aus Indien". *BAMF*, German National Contact Point for the European Migration Network (EMN). *Working paper* 26: 1–234.

Parek, B. G. Singh and S. Vertoveč. eds. 2003. *Culture and Economy in the Indian Diaspora*. London: Routledge.

Pavone, J. 1980. *Implicational Scales and English Dialectology*. Ann Arbor: University Microfilm International.

Pettorino, M., M. Maffia, E. Pellegrino, M. Vitale and A. De Meo. 2013. "VtoV: A perceptual cue for rhythm identification". In P. Mertens and A. C. Simon, eds, *Proceedings of the Prosody-Discourse Interface Conference*. Leuven, Belgium, 101–6.

Pettorino, M. and E. Pellegrino. 2016. "%V and VtoV: An acoustic perceptual approach to the rhythmic classification of languages". In C. Bardel and A. De Meo, eds, In *Parler les langues romanes/Parlare le lingue romanze/Hablar las lenguas romances/Falando línguas românicas*. Naples: Il Torcoliere, 13–28.

Pickering L. and C. Wiltshire. 2000. "Pitch accent in Indian-English teaching discourse". *World Englishes* 19: 173–83.

Pike, K. 1967. *Language in Relation to a Unified Theory of Structure of Human Behaviour*. The Hague: Mouton.

Podesva, R. J. and D. Sharma. eds. 2013. *Research Methods in Linguistics*. Cambridge: Cambridge University Press.

Podesva, R. J. and E. Zsiga. 2013. "Sound recordings: Acoustic and articulatory data". In R. J. Podesva and D. Sharma, eds, 169–94.

Preston, D. R. 1981. "Perceptual dialectology. Mental maps of United States dialects from a Hawaiian perspective (summary). In H. Warkentyne, ed., *Methods IV/Méthodes IV (Papers from the Fourth International Conference on Methods in Dialectology)*. University of Victoria, British Columbia, 192–98.

Preston, D. R. 1982. "Perceptual dialectology: Mental maps of United States dialects from a Hawaiian perspective". *Hawaii Working Papers in Linguistics* 14: 5–49.

Preston, D. R. 1989. *Perceptual Dialectology: Nonlinguists' Views of Areal Linguistics*. Dordrecht, Holland Providence R.I., US: Foris.

Preston, D. R. 1996. "Whaddayaknow?: The modes of folk linguistic awareness". *Language Awareness* 5: 40–74.

Preston, D. R. ed. 1999. *Handbook of Perceptual Dialectology, Vol. 1*. Amsterdam: Benjamins.

Preston, D. R. 2010. "Language, people, salience, space. Perceptual dialectology and language regard". *Dialectologia* 5: 87–131.

Preston, D. R. and G. M. Howe. 1987. "Computerized studies of mental dialect maps". In K. Denning, S. Inkelas, F. C. McNair-Knox and J. R. Rickford, eds, *Variation in language: NWAV-XV at Stanford*. Department of Linguistics: Stanford University, 361–78.

Punch. K. F. 1998. *Introduction to Social Research: Quantitative and Qualitative Approaches*. London: Sage.

Punnamparambil, J. 2008. "Indische Migration nach Deutschland". *Meine Welt. Heimat in der Fremde: Migrationsgeschichten von Menschen aus Indien in Deutschland*. Heidelberg: Draupadi, 15–23.

Ramus, F., M. Nespor, and J. Mehler. 1999. "Correlates of linguistic rhythm in the speech signal". *Cognitorium* 73: 265–92.

Rathore, C. 2014. "East African Indian twice migrants in Britain. Phonological variation across generations". In M. Hundt and D. Sharma, eds, 55–83.

Récanati, F. 1991. "The pragmatics of what is said". In S. Davis, ed., *Pragmatics: A Reader*. Oxford: Oxford University Press, 97–120.

Regnoli, G. 2016. "Indexicality and contextualisation. Linguistic, cultural and social stances of Indian English speakers in Heidelberg". M.A. unpublished thesis. University of Naples L'Orientale.

Regnoli, G. 2019a. "Attitudinal alignment and meta-linguistic awareness in Indian English migrant varieties". In V. Bonsignori, G. Cappelli and E. Mattiello, eds, *Worlds of Words: Complexity, Creativity, and Conventionality in English Language, Literature and Culture, Vol. 1: Language*. Pisa: Pisa University Press, 449–60.

Regnoli, G. 2019b. "Local and global ideologies in transient contact zones: Evidence from an Indian student community". In M. M. Coppola, F. Di Blasio and S. Francesconi, eds, *Contact Zones: Cultural, Linguistic and Literary Connections in English*. Quaderni: Labirinti, 179, 143–61.

Regnoli, G. 2019c. "Translanguaging as an expression of transnational identity. Ethnicity renegotiation in the Indian diaspora". *Translation and Translanguaging in Multilingual Contexts* 5:165–84.

Regnoli, G. (forthcoming) "Rhythmic contrast in Marathi English and Telugu English". In R. Fuchs, ed., *Speech Rhythm in L2 and Learner Varieties of English*. Singapore: Springer.

Rice, S. 2010. "Sampling in geography". In N. Clifford and G. Valentine, eds, *Key Methods in Geography*. London: Sage, 230–52.

Richards, K. 2003. *Qualitative Inquiry in TESOL*. London: Palgrave Macmillan.

Rickford, J. R. 1986. "Concord and contrast in the characterization of the speech community". *Sheffield Working Papers in Language and Linguistics* 3: 87–119.

Rickford, J. R. 2002. "Implicational Scales". In J. K. Chambers, P. Trudgill and N. Schilling-Estes, eds, 142–67.

Romaine, S. 1994. *Language in Society: An Introduction to Sociolinguistics*. Oxford: Blackwell.Sailaja, P. 2009. *Dialects of English. Indian English*. Edinburgh: Edinburgh University Press.

Sailaja, P. 2012. "Indian English: Features and sociolinguistic aspects". *Language and Linguistics Compass* 6: 359–70.

Sakel, J. and D. Everett. 2012. *Linguistic Fieldwork*. Cambridge: Cambridge University Press.

Salkind, N. ed. 2010. *Encyclopedia of Research Design*. Thousand Oaks, CA: Sage.

Sanders, C. 2004. *The Cambridge Companion to Saussure*. Cambridge: Cambridge University Press.

Sankoff, G. 1974. "A quantitative paradigm for the study of communicative competence". In R. Bauman and J. Sherzer, eds, *Explorations in the Ethnography of Speaking.* Cambridge: Cambridge University Press, 18–49.

Sankoff, G. 1980. "A quantitative paradigm for the study of communicative competence". In G. Sankoff, ed., *The Social Life of Language*. Philadelphia: University of Philadelphia Press, 47–79.

Sapir, E. [1921] 1949. *Language: An Introduction to the Study of Speech.* New York: Harcourt, Brace and Company.

Saravanan, V. S., S. Saravanan and C. Butsch. 2018. *A Home away from Home: An Overview of Indian Associations in Germany.* Department of Political and Cultural Change, Centre for Development Research (ZEF). Bonn: University of Bonn.

Schilling, N. 2013. "Surveys and interviews". In R. J. Podesva and D. Sharma, eds, 96–115.

Schlieben-Lange, B. 1991. *Soziolinguistik: Eine Einführung.* Stuttgart: Kohlhammer.

Schmied, J. 2008. "East African English (Kenya, Uganda, Tanzania): Phonology". In R. Mesthrie, ed., *Varieties of English, Vol. 4: Africa, South and Southeast Asia*. Berlin: de Gruyter 150–63.

Schneider, E. W. 2003. "The dynamics of New Englishes: From identity construction to dialect birth". *Language* 79: 233–81.

Schneider, E. W. 2007. *Postcolonial English: Varieties around the World.* Cambridge: Cambridge University Press.

Schneider, E. W. 2017. "Models of English in the world". In M. Filppula *et al.*, eds, 35–57.

Schnepel, B. 2004. "Inder in der Fremde". *Orientwissenschaftliche Hefte* 13: 115–141.

Schreirer, D. 2014. "On cafeterias and new dialects: The role of primary transmitters". In S. Buschfeld, T. Hoffmann, M. Huber and A. Kautzsch, eds, *The Evolution of Englishes: The Dynamic Model and Beyond*. Amsterdam: Benjamins, 231–48.

Schuchardt, H. [1885] 1972. "On sound laws: Against the neogrammarians. In T. Vennemann and T. Wilbur, eds, *Schuchardt, the Neogrammarians, and the Transformational Theory of Phonological Change.* Frankfurt: Athenaeum, 39–72.

Schütze, C. T. and J. Sprouse. 2013. "Judgment data". In R. J. Podesva and D. Sharma, eds, 27–50.

Setter, J. and J. Jenkins. 2005. "Pronunciation". *Language Teaching* 38: 1–17.

Sharma, D. 2005. "Dialect stabilization and speaker awareness in non-native varieties of English". *Journal of Sociolinguistics* 9: 194–224.

Sharma, D. 2009. "Typological diversity in new Englishes". *English World-Wide* 30: 170–95.

Sharma, D. 2014. "Translational flows, language variation, and ideology". In M. Hundt and D. Sharma, eds, 215–42.

Sharma, D. 2017. "World Englishes and sociolinguistic theory". In M. Filppula *et al.*, eds, 232–51.

Sharma, D. and L. Sankaran. 2011. "Cognitive and social forces in dialect shift: Gradual change in London Asian speech". *Language Variation and Change* 23: 399–428.

Sharma, R. and E. Annamalai. eds. 2003. *Indian Diaspora: In Search of Identity.* Mysore: Central Institute of Indian Languages.

Sharma, U. eds. 2008. *Festivals in Indian Society.* Two volumes. New Delhi: Mittal.

Shin, S. J. 1998. "Paibu dollar please! Bilingual Korean American children in New York City". *Bilingualism: Language and Cognition* 2: 147–67.

Shuck, G. 2004. "Conversational performance and the poetic construction of an ideology". *Language in Society* 33: 195–222.

Silverstein, M. 1979. "Language structure and linguistic ideology". In R. Cline, W. Hanks and C. Hofbauer, eds, *The Elements: a Parasession on Linguistic Units and Levels.* Chicago: Chicago Linguistic Society.

Silverstein, M. 1981. "The limits of awareness". *Sociolinguistic Working Paper 84.* Austin, TX: Southwest Educational Development Laboratory.

Silverstein, M. 1996. "Encountering languages and languages of encounter in North American ethnohistory". *Journal of Linguistic Anthropology* 6:126– 44.

Simo Bobda, A. 2001. "East and Southern African English accents". *World Englishes* 20: 269–284.

Singh, A. D. and S. I. Rajan. 2016. *Politics of Migration: Indian Emigration in a Globalised World.* New Delhi: Routledge.

Singhvi, L. M. ed. 2001. *Report of the High-Level Committee on the Indian Diaspora.* New Delhi: MEA.

Singler, J. V. 1996. "An OT account of pidgin phonology: Coda consonants in Vernacular Liberian English". In J. Johnson, M. L. Juge and J. L. Moxley, eds, *Proceedings of the Twenty-Second Annual Meeting of the Berkeley Linguistics Society.* Berkeley, CA: Berkeley Linguistics Society, 375–86.

Sirsa, H. and M. A. Redford. 2013. "The effects of native language on Indian English sounds and timing patterns". *Journal of Phonetics* 41: 393–406.

Skutsch, C. 2005. *Encyclopedia of the World's Minorities*. London: Routledge.

Smit, U. 1996. *A New English for a New South Africa? Language Attitudes, Language Planning and Education*. Wien: Braumüller.

Spencer-Rodgers J. and T. McGovern. 2002. "Attitudes toward the culturally different: The role of intercultural communication barriers, affective responses, consensual stereotypes, and perceived threat". *International Journal of Intercultural Relations* 26: 609–31.

SRH = Hochschule Heidelberg <https://www.hochschule-heidelberg.de> (last accessed: 16/10/2020).

Sridhar, K. K. 2008. "South Asian diaspora in Europe and the United States". In B. B. Kachru, Y. Kachru and S. N. Sridhar, eds, *Language in South Asia*. Cambridge: Cambridge University Press, 515–533.

Stadt Heidelberg. <https://www.heidelberg.de/hd,Lde/HD.html> (last accessed: 28/10/2020).

Stalkner, R. C. 1978. "Assertion". In P. Cole, ed. *Syntax and Semantics 9: Pragmatics*. New York: Academic Press, 315–32.

Stangor, C. and J. E. Lange. 1994. "Mental representations of social groups: Advances in understanding stereotypes and stereotyping". In M. P. Zanna, ed., *Advances in Experimental Social Psychology, Vol. 26*. San Diego: Academic Press, 357–416.

Stanlaw, J., N. Adachi and Z. Salzmann. 2018. *Language, Culture, and Society: An Introduction to Linguistic Anthropology*. Westview: New York.

Sturtevant, E. 1947. *An Introduction to Linguistic Science*. New Haven: Yale University Press.

Tagliamonte, S. 2006. *Analysing Sociolinguistic Variation*. Cambridge: Cambridge University Press.

Tajfel, H. ed. 1978. *Differentiation Between Social Groups: Studies in The Social Psychology of Intergroup Relations*. London: Academic Press.

Tajfel, H. 1981. *Human Groups and Social Categories*. Cambridge: Cambridge University Press.

Tajfel, H. 1982. "Introduction". In H. Tajfel, ed., *Social Identity and Intergroup Relations*. Cambridge: Cambridge University Press, 1–11.

Takeyasu, H. and N. Hattori. 2011. "Language discrimination using low-pass filtered songs: Perception of different rhythm classes". *International Conference of Phonetic Sciences XVII*. Hong Kong, 1946–9.

Thakerar, J. N. and H. Giles. 1981. "They are – so they spoke: Noncontent speech stereotypes". *Language & Communication* 2/3: 255–61.

Tôjô, M. 1938. *Hôgen to Hôgengaku* [Dialects and Dialectology]. Tokyo: Shunyôdô.

Tôjô, M. ed. 1954. *Nihon hôgengaku* [Japanese Dialectology]. Tokyo: Yoshikawa Kôbundô.

Tomokiyo, L. M., A. W. Black and K. A. Lenzo. 2005. "Foreign accents in synthetic speech: Development and evaluation". *Interspeech* 9: 1469–72.

Trudgill, P. 1972. "Sex, covert prestige, and linguistic change in the urban British English of Norwich". *Language in Society* 1: 179–95.

Trudgill, P. 1974. *The Social Differentiation of English in Norwich.* Cambridge: Cambridge University Press.

Trudgill, P. 1983. *On Dialect: Social and Geographic Factors.* Oxford: Blackwell.

Trudgill, P. 1986. *Dialects in Contact.* Oxford: Blackwell.

Trudgill, P. 1999. "Standard English: What it isn't". In T. Bex and R.J. Watts, eds, 117–28.

Trudgill, P. 2000. *Sociolinguistics: An Introduction to Language and Society.* Harmondsworth: Penguin.

Trudgill, P. 2017. "The spread of English". In M. Filppula *et al.*, eds, 14–34.

Trudgill, P. and J. Hannah. 2002. *International English.* London: Arnold.

Turner, J. C. 1982. "Towards a cognitive redefinition of the social group". In H. Tajfel, ed., 15–40.

Uffmann, C. 2017. "World English and Phonology". In M. Filppula *et al.*, eds, 63–83.

UN DESA = United Nations Department of Economic and Social Affairs. 2015. <https://www.un.org/en/development/desa/population/migration/data/estimates2/estimates15.shtml> (last accessed: 04/11/2020).

Universität Heidelberg. 2017. *Studierendenstatistik Wintersemester 2017/2018.* Division of Student Affairs and Teaching, 1–76.

Universität Heidelberg. 2018. *Studierendenstatistik Sommersemester 2018.* Division of Student Affairs and Teaching, 1–52.

Venema, M. 2004. *Green Card für Ausländishe IT-Fachleute.* Offenbach: Marplan.

Vertovеč, S. 1999. "Three meanings of 'diaspora', exemplified among South Asia religions". *Diaspora* 6: 277–300.

Voigt, J. H. 1999. "Deutsch-indische Beziehungen im 20. Jahrhundert". *Indien in der Gegenwart* 4: 1–28.

Walker, J. A. 2013. "Variation analysis". In R. J. Podesva and D. Sharma, eds, 440–59.

Wardhaugh, R. 1986. *An Introduction to Sociolinguistics.* Oxford: Blackwell.

Wassink, A. B. and A. Curzan. 2004. "Addressing ideologies around African American English". *Journal of English Linguistics* 32: 171–85.

Weinreich, U., W. Labov and M. Herzog. 1968. "Empirical foundations for a theory of language change". In W. Lehmann and Y. Malkiel, eds, *Directions for Historical Linguistics: A Symposium*. Austin: University of Texas Press.

Wells, J. C. 1982. *Accents of English*. Three volumes. Cambridge: Cambridge University Press.

Wells, J. C. 2006. *English Intonation: An Introduction*. Cambridge: Cambridge University Press.

Wenker, G. 1877. *Das Rheinische Platt. Den Lehrern des Rheinlandes Gewidmet*. Düsseldorf: Selbstverlag.

Westerhoff, H. D. 2007. *Die Greencard. Zur Wirtschaftspolitik der Rot-grünen Bundesregierung*. Fachbereich Wirtschaftswissenschaften, University of Duisburg-Essen.

White, L. and S. L. Mattys. 2007. "Calibrating rhythm: First language and second language studies". *Phonetics* 35: 501–22.

Williams, A., P. Garrett and N. Coupland. 1999. "Dialect recognition". In D. Preston, ed., 345–58.

Wiltshire, C. 2005. "The 'Indian English' of Tibeto-Burman Language Speakers". *English World-Wide* 26: 291–303.

Wiltshire, C. and J. D. Harnsberger. 2006. "The influence of Gujarati and Tamil L1s on Indian English: A preliminary study". *World Englishes* 25: 91–104.

Wiltshire, C. and R. Moon. 2003. "Phonetic stress in Indian English vs. American English". *World Englishes* 22: 291–303.

Winford, D. 1978. "Phonological hypercorrection in the process of decreolization. The case of Trinidadian English". *Journal of Linguistics* 14: 277–91.

Winford, D. 2017. "World Englishes and creoles". In M. M. Filppula *et al.*, eds, 194–210.

Wolfram, W. and R. W. Fasold. 1974. *The Study of Social Dialects in American English*. Englewood Cliffs, NJ: Prentice-Hall.

Wolfson, N. 1976. "Speech events and natural speech: Some implications for sociolinguistic methodology". *Language in Society* 5: 189–209.

Wogart, J. P. and M. Schüller. 2011. "The EU's blue card: Will it attract Asia's highly skilled?". *German Institute of Global and Area Studies* 3: 1–8.

Woolard, K. A. 1985. "Language variation and cultural hegemony: Toward an integration of sociolinguistic and social theory". *American Ethnologist* 12: 738–49.

Zipp, L. 2014. "Indo-Fijan English: Linguistic diaspora or endonormative stabilization?". In M. Hundt and D. Sharma, eds, 187–214.

Zwickl, S. 2002. *Language Attitudes, Ethnic Identity and Dialect Use across the Northern Ireland Border: Armagh and Monaghan*. Belfast: Cló Ollscoil na Banríona.

8 Appendix: Research Instruments

8.1 Written Questionnaires

8.1.1 Survey I: Language Background and Language Use

I.1 General Details

1. Name and Surname: ....
   Gender: ....
   Age: ....
   First Language: ....
   Years in Heidelberg: ....
   Faculty:
2. Please list below what languages you know and tell how well you understand, speak, read and write these languages by writing the appropriate number corresponding to the following:
   1= well
   2= some
   3= not much
   e.g. 1) ENGLISH Understand: 2; Speak: 2; Read: 3; Write: 3.
   2) HINDI Understand: 3; Speak: 2; Read: 2; Write 1.
   3) ...
3. What was the first language that you learnt as a child? You may list more than one.
4. What is the language that you speak more often now? You may list more than one.
5. How often do you use your first language now?

   all the time • • • • • never

6. Who was the main caregiver who raised you when you were a child?
   • Mother • Father • Grandmother • Grandfather
   • Other family member • Non-related person

7. Which language(s) do/did you speak when you talk/ed to:
   Mother: ....
   Father: ....
   Brother: ....
   Sister: ....
   Grandmother: ....
   Grandfather: ....
   Other family member: ....
8. Do/Did the person who mainly raised you speak English? Please tick the most appropriate answer. If more than one person raised you, base your answer on the person who spoke the language most fluently.
   • No, he/she does/did not speak English
   • Yes, he/she can/could say words and simple sentences
   • Yes, he/she can/could have a conversation in limited situations
   • Yes, he/she can/could have a conversation about everything in all situations
   • Unsure
9. Which language do you most strongly identify with?
10. In relation to the last question (no.9), please tell me who in your family is associated with this language by ticking the appropriate box.
    • Mother • Father • Grandmother • Grandfather • Other family member • Spouse • Non-related person (this language in only associated with when I have grown up/have lived/other)
11. Did you grow up in the area where this language is spoken (see question no. 9) • Yes • No • Unsure
12. How well do you speak this language? (see question no. 9)
    • I do not speak the language at all.
    • I can say some words and simple sentences.
    • I can have a conversation in limited situations.
    • I can have a conversation about everything in all situations.
13. Do you use this language more often, less often, or the same amount as when you were in India? (see question no. 9)

    all the time • • • • • never

14. If you use this language (see question no. 9) more often or less often that you did when you were in India, please list the reasons which you think your language use has changed. If your language use has not changed, what do you think helped keep it the same?

15. When did you learn this language? (see question no. 9)
    • As a child • As a teenager • As an adult

16. How did you learn this language? (see question no. 9)
    • From my parents • From my grandparents • At school • On my own • Other: ....

17. When I take into consideration all the situations in which I use language (my home life, my social life, my university life, etc.), I would say that, overall, I'm most comfortable:
    understanding: ....
    speaking: ....
    reading: ....
    writing: ....

I.2 General Use of English

1. Use of English in personal interactions

Family	all the time	•	•	•	•	•	never
Friends	all the time	•	•	•	•	•	never
Professors	all the time	•	•	•	•	•	never
Social Networks	all the time	•	•	•	•	•	never

2. General preference for models of English
   • British English • American English • Indian English • unsure

3. Faculty preference for models of instruction
   • British English • American English • Indian English • unsure

4. Reasons for studying English
   • To understand textbooks assigned in universities or other institutions of higher education better
   • To get along within and outside India
   • To become broadly educated
   • To get a job which pays more
   • It yields personal satisfaction
   • To begin to think and behave as the British/Americans do
   • To learn about different cultures
   • Because English is the language of the globalised world

5. How do you label your own spoken variety of English?
   • British English • American English • Indian English • 'Mixture' of all three
   • 'Good' English • unsure

6. Interactions with native English speakers
   all the time • • • • • never

7. In which language(s) did you study in India?
   • English • Other: ....

8. Which schools did you attend?
   • Public/Government schools • Private schools • Both

9. What is the highest educational level you have achieved?
   • Primary school • Secondary school • Undergraduate (Bachelor's)
   • Graduate (Master's) • Ph.D. • Post-doc

10. How do/did you usually interact in India?

	English	**Mother Tongue**	**State/local language**	**Hindi**
Family	•	•	•	•
Friends	•	•	•	•
Neighbours who can speak your language	•	•	•	•
Professors	•	•	•	•
Strangers to ask for information	•	•	•	•
Grocery shop owners	•	•	•	•
Office and bank employees	•	•	•	•
Political and technical discussions	•	•	•	•
While visiting a Northern state in India	•	•	•	•
While visiting a Southern state in India	•	•	•	•

11. Use of English in reading general literature

Web	all the time	•	•	•	•	•	never
University texbooks	all the time	•	•	•	•	•	never
Newspapers and magazines	all the time	•	•	•	•	•	never
General reading	all the time	•	•	•	•	•	never

I.3 Language Use in Heidelberg

1. How often do you speak English in Heidelberg?

all the time • • • • • never

2. How do you usually interact in Heidelberg?

	English	**German**	**Mother Tongue**	**Hindi**
Indian friends	•	•	•	•
German friends	•	•	•	•
International friends	•	•	•	•
Professors	•	•	•	•
Strangers to ask for information	•	•	•	•
Grocery shop owners	•	•	•	•
Office and bank employees	•	•	•	•
Political and technical discussions	•	•	•	•
While visiting another city in Germany	•	•	•	•

3. Keeping my Indian languages strong in Heidelberg is important to me. Please indicate whether you agree or disagree with the following statements by ticking the appropriate answer.

strongly agree • • • • • strongly disagree

4. It is important for Indians living here to pass their language knowledge to future generations.

   strongly agree • • • • • strongly disagree

5. The use of my background languages is a strong part of my identity in Heidelberg as well as among other Indians.

   strongly agree • • • • • strongly disagree

8.1.2 Survey II, Part I: Accent and Identity and part II: Accent Identification Task

II.1 Accent and Identity

1. Name and Surname: ....
   Gender: ....
   Age: ....
   First Language: ....
   Years in Heidelberg: ....
   Faculty: ....
2. Do you think you have an accent?
   • Yes • No • Unsure
3. If yes, what accent do you think you have?
4. In your opinion, is your accent different from the accent of nearby towns and cities, or of other parts of India? Can you think of any specific ways in which it is different? For instance, are there different words and/or words which are pronounced differently?
5. Are you proud of your accent or would you rather not have any accent at all?
6. Would you prefer to have a different accent? If so, which one? Why?
7. Do you think it is good to have an accent? Why or why not?
8. Have you ever felt embarrassed about your accent? When? Why?
9. I am prepared to spend money on taking courses to improve my accent. When there is a scale 1 is high (e.g., 'Yes, definitely; 'most friendly'), 5 is low (e.g., 'Absolutely not'; 'least friendly').

   1 • • • • • 5

10. Are there different accents in India?
    • Yes • No • Unsure
11. If there are, what are they? Do you like them? Can you tell them apart easily?
12. In which Indian state/city/town are people generally more friendly? Why?
13. In your opinion, is it necessary to speak with a local accent to 'belong'?
14. Do you know some Indians who changed their accent when they moved to Heidelberg?
    • Yes • No • Unsure
15. If so, why do you think they did so?

II.1 Accent Identification Task

You will now hear a number of voices reading the same passage. On the basis of your reaction to the voice alone, please answer the following questions. When there is a scale 1 is high (e.g., 'most friendly'), 5 is low (e.g., 'least friendly').

1. Identify the ethnicity of the following speaker and assign each voice to the site it belongs on the map provided.
2. How sure are you?
   extremely sure • • • • • extremely unsure
3. What cues/clues did you consider to identify the speaker's origin?
4. To what degree does this accent differ from your own?
   same • • • • • unintelligible
5. How pleasant do you think the speaker is?
   1 • • • • • 5
6. How correct do you think the speaker is?
   1 • • • • • 5
7. How intelligent do you think the speaker is?
   1 • • • • • 5
8. How friendly do you think the speaker is?
   1 • • • • • 5

9. How polite do you think the speaker is?

   1 • • • • • 5

10. How educated do you think the speaker is?

    1 • • • • • 5

11. How attractive do you think the speaker is?

    1 • • • • • 5

12. How ambitious do you think the speaker is?

    1 • • • • • 5

13. How confident do you think the speaker is?

    1 • • • • • 5

14. What kind of job do you think this speaker has, or would do have in the future?
15. This speaker should spend money on taking courses to improve his/her accent.

    strongly agree • • • • • strongly disagree

8.2 Cognitive Map Sample

Name and Surname: ....
First Language: ....
Draw boundaries on the blank map below around areas where you believe English accents are different.

8.3 Oral Questionnaire: Interview guideline

Mod. I. Demography

1. Let's start by introducing yourself….
2. When where you born?
3. Have you lived in different places in India?
4. When were your parents born or raised? Which languages can they speak?
5. Which languages can you speak besides English?
6. With whom?
7. Which schools did you attend?

8. What did you study in India and what are you studying now?
9. Have you travelled very much outside of your hometown? Where?
10. In which languages do you usually communicate in India?

Mod. II. Accent and Identity; Language Attitudes and Regard

1. What do you think about this accent recognition test? Was it difficult?
2. Were you able to discriminate speakers geographically just from the audio clip?
3. Which cues/clues did you use to discriminate speakers?
4. Many people from the Indian community say that Southern Indians have a peculiar speech. What do you think about that? Is it true in your opinion? Why?
5. Can you tell if someone's from the South of India by the way he talks? How can you tell?
6. Do you like the way people from the South of India sound? What do you like about it? What don't you like about it?
7. How about in comparison to say, Northern India?
8. (if the speaker is from the South) Has anyone ever told you that you sound like a Southern Indian? Did you (would you) take it as a compliment?(if the speaker is from the North) If you told someone that he sounded like he came from Southern India, would you mean it as a compliment?
9. Do you think people in your town sound different from people in other parts of India? How so?
10. Where in India do you think they speak the best English?
11. Have you ever tried to change anything about the way you talk? What?
12. Has anyone else ever tried to make you change something about the way you talk? What?(teachers; parents; friends)
13. Do you think people should try to improve their speech?
14. Well, if you could change the way you talk, what would you change?
15. If you were a teacher in India, would you try to improve the way kids talk? What would you improve?
16. What did you think about the question about Indians who changed their accent when they moved to Heidelberg?

Mod II. Heidelberg and Networking

1. Tell me, when and why did you decide to come to Heidelberg?
2. How long have you been living in Heidelberg?
3. How long are you planning on staying here?

4. Do you know many Indians residing in Heidelberg?
5. Why, do you think, Indians come to Heidelberg?
6. Did you make friends with some of them here?
7. Are there some that you see almost every day?(Get ethnicity, age, first language)
8. Where do you guys hang out around here?
9. What do you usually do together?
10. Do you know HISA? Do you usually go to its cultural events? What do you think of it?
11. What are your plans for the future? Are you planning to go back to India at some point of your life?

8.4 Recorded Reading Passage

Excerpt from Desai (2001:5 [1980])

'That is the risk of coming home to Old Delhi', she announced in the hard voice that had started up the prickle of distrust that ran over the tips of the hairs of Tara's arms, rippling them. 'Old Delhi does not change. It only decays. My students tell me it is a great cemetery, every house a tomb. Nothing but sleeping graves. Now *New* Delhi, they say is different. That is where things happen. The way they describe it, it sounds like a nest of fleas. So much happens there, it must be a jumping place. I never go. Baba never goes. And here, here nothing happens at all. Whatever happened, happened long ago. in the time of the Tughlaqs, the Khiljis, the Sultanate, the Moghuls – that lot'. She snapped her fingers in time to her words, smartly. 'And then the British built New Delhi and moved everything out. Here we are left rocking on the backwaters, getting duller and greyer, I suppose. Anyone who isn't dull and grey goes away – to New Delhi, to England, to Canada, the Middle East. They don't come back'.

VarioLingua
Nonstandard – Standard – Substandard

Band 1 Klaus J. Mattheier / Edgar Radtke (Hrsg.): Standardisierung und Destandardisierung europäischer Nationalsprachen. 1997.

Band 2 Evelyn Ziegler: Sprachgebrauch – Sprachvariation – Sprachwissen. Eine Familienfallstudie. 1996.

Band 3 Göz Kaufmann: Varietätendynamik in Sprachkontaktsituationen. Attitüden und Sprachverhalten rußlanddeutscher Mennoniten in Mexiko und den USA. 1997.

Band 4 Rolf Kailuweit: Vom EIGENEN SPRECHEN. Eine Geschichte der spanisch-katalanischen Diglossie in Katalonien (1759-1859). 1997.

Band 5 Arno Scholz: Neo-standard e variazione diafasica nella canzone italiana degli anni Novanta. 1998.

Band 6 Jannis K. Androutsopoulos: Deutsche Jugendsprache. Untersuchungen zu ihren Strukturen und Funktionen. 1998.

Band 7 Jannis K. Androutsopoulos / Arno Scholz (Hrsg.): Jugendsprache – langue des jeunes – youth language. Linguistische und soziolinguistische Perspektiven. 1998.

Band 8 Verena Krus-Bühler: Strukturen des Wortschwunds in Lincolnshire: *Real-time* und *Apparent-time*. 1999.

Band 9 Michael Schreiber: Textgrammatik – Gesprochene Sprache – Sprachvergleich. Proformen im gesprochenen Französischen und Deutschen. 1999.

Band 10 Szilvia Deminger / Thorsten Fögen / Joachim Scharloth / Simone Zwickl (Hrsg.): Einstellungsforschung in der Soziolinguistik und Nachbardisziplinen – Studies in Language Attitudes. 2000.

Band 11 Francesca Sboarina: Il lessico medico nel *Dioscoride* di Pietro Andrea Mattioli. 2000.

Band 12 Klaus Mattheier (ed.): Dialect and Migration in a Changing Europe. 2000.

Band 13 Christian Timm: Das dreigliedrige Allokutionssystem des Italienischen in Neapel. 2001.

Band 14 Anne Cammenga-Waller: Substandard im Deutschen und Französischen. Lexikologische Studien zur zeitgenössischen Konsumliteratur. 2002.

Band 15 Thomas Krefeld (ed.): Spazio vissuto e dinamica linguistica. Varietà meridionali in Italia e in situazione de extraterritorialità. 2002.

Band 16 Pietro Maturi: Dialetti e substandardizzazione nel Sannio Beneventano. 2002.

Band 17 Christiane Wössner: *Qua parlón fa noantri!* Spracherhalt und ethnische Identität in Chipilo - einer Sprachinsel des Veneto in Mexiko. 2002.

Band 18 Jannis K. Androutsopoulos / Evelyn Ziegler (Hrsg.): „Standardfragen". Soziolinguistische Perspektiven auf Sprachgeschichte, Sprachkontakt und Sprachvariation. 2003.

Band 19 Christel Schlindwein: *...je ne me lasse point de te lire.* Zur Sprachgeschichte des Alltags in französischen Briefen in Deutschland (1792–1813). 2003.

Band 20 Alexandra N. Lenz / Edgar Radtke / Simone Zwickl (Hrsg.): Variation im Raum. Variation and Space. 2004.

Band 21 Szilvia Deminger: Spracherhalt und Sprachverlust in einer Sprachinselsituation. Sprache und Identität bei der deutschen Minderheit in Ungarn. 2004.

Band 22 Dirk Deissler: Die entnazifizierte Sprache. Sprachpolitik und Sprachregelung in der Besatzungszeit. 2., korrigierte und ergänzte Auflage. 2006.

Band 23 Alexandra N. Lenz / Klaus J. Mattheier (Hrsg.): Varietäten – Theorie und Empirie. 2005.

Band 24 Danielle A. V. Löw-Wiebach: Language Attitudes and Language Use in Pitmedde (Aberdeenshire). 2005.

Band 25 Claudia Bluhm-Faust: Die Pädagogisierung der deutschen Standardsprache im 19. Jahrhundert am Beispiel Badens. 2005.

Band 26 Rembert Eufe: *Sta lengua ha un privilegio tanto grando.* Status und Gebrauch des Venezianischen in der Republik Venedig. 2006.

Band 27 Nina Berend / Elisabeth Knipf-Komlósi (Hrsg.): Sprachinselwelten – The World of Language Islands. Entwicklung und Beschreibung der deutschen Sprachinseln am Anfang des 21. Jahrhunderts.The Developmental Stages and the Description of German Language Islands at the Beginning of the 21st Century. 2006.

Band 28 Winifred V. Davies / Nils Langer: The Making of Bad Language. Lay Linguistic Stigmatisations in German: Past und Present. 2006.

Band 29 Christian H. Münch: Sprachpolitik und gesellschaftliche Alphabetisierung. Zur Entwicklung der Schreibkompetenz in Katalonien seit 1975. 2006.

Band 30 Janet Spreckels: *Britneys, Fritten, Gangschta und wir:* Identitätskonstitution in einer Mädchengruppe. Eine ethnographisch-gesprächsanalytische Untersuchung. 2006.

Band 31 Isolde Opielka: *Residencia tomada a los jueces de apelación, por Alonso de Zuazo,* Hispaniola, 1517. Partielle kommentierte Edition, diskurstraditionelle und grapho-phonologische Aspekte. 2008.

Band 32 Brigitte E. Lambert: Family Language Transmission. Actors, Issues, Outcomes. 2008.

Band 33 Doris Schüpbach: Shared Languages, Shared Identities, Shared Stories. A Qualitative Study of Life Stories by Immigrants from German-speaking Switzerland in Australia. 2008.

Band 34 Annalisa Buonocore: Varietà dialettali microareali della Costiera Amalfitana. 2009.

Band 35 Ellen Rötterink: Parler scout en réunion. Analyse du style communicatif d'un groupe de jeunes. 2009.

Band 36 Jo-anne Hughson: Diversity and Changing Values in Address. Spanish Address Pronoun Usage in an Intercultural Immigrant Context. 2009.

Band 37 Peter Gilles / Joachim Scharloth / Evelyn Ziegler (Hrsg.): Variatio delectat. Empirische Evidenzen und theoretische Passungen sprachlicher Variationen. Herausgegeben von Peter Gilles, Joachim Scharloth und Evelyn Ziegler für Klaus J. Mattheier zum 65. Geburtstag. 2010.

Band 38 Csilla Anna Szabó: Language shift und Code-mixing. Deutsch-ungarisch-rumänischer Sprachkontakt in einer dörflichen Gemeinde in Nordwestrumänien. 2010.

Band 39 Till Stellino: Kommunikations- und Sachwandel in der süditalienischen Weinproduktion. Eine Neukonzeption von *Wörter und Sachen.* 2010.

Band 40 Alexandra N. Lenz / Albrecht Plewnia (eds.): Grammar between Norm and Variation. 2010.

Band 41 Silvia Natale / Daniela Pietrini / Nelson Puccio / Till Stellino (a cura di / Hrsg.): "Noio volevàn savuàr". Studi in onore di Edgar Radtke per il suo sessantesimo compleanno. Festschrift für Edgar Radtke zu seinem 60. Geburtstag. A cura di Silvia Natale, Daniela Pietrini, Nelson Puccio e Till Stellino. Herausgegeben von Silvia Natale, Daniela Pietrini, Nelson Puccio und Till Stellino. 2012.

Band 42 Eva Bernhardt: Variación diafásica en una conversación polémica y pública. Análisis de un talk show de la television española. 2012.

Band 43 Anna Kessler: Interkorrelationen von generationsspezifischen Varietäten und Identitätsprofilen. Eine statistische Analyse in Padua. 2013.

Band 44 Zeichen und Stil. Der Mehrwert der Variation. Festschrift für Beate Henn-Memmesheimer. Herausgegeben von Georg Albert und Joachim Franz. 2013.

Band 45 Mark Möst: Grammatik des Kreolischen von Mauritius. 2014.

Band 46 Maria Gabriella Conte: Dialetti in contatto nella Valle del Mércure. La variazione microdialettale e la sua percezione nell'Area Lausberg. 2014.

Band 47 Tiziana Roncoroni: Argumentative Strategien in deutschen und italienischen wissenschaftlichen Artikeln. Am Beispiel der Soziologie und der Sprachwissenschaft. 2015.

Band 48 Heike Susanne Jauch: Das Frankoprovenzalische in Italien, Frankreich und der Schweiz. Sprachkontakt und Mehrsprachigkeit im Dreiländereck. 2016.

Band 49 Kathrin Wenz: *Bloguer sa vie*. Linguistische Studie über die Kommunikation in französischen Weblogs im Spannungsfeld zwischen Individualität und Gruppenzugehörigkeit. 2017.

Band 50 Vladislava Warditz: Varianz im Russischen. Von funktionalstilistischer zur soziolinguistischen Perspektive. 2018.

Band 51 Elisabeth Klein: Nonstandard im semantischen Raum. 2019.

Band 52 Sara Matrisciano: Neapel und das Neapolitanische als diskursiv konstruierter Mythos. Eine variationslinguistische Analyse. 2020.

Band 53 Giuliana Regnoli: Accent Variation in Indian English. A Folk Linguistic Study. 2021.

www.peterlang.com

www.ingramcontent.com/pod-product-compliance
Ingram Content Group UK Ltd.
Pitfield, Milton Keynes, MK11 3LW, UK
UKHW021420091026
15624UKWH00010B/265

9 783631 857427